ORTHOPAEDICS AND ACCIDENTS

Best Wishes,

From Ward 7.

D1799420

MODERN NURSING SERIES

General Editors
A. J. HARDING RAINS M.S., F.R.C.S.
MISS VALERIE HUNT S.R.N., S.C.M., R.N.T.

AT PRESENT AVAILABLE AS PAPERBACKS

Anaesthesia, Recovery and Intensive Care
D. A. BUXTON HOPKIN F.F.A., M.D., M.R.C.S.

Obstetrics and Gynaecology for Nurses
GORDON W. GARLAND M.D., F.R.C.O.G.
JOAN M. E. QUIXLEY S.R.N., R.N.T.
MICHAEL D. CAMERON M.A , M.B., B.chir., F.R.C.S., M.R.C.O.G.

Ophthalmology
I. M. DUGUID M.D., Ph.D., F.R.C.S., D.O.
A. A. BERRY S.R N., O.N.D., BTA Cert., C.M.B. Part 1 Middle Management Cert.

Principles of Medicine and Medical Nursing
J. C. HOUSTON M.D., M.R.C.P.
MARION STOCKDALE S.R.N.

Principles of Surgery and Surgical Nursing
SELWYN TAYLOR D.M., M.ch., F.R.C.S.

Physiology for Nurses
DERYCK TAVERNER M.B.E., M.D., F.R.C.P.

Venereology for Nurses
R. D. CATTERALL M.R.C.P.(Edin).

Psychology and Psychiatry for Nurses
PETER DALLY M.B., F.R.C.P., D.P.M.
HEATHER HARRINGTON S.R.N., R.M.N.

Emergency and Acute Care
A. J. HARDING RAINS M.S., F.R.C.S.
VALERIE HUNT S.R.N., S.C.M., R.N.T.
KEITH REYNOLDS M.S., F.R.C.S.

The Nursing of Accidents
RAYMOND FARROW F.R.C.S.

Community Health and Social Services
J. B. MEREDITH DAVIES M.D.(London), D.P.H.

Therapeutics
J. G. LEWIS M.D., M.R.C.P.

ORTHOPAEDICS AND ACCIDENTS

MARGARET MILLER
R.G.N., S.C.M.
Formerly Ward Sister, Orthopaedic and Accident Unit, Glasgow Royal Infirmary

JAMES H. MILLER
M.B., Ch.B., F.R.C.S. Glas., F.R.C.S. Edin.
Consultant Orthopaedic and Accident Surgeon, Glasgow Royal Infirmary;
Appointed Examiner for British Orthopaedic Nursing Certificate

HODDER AND STOUGHTON
London Sydney Auckland Toronto

ISBN 0 340 12482 2 Boards
ISBN 0 340 12483 0 Paperback

First published 1972. Reprinted 1976

Copyright © 1972 M. Miller and J. H. Miller
All rights reserved. No part of this publication
may be reproduced or transmitted in any form
or by any means, electronic or mechanical,
including photocopy, recording, or any information
storage and retrieval system, without permission
in writing from the publisher.

Printed in Great Britain for
Hodder and Stoughton Educational,
a division of Hodder and Stoughton Limited,
Mill Road, Dunton Green, Sevenoaks, Kent
by Biddles Ltd, Guildford, Surrey

EDITOR'S FOREWORD

Orthopaedics and Accidents is a welcome addition to this popular series which has been designed to provide a range of textbooks written specially for students of nursing, midwifery, physiotherapy, radiography, speech training and hygiene. In assembling these texts care has been taken to maintain a reasonably uniform level of presentation with theory and practice kept in balance. Terminology is as rational as possible, and where necessary simple definitions of technical terms are included.

The series is designed to cover the requirements of the State Registration Examinations conducted by the General Nursing Council. Among the many additions to the series will be found useful books for those wishing to continue a career ancillary to a particular specialty or discipline of medicine, e.g. Psychiatry, Ophthalmology, Midwifery, Neurology, Anaesthesia, Venereology and Public Health.

The editors and publishers hold the view that these texts should as far as possible be written by a physician or surgeon in conjunction with a nursing sister or tutor. This is with the deliberate intention of stressing the close association between clinical medicine and nursing. Now as far as *Orthopaedics and Accidents* is concerned, I am glad to tell our readers that the rôles of author have been reversed for here is a book written by a former ward sister with considerable clinical experience in conjunction with a consultant orthopaedic and accident surgeon from one of the best organised units in the United Kingdom. Our readers will also be pleased to note that the surnames of the authors are the same—for this is a husband and wife team.

In writing this book the authors have been afforded support and advice by a large number of consultants and colleagues representing orthopaedic and accident surgery, anaesthesia, paediatrics, plastic surgery, pathology and bacteriology, physiotherapy, radiography, and medical social workers—the whole spectrum of service applied to the care of the whole patient.

This book fills a special need in the Modern Nursing Series and I am sure it will be an ever-popular text amongst general and orthopaedic nurses and also physiotherapists.

A. J. HARDING RAINS

PREFACE

Existing books on orthopaedics and accident surgery have a strong medical bias and are not always well orientated to nursing. There is a need now for a book which will not only give simple explanations of the common conditions and their nursing care, but also indicate the progressive, exciting new techniques and developments in this field. This book is intended to give the nurse confidence in the management of patients in the orthopaedic and accident wards. The student nurse seeks a book for explanation, the trained nurse for instruction, the specialised sister for information and the tutor for a means of re-illumination of the subject and a basis for discussion. These are the reasons which prompted us to write this book. It differs from many other books on the nursing of orthopaedic and accident surgery in that it is written by a nurse for nurses, with the advice of an orthopaedic and accident surgeon.

MARGARET MILLER
JAMES H. MILLER

ACKNOWLEDGMENTS

The Authors would like to thank the following people for help given in the preparation of this book.

For the provision of material or helpful suggestions, we are indebted to Mr. D. A. MacPherson, Consultant Orthopaedic Surgeon, The Royal Hospital for Sick Children and the Western Infirmary, Glasgow, to Dr. D. Campbell, Consultant Anaesthetist, Honorary Clinical Lecturer in the University Department of Anaesthetics, Glasgow Royal Infirmary, to Sister M. Gilchrist, Ward Sister, Royal Hospital for Sick Children, Glasgow, to Sister E. Macallan, Ward Sister, Glasgow and West of Scotland Regional Plastic Surgery Unit, to Miss M. Burns, Matron, Lightburn Geriatric Hospital, to Miss A. Fotheringham, Theatre Superintendent, Stirling Royal Infirmary, to Mr. D. Anderson, Principal Tutor, School of Physiotherapy, to Mrs. M. Cathro, Superintendent, and to Mr. T. Anderson, Physiotherapist, of the Physiotherapy Department, to Miss B. Brodie, Chief Occupational Therapist, to Mr. A. McDonald, Superintendent Radiographer, Orthopaedic and Accident Division and to Mrs. M. Hill, Medical Social Worker, Orthopaedic and Accident Division, all of Glasgow Royal Infirmary.

We are very much obliged to Mr. J. T. Brown, Consultant Orthopaedic Surgeon, Glasgow Western Infirmary, to Mr. J. White, Chairman, Orthopaedic and Accident Division and to Sister E. F. McPherson, Sister in Charge, Respiratory Intensive Care Unit, both of Glasgow Royal Infirmary, for their criticisms and valuable suggestions.

We thank Sir David P. Cuthbertson, University Department of Pathological Biochemistry, Glasgow Royal Infirmary, Mr. Derek Henderson, Consultant Oral Surgeon, Canniesburn Hospital, Dunbartonshire, Mr. J. Garden, Consultant in Charge, Orthopaedic and Accident Department, Law Hospital, Lanarkshire, Dr. T. A. McAllister, Consultant in Charge of the Bacteriological Departments of the Royal Hospital for Sick Children and the Queen Mother's Hospital, Glasgow, and Mr. W. R. Cox, B.Sc., M.I.C.E., Chartered Engineer for advice given on specific points in this book.

Our thanks are also due to the members of staff of Glasgow Royal Infirmary School of Nursing who gave us such encouragement in the production of this book.

We are extremely grateful to Mrs. J. H. Blackie, Headmistress, Pinewood Primary School, Glasgow for advice and guidance in English Language and Grammar.

We extend our sincere thanks to Miss A. Taggart and to Miss S. Masson of the Orthopaedic and Accident Division, Glasgow Royal Infirmary who typed the manuscript. It was a pleasure to work with two such interested and enthusiastic people.

The illustrations are the work of Miss Jean MacDonald, D.A. (Glas) A.I.M.I., Medical Artist, University Department of Surgery, Royal Infirmary, Glasgow. We feel these make an excellent contribution to our book. We should like also to express our appreciation to our parents and other relatives who devoted so much of their time to entertaining our two small children, Valerie and Eric, and without whose assistance we should not have been able to complete this work.

From A. J. Harding Rains, M.S., F.R.C.S., Professor of Surgery, Charing Cross Hospital Medical School, Honorary Consultant Surgeon, Charing Cross Hospital and General Editor to the Publishers, we have received guidance and encouragement which have helped us considerably in our approach to this textbook. We are most grateful to him not only in this respect but also because he has kindly agreed to write the Foreword.

Lastly, we must acknowledge the advice given and the patience and consideration shown by the publishers during our preparation of this book.

CONTENTS

PART II BASIC ORTHOPAEDIC NURSING TECHNIQUES
AND REHABILITATION

INTRODUCTION

Orthopaedic surgery deals with conditions affecting the locomotor system. These may be congenital, or acquired through habit or disease. Although some of these conditions present in an acute form many follow a more chronic course and their treatment is continued over a prolonged period.

Accident surgery, however, deals with injury to the locomotor and associated systems, leading to emergency situations requiring more urgent measures in their treatment. The nature and extent of injury determine whether a patient requires short or long term treatment.

The scope of orthopaedic and accident management and nursing covers the care of patients of both sexes and all ages, over either a short or long term period of hospitalisation. There are three main pillars of treatment; RESTRICTION or IMMOBILISATION, SURGERY and REHABILITATION.

This book is written in two parts. PART I gives a simple description of the management of some common orthopaedic and traumatic conditions. It is sub-divided into three sections. In Section I the conditions are classified according to their pathology. A regional grouping and explanation of other affections of the locomotor system is given in Section II. Section III is confined to traumatology, commencing with the principles of fracture treatment and finishing with the reception of casualties. It includes a chapter on major multiple injuries, the first part of which deals with reception, resuscitation and diagnosis of the injured while the second part describes the treatment and special nursing management.

The division between orthopaedics and trauma can be difficult, e.g. dislocation of the shoulder, torn cartilage in the knee joint. Some such lesions are therefore included in the orthopaedic section while others are discussed under trauma. We have done this by using the wards to which these conditions are usually admitted, i.e. orthopaedic or traumatic, as a guide to the section of the book in which they should be described. Dislocation of the shoulder therefore appears in the trauma section while recurring dislocation of the shoulder and tears of the menisci are described in orthopaedic chapters.

PART II of the book centres almost entirely on nursing. The principles of the application and care of traction and plaster of Paris are explained in detail. A brief description of the more common operations and the post-operative management of the patient is given. Specific mention is made of the positioning of patients after surgery or following trauma. Some of the factors which influence satisfactory wound healing are discussed. A short chapter on the important aspect of pain appreciation in patients following surgery or trauma is included. A brief explanation of what is meant by the metabolic response to injury is given. No book on orthopaedics and accidents would be complete if it failed to mention the problems involved in nursing the young and the elderly. In the orthopaedic and accident unit, radiography forms an integral part of the diagnosis and surgical treatment. For this reason, a short chapter is included to explain some of the important features of this specialty. As teamwork is essential in the orthopaedic and accident departments some insight is necessary into the work of the ancillary services such as physiotherapy, occupational therapy and medical social work, all of which are important in the total rehabilitation of the patient. An outline of this work is given in the final chapters.

Common Orthopaedic Conditions and the Management of Trauma

SECTION I

GENERAL ORTHOPAEDICS

1 POSTURE AND ITS VARIATIONS

Posture means the relative disposition of the various parts of the body, i.e. the position or carriage of the body as a whole. It is the basis of all movement as each movement begins in one postural position and ends in another. It is difficult to state specifically what constitutes a 'normal posture.' **Postural attitudes** are influenced by many factors such as **physique, occupation, habit** and **environment.**

The formation and arrangement of the bones of the skeleton are such that the heavier, larger bones are situated in the lower trunk, pelvis and limbs to act as a support to the body in the erect position. The joints are constructed to provide for an extensive range of movement where this is required, e.g. the hip and shoulder joints. In other instances the emphasis is on strength and stability rather than mobility, e.g. the intervertebral joints of the spine. The skeletal muscles vary according to their situation and the amount of movement that is allowed by a particular joint, e.g. large muscles round the hip and shoulder joints. Muscle contraction is dependent on nerve stimulation to produce the required movements at the desired moment. The ligaments act as stabilisers, controlling gross extremes of movement and affording added strength to a joint.

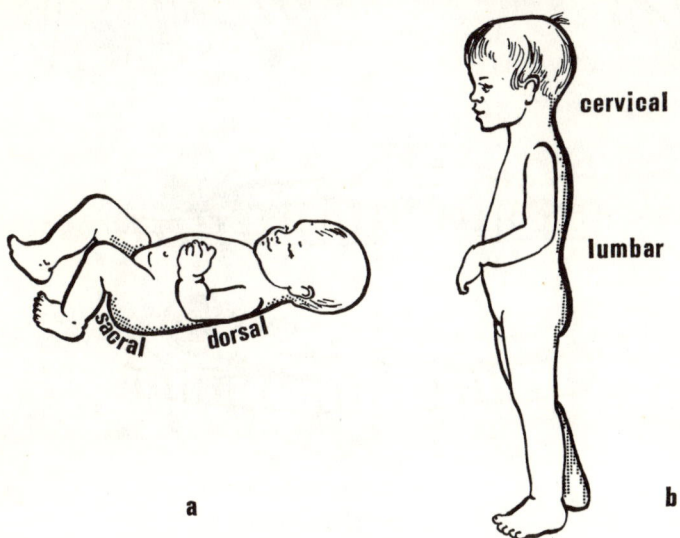

FIG. 1 (a) Primary spinal curves—dorsal and sacral
(b) Secondary spinal curves—cervical and lumbar

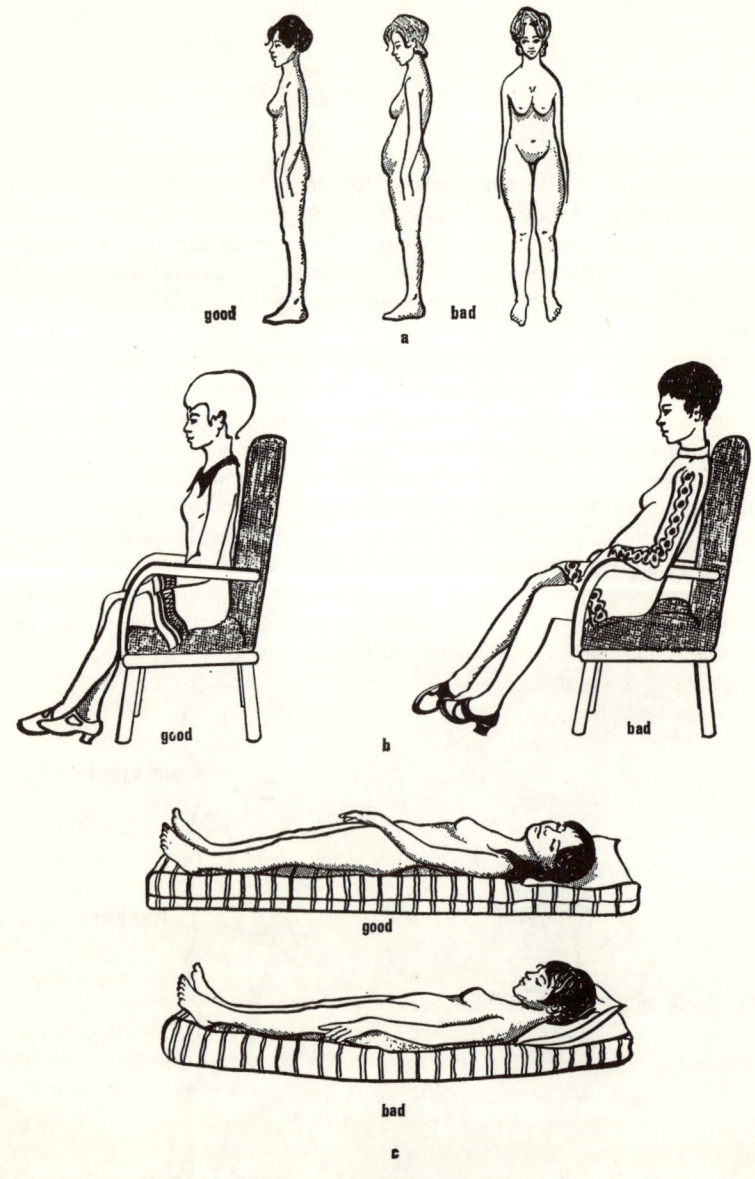

FIG. 2 Correctable postural defects
(a) Standing
(b) Sitting
(c) Lying

A **baby** at birth has two **primary** or **fixed spinal curves,** the **dorsal** and **sacral** (*Fig. 1a*). The ability of the child to sit and later to stand erect predisposes to the development of the further **compensatory mobile curves,** the **cervical** and **lumbar** (*Fig. 1b*). The development and function of all these structures, therefore, determine one's posture.

Variations of posture include correctable postural defects, transient changes in growth pattern and structural deformities produced by congenital abnormalities, disease or injury to bone, joint, muscle, ligaments or nerve tissue. Age is also an influencing factor. Bones undergo softening or osteoporosis, joints stiffen, muscles lose tone and discs degenerate. These changes produce associated disturbances or deformities of posture.

CORRECTABLE POSTURAL DEFECTS
A 'postural' deformity is distinct from a 'structural' one in that although there is deviation from the normal axis it is correctable by voluntary muscular effort; there is **no underlying bony deformity** (*Fig. 2a, b and c*).

TRANSIENT VARIATIONS IN GROWTH PATTERN
These are seen in early childhood, usually soon after the child has begun to walk. The deformity is noticed by the parents who are anxious for advice. In most instances, however, they can be reassured that this is a physiological stage in development which will correct without treatment. A very small proportion of these children return at a later date with a persistent deformity. Knock knees and bowed legs (**genu valgum** and **genu varum**) are perhaps the more common deformities encountered. The knees tend to bump together on walking or the legs are bowed or bent. This makes walking awkward but symptomless unless there are other associated deformities, e.g. congenital hip dislocation.

It is important to **exclude** by means of clinical, X-ray and blood examination, **disease or injury**, e.g. softening of the bones in rickets, muscle spasm in spastic paraplegia, damage to the growing epiphyses of the long bones of the lower limbs by injury or skeletal deformity in chronic renal disease (renal rickets).

Treatment is unnecessary in the purely physiological case. If the parents are over-anxious they may be shown how to do daily passive corrective exercises of the child's limbs. Where the deformity is acquired by disease or injury, initial treatment will be related to the **primary condition,** e.g. vitamins in rickets or walking calipers in spastic paraplegia. Correction of the deformity by osteotomy may be considered later. If the condition persists, osteoarthritis of the knees and associated joints may be a late complication.

Children may also suffer from **flat feet.** This is again due to lack of development of the arches of the feet and the mobility of the joints. As growth proceeds this condition corrects itself. Other variations of posture, such as kyphosis and lordosis, may be associated with the growing period. In the toddler there is often a marked lordosis, protuberant abdomen and a pelvic tilt which corrects as muscles develop and balance improves. Postural scoliosis, present on sitting and stand-ing, is yet another correctable deformity found in the child or adolescent, which soon disappears with the help of instruction in good posture and postural exercises.

VARIATIONS OF POSTURE DUE TO DISEASE OR INJURY

The deformity produced is structural and fixed, therefore it is **incorrectable by voluntary effort**: there may be **underlying bony deformity**. In this chapter the structural forms of torticollis, kyphosis, lordosis, scoliosis and flat feet are discussed.

Torticollis or Wry Neck

In this condition the neck is deviated from the midline. The cause may be **con-genital, traumatic** or **degenerative**. At birth a child may present with a non-inflammatory mass or swelling in one sterno-mastoid muscle. This progresses to fibrosis and contracture, so pulling the head and neck out to one side. Maldevelop-ment of the cervical vertebrae produces a structural deformity resulting in wry neck. Damage to the cortex of the brain, as in the athetoid spastic child, or de-generative changes in the basal nuclei in the adult, as in paralysis agitans or Parkinsonism, give rise to a spasmodic torticollis. Trauma to the small joints in the neck may, depending on the degree of protective muscle spasm, predispose to wry neck. Disease of the joints in the rheumatoid arthritic may produce a shift from the midline. Once this is established the weight of the head may contribute to the progression of the deformity.

The **clinical features** in the infantile variety are only those of deformity. In the adult there is **obvious deformity, awkward posture, limitation of move-ment and pain.**

Investigations include **neurological examination** to exclude neurological disease, **X-ray examination** to reveal any existing bony abnormalities, damage or disease, and **blood examination** (e.g. E.S.R.) for the suggestion of inflam-matory or arthritic conditions.

Treatment. The treatment of **infantile** torticollis is **operative division**, under general anaesthetic, of the **sterno-mastoid muscular attachment** to the clavicle. The neck is then manipulated into the over-corrected position. A firm bandage is applied and adjusted daily to maintain this position. Immediate and prolonged **physiotherapy** is necessary, passive movements initially, progressing to active exercises later. Regular clinical examination will avoid or detect any recurrence. Operation may have to be repeated in some cases.

In the **adult** the aim is to treat the cause if possible. A **cervical collar** (*see* Appendix, *Fig.* 51a) is fitted in the outpatient department when the condition is mild. In more severe cases the patient is admitted to hospital, nursed on a firm bed and **head halter traction** applied to relieve pain and muscle spasm. **Physio-therapy** is necessary to increase movement and strengthen muscle. If conservative treatment fails **operative fusion** of the **affected vertebrae** is performed to prevent movement.

Anti-rheumatic drugs are given for the rheumatoid wry neck. A cervical collar supports the neck; physiotherapy is given to maintain and improve the range of movement. A firm bed and head halter traction may be required in some cases. Where the condition is extreme, with the head tilting increasingly towards one shoulder, **operative fusion** of the **head to the spine** in the corrected position may be considered in a fit patient.

For the spasmodic neurological wry neck, **injection** of the basal nuclei in the deeper parts of the brain with **alcohol** may relieve the troublesome spasms and jerking of the head and neck.

The **complications** associated with the condition are **deformity** of the **face** and **head** on the affected side in longstanding cases, and **osteoarthritis** and **spondylosis** of the joints of the neck.

Kyphosis

Kyphosis is the name given to an exaggerated dorsal curve. The deformity results from a wedging of an individual vertebra or several vertebrae. The vertebra is composed of softer bone anteriorly, with compact bone posteriorly, and once weakened by some predisposing factor the vertebra collapses anteriorly and becomes wedge-shaped (*Fig. 3a*).

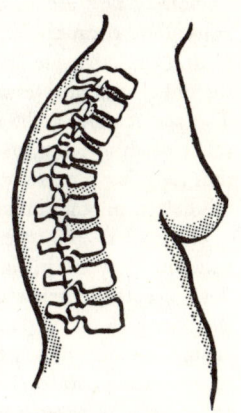

The lesion causing this condition may be of **congenital, traumatic, inflammatory, degenerative, metabolic** or **neoplastic** origin. In adolescence it may be the result of a **non-inflammatory** affection of unknown cause and is known as **adolescent kyphosis.**

The **symptoms** are those of **pain, limitation of movement** and in addition those associated with the particular underlying cause. **Investigation** by means of X-ray examination is routine, and blood examination and bone biopsy may be required to complete the diagnosis.

FIG. 3A Kyphosis

Treatment. Where the condition is symptomless and correctable, as in the growing child, treatment is unnecessary. Participation in sport, gymnastics, swimming, etc., is an effective way of overcoming the problem and is less obvious to the child than physiotherapy in a special centre.

In the **painful kyphosis** where there is associated limitation of movement, **rest and immobilisation** may be required, e.g. in adolescent kyphosis. Where there has been recent injury, bed rest and general nursing care for about three weeks followed by more active physiotherapy is the method of treatment. Occasionally a supportive brace may be required. In an acute or chronic inflammatory lesion the appropriate **anti-inflammatory treatment** is carried out. In neoplasm, palliative treatment in the form of bed rest, **deep X-ray therapy** and perhaps fitting the patient with a **protective spinal brace** may give him some comfort.

Lordosis

This is the name given to an exaggerated lumbar curve. It is usually **compensatory** to some other established deformity, such as a dorsal kyphosis, or the exaggerated tilt of the pelvis in congenital hip dislocation. It is symptomless and correctable initially. Later, pain due to muscle fatigue and ligamentous strain, and a fixed deformity, develop. X-ray examination shows the spinal deformity clearly. The **treatment** is to **cure** the **primary condition** where possible, remembering that the lordosis is a compensatory mechanism. Degenerative changes of spondylosis and osteoarthritis in the spine are later complications.

Scoliosis

Scoliosis is a sideways or lateral curvature of the spine. It is **transient** when postural in origin or **structural** where there is malformation of the vertebrae, particularly the vertebral bodies. In structural scoliosis the deformity persists when the patient attempts to touch his toes. The causes are varied and sometimes not obvious. They are usually grouped as **congenital** or osseous, **neurological, muscular, thoracic** and **idiopathic.** The bony abnormality may be present at birth. Nerve damage paralysing muscles as in anterior poliomyelitis, or disease of the muscles themselves such as muscular dystrophies, can produce this deformity. Thoracic scoliosis is the result of damage to lung tissue. The lung collapses as the result of an infection in the pleural cavity producing severe scarring or fibrosis, thus reducing the size of the cavity. The spine curves laterally to compensate for this defect. In other instances of scoliosis there is no apparent cause.

There are several types of structural or regional scoliosis which form consistent patterns. They are **initially painless**; the pain only develops with the complications of **osteoarthritis** and **spondylosis** in later life. The deformed shape of the chest may, however, interfere with **pulmonary** and **cardiac function.** The picture of the scoliotic patient shows a 'hump' or **angulation** of the spine and ribs **to one side posteriorly,** with **prominence** of the rib cage to the opposite side **anteriorly.** In an attempt to maintain an erect position, **secondary curves** are formed above and below the primary one. The arm on the same side as the convexity of the curve is close to the chest, whilst that on the opposite or concave side hangs away from the chest and may appear longer. **Spinal movements are restricted.**

Investigation is by means of initial X-rays to show the site and nature of the deformity and serial X-ray examination at three monthly intervals to determine any progression in the curvature. **Respiratory function tests** determine the degree of lung damage in the thoracic type.

Treatment. The treatment of structural scoliosis is concentrated on **prevention** of the **progression** of the deformity and on **correction** of the **fixed deformity** as much as possible. Correction of the deformity is either by **external splintage** or **internal operative** means. Externally, a special plaster cast, a Risser jacket (*Fig. 3b*), or an adjustable Milwaukee brace (*Fig. 3c*) is used. Internally, spinal

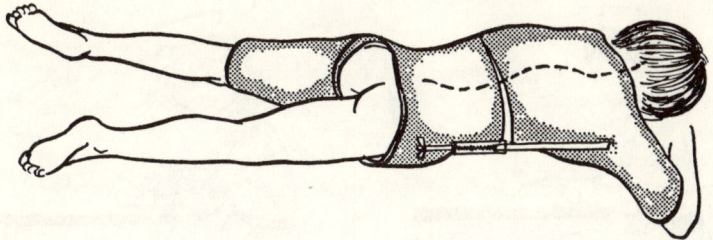

FIG. 3B Risser jacket

fusion or internal fixation of the spine in the corrected position by the use of metal struts or rods may be carried out.

Flat Foot
Pes planus or pes valgus is a condition recognised by a **failure in development of the longitudinal arch** in the foot. In the infant these arches are undeveloped and all the joints are mobile. The adult foot has the longitudinal and transverse arches developed but the foot is less mobile. Perhaps standing and walking as well as the wearing of shoes contribute to such development.

The deformity is classified into three types: postural or mobile; structural or rigid; spastic flat foot. **Postural** flat foot is seen in adolescents as part of the general 'postural slump' position. The **foot remains mobile** but the **arches sag** due to weak muscles and slack ligaments. **Structural** flat foot is seen in adult life about middle age. The deformity arises as a result of the **chronic strain** of excessive walking and standing, or of obesity. The muscles tire, ligaments stretch and the arches sag. If uncorrected, **adaptive changes** to the altered position occur in the structure of the **bones,**

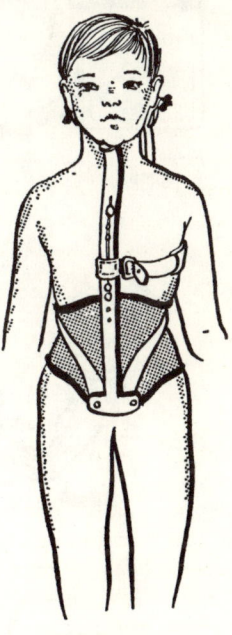

FIG. 3C
Milwaukee brace

thus interfering with the smooth movements of the joints. The deformity is then **rigid** and the foot stiff and flat. Osteoarthritis is, therefore, an associated condition. Fractures of the bones of the foot or diseases such as rheumatoid arthritis may destroy the arches and result in flat foot.

Disease or congenital abnormality involving fusion of the os calcis and navicular, or os calcis and talus, may be responsible for the stiff **spastic flat foot,** a condition unrelated to spastic paralysis. The patient is often a **young child** of nine or ten years who complains of pain in one foot, particularly when walking on uneven ground. On examination both feet look flat but whereas the symptomless foot is fully mobile the painful one is **stiff** with extensor muscle spasm. Spastic flat foot

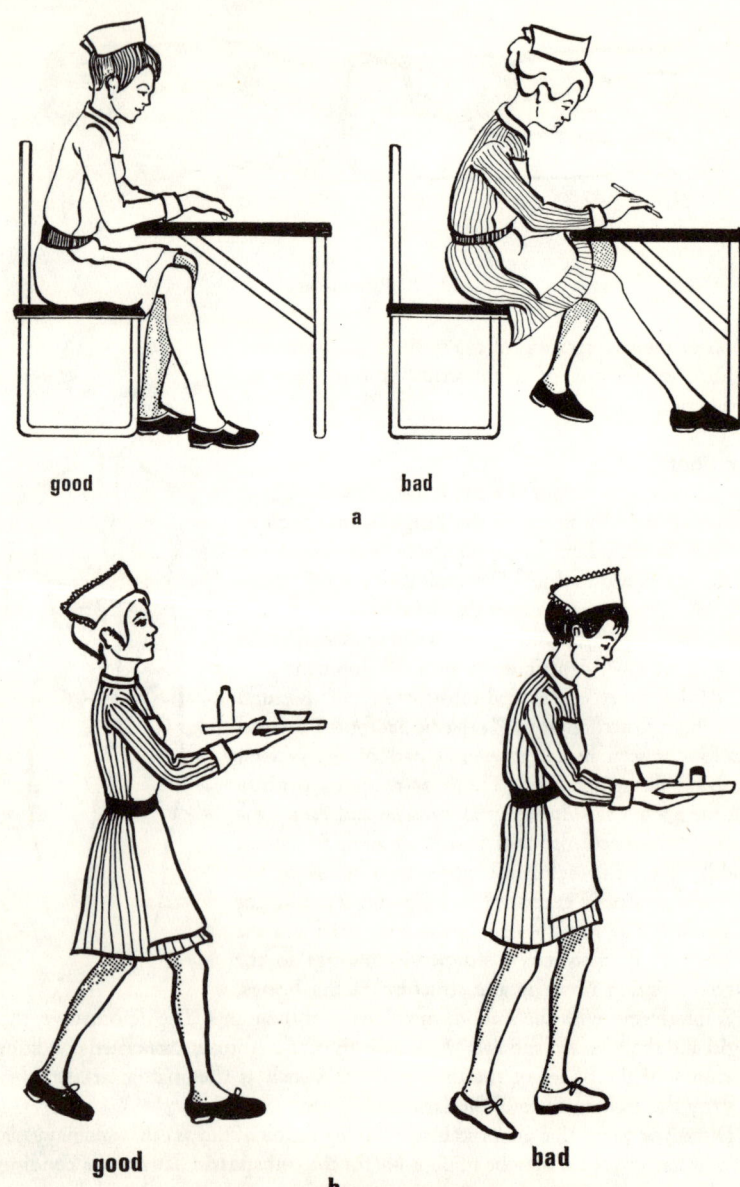

good   bad

a

good   bad

b

FIG. 4 Posture and the nurse
(a) Sitting
(b) Standing or carrying

can, however, exist for no obvious reason. X-ray investigation confirms the type of flat foot deformity.

Treatment. Physiotherapy may improve the muscle tone, but **modification** of the soles of the **shoes,** sometimes with additional **arch supports** inside the shoe, may give temporary support until the muscles strengthen (*see* Appendix, *Fig. 50d*). In the structural type a rigid arch support is required permanently. The patient should have a **sedentary occupation.** In spastic flat foot, conservative measures may suffice. These include arch supports or a below-knee walking caliper which holds the foot in such a position that the longitudinal arches are supported. Sometimes **excision** of **bony connections** which have persisted after birth, e.g. between the os calcis and navicular, may be curative. If this fails, there is the necessity in later life for **triple arthrodesis** which fuses the main joints in the foot and makes the arches rigid. This limits movement but relieves pain.

POSTURE AND THE NURSE

In the course of her work the nurse is subjected to an unusual amount of walking, standing and lifting. This is particularly so in the nursing of patients partially or completely immobilised in plaster of Paris or splints, and in the case of the chronic sick. A knowledge of how to protect her body from unnecessary mechanical strain is therefore important. A simple rule worth observing is '**Anything that keeps the back straight is good for it, anything which bends the back is therefore bad and should be avoided** (*Fig. 4a and b*).

Where a **mechanical lifting device** is available it should always be utilised in preference to manual lifting. Such devices can be used for changing the patient's position while in bed, from bed to chair, from chair to bath and vice versa.

Changing the patient's position in bed without the use of a mechanical device requires two nurses at least, more when the patient is unconscious and unable to co-operate (*Fig. 5*).

Assisting patients on to plinths or into bed need not present a problem. Most patients given clear and proper instruction manage with assistance rather than being actually lifted by the nurse. The patient turns his back to the plinth and uses a foot stool to allow him to ease his buttocks on to it, with the assistance of the nurse. The process is similar when the patient steps down from the plinth, the sequence being in the reverse order.

In theatre, heavy patients who are unconscious have to be transferred quickly from table to trolley or bed, and vice versa. Fortunately, many theatres have male theatre staff to relieve the nurse of this job. Where a stretcher canvas is available it is rolled under the patient as he is turned to either side. The poles are put in position and, where possible, four lifters, keeping their arms close to their sides and their backs straight, transfer the patient to the trolley. If a stretcher canvas is not used, or where a patient in a hip spica or plaster bed is being transferred directly to his bed from the theatre table the procedure illustrated in Figure 6 is important.

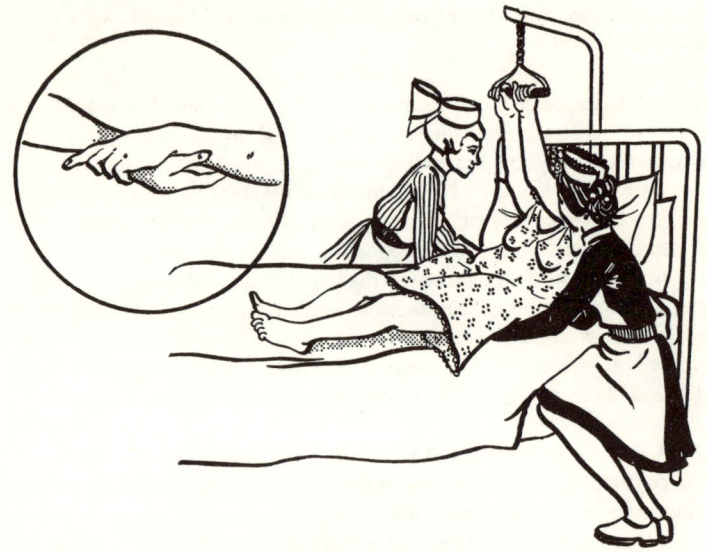

FIG. 5 Changing the patient's position

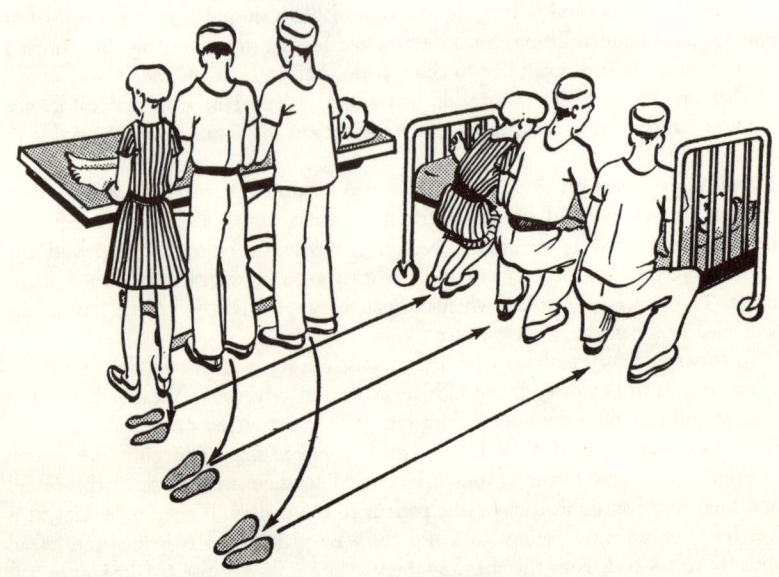

FIG. 6 Lifting and transferring a helpless patient

THE NURSING OF PATIENTS WITH EXISTING POSTURAL DEFORMITIES

If the deformity is fixed, e.g. structural kyphoscoliosis, a very firm bed will fail to support the more mobile compensatory curves in the back, and these are therefore subject to strain. The use of **fracture boards,** a good **interior sprung mattress** and **supporting pillows** cradling the deformity allow the patient to lie comfortably. The skin over the apex of the curve is in this way free from pressure. Many patients prefer to lie in the lateral position. It is particularly important to **support** the **head** and **neck.** When seating the patient in a chair enough pillows should be used to **accommodate** the **deformity.** A patient with ankylosing spondylitis demands regular postural observation. If his neck is over-supported and his dorso-lumbar spine poorly supported he will develop a fixed 'C' curve and be unable to see ahead when walking. Postural exercises are of little use in fixed deformities but **breathing exercises** should be encouraged. Where a patient is admitted wearing a **surgical appliance** it is important that it is not forgotten when he once again becomes mobile.

Valgus or **varus deformities** of the limbs will probably give little trouble while the patient is confined to bed or sitting in a chair. These deformities are more troublesome when he starts to walk. Sticks, crutches or other **walking aids** may be of use during the convalescent period. The patient should be advised to wear **comfortable shoes** which adequately support the foot and ankle. **Arch supports** may be required if he has been non-weight-bearing for a time, or where there is valgus deformity of the feet. Callosities, corns and other minor foot problems which could make early ambulation uncomfortable for the patient can be treated by a **chiropodist.**

2 CONGENITAL AND DEVELOPMENTAL DISORDERS

Congenital abnormalities are those which are present at or before birth. The cause of the abnormality may be a **defective gene,** i.e. an inherited characteristic passed on from one or other parent. It is possible therefore that in subsequent generations such genetic congenital deformities may be reproduced. Congenital disorders, however, may not be genetic in origin. It is known that there are **environmental factors** which are associated with foetal abnormality, i.e. an unprotected pregnant woman exposed to the virus of Rubella during the first eight weeks of pregnancy. Further, it is thought that in some instances maldevelopment of the foetus may be related to a **defect within the uterus.** Treatment of an inherited defect or developmental disorder is not yet possible but there has been continued progress in the **management of the resultant deformity.**

The word *orthopaedic* means *straight child.* This is exactly the result aimed at by the orthopaedic surgeon treating children's deformities. Treatment is, therefore, concentrated on enabling the child to stand up straight, walk and run normally. The vast difference in the management of orthopaedic problems in children from that of adults is the **growth factor.** In congenital abnormalities Nature appears to be opposing the surgeon continuously during the whole period of growth, making relapse of the condition a common occurrence and resistance to treatment considerable. Fortunately, this conflict applies mainly to the treatment of deformities, and examples of Nature assisting the surgeon are seen in the treatment of trauma and infection.

Deformities in children may be manifest in many different ways, varying from a minor single disorder to multiple and sometimes gross anomalies, severely crippling the child both physically and mentally. Simple anatomical classifications of such derangements can be made:

1 **Absence of a part.** Phocomelia, for example, is the absence of limbs producing a 'seal-like' deformity.
2 **Maldevelopment of a part.** Congenital high scapula (Sprengel's shoulder) is an example of an incomplete developmental disorder, which consists of an abnormally high and permanently elevated shoulder.
3 **An extra part.** Polydactilism, for example, is the presence of more than five digits on either hand or foot.

In this chapter only three of the more common affections of the child will be described: club foot, congenital dislocation of the hip and spina bifida cystica.

CLUB FOOT

The medical term for this condition is **congenital talipes equino varus** and although it may seem rather formal to use this terminology it is one occasion when the name completely describes the deformity. The word *congenital* means *born with*. *Talipes* is derived from the words *talus*, the bone in the ankle joint, and *pes* meaning *foot*. In club foot the head of the talus projects on the outer side of the foot, and if the deformity remained uncorrected the child would walk on this projection, i.e. a *talus foot*. *Equinus* comes from the Latin word meaning *horse*. A horse's heel is high and poorly developed, and the toes (hoof) point towards the ground. The word *varus* describes the position of the sole of the foot in the deformity. It faces in an upward direction.

Treatment

The sooner this is started the better the result is likely to be. Some authorities suggest that treatment should be started immediately. Others advise waiting until the baby is about **two weeks old.** There are several reasons for the latter sugges- tion. Firstly, it allows the baby to become accustomed to his new environment, that is a separate existence outside the uterus. Secondly, by this time the mother has recovered from the birth and can visit the child in hospital. She can also continue to breast feed the baby if this has been established. Thirdly, it is thought that the results are equally good as long as the treatment is started within the first three weeks of life. The baby is admitted to the children's ward so that initial treatment may be intensive, continuous and under the close supervision of staff skilled in the management of babies and their splints.

Correction of the deformity is produced by manipulative stretching of the tight tissues on the inner side of the foot and the back of the leg. This stretching is done gently but firmly, stopping short of complete rupture of the part. Although anaesthesia is not required, stretching of the tight and shortened tissues on the inner side of the foot is painful, hence the reason for gentleness and care in the manipulation. Rough handling can produce surgical shock and a baby may even collapse. Skill and experience in the procedure are required and can only be gained by practice under the guidance of a skilled supervisor.

The correction obtained by the mani- pulation has to be maintained by **splintage.** The splint most frequently used is the **Dennis Browne** metal splint, suitably padded to prevent pressure sores occurring (*Fig. 7*). The foot is held in the splint by 1 inch (2.5 cm) Elastoplast strapping. Stretching of the tissues causes reactionary swelling of the foot, and the toes must be examined carefully for any change in circulation. Hence in this procedure

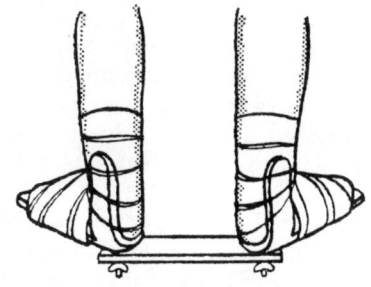

FIG. 7 Dennis Browne's splint

Elastoplast is often preferred to adhesive strapping. It allows for some elastic expansion to accommodate swelling and avoids a 'tourniquet-like' effect. The child requires constant supervision, preferably in hospital, during the first week of treatment. Manipulation and splintage are repeated daily for seven to ten days when over-correction of the deformity is usually obtained. At this stage reactionary swelling has settled and the baby can be allowed home.

Splintage is further maintained for about one year. The child attends as an outpatient at fortnightly intervals to have the splint changed. By the age of one year the child is ready to walk and fixed splintage is discarded. **Specially adapted boots** are then substituted. The adaptations to the boots are simple and are aimed at maintaining the correction which has been obtained by the previous regime. The heels are removed in an attempt to stretch the calf muscles when the child puts his foot on the ground. An outer raising of about ⅛-in. (0·3 cm) is applied to the sole in order to keep the foot in the valgus position, which is that opposite to the original varus deformity.

While in bed the child wears a pair of boots to which is attached a metal bar, holding the feet in the over-corrected position. In this way, treatment is continuous twenty-four hours per day. Without **night boots,** relapse would occur as the normal position of the feet in bed is one of equinus and varus.

It has been shown that after one year of treatment about 60 per cent of club foot deformities are corrected. This, unfortunately, leaves a large percentage of children requiring further treatment. When conservative treatment has failed, operation is necessary. Relapse of the deformity is usually obvious by the age of two years. It is at this age that a **soft tissue release operation** is undertaken. This consists of removing the tight subcutaneous tissue on the inner side of the foot, lengthening the short muscles and mobilising the joints. The foot can then be placed in the corrected position and held for three to four months, until the growth is normal on both sides. By this operative procedure a further 20 per cent of deformities are corrected and remain satisfactory.

In children with persistent deformity additional operative procedures are required. At the age of five or six, the child may be admitted to hospital for the operative removal of a wedge of cartilage from the calcaneo-cuboid joint on the lateral side of the foot (**Delwyn Evan's operation**). This allows for eversion of the foot and correction of the varus deformity. Further operation may be necessary to correct a persistent equino-varus deformity, but is usually withheld until the child is nine or ten years of age. **Triple arthrodesis** involves correction of the deformity and fusion of the three main joints of the foot, i.e. the sub-taloid, the calcaneo-cuboid and the talo-navicular joints. Thus the foot is stabilised in the normal plantigrade position.

Post-operative Management of Corrective Operation

The child's limb is immobilised in a **plaster cast** for two weeks. Stitches are removed under a general anaesthetic and, at the same time, the foot is re-manipulated if necessary. Thereafter, a walking plaster is applied after which the child is allowed to go home. The plaster is changed as required but immobilisation is maintained for **three months.** This regime allows a child to return to school if he is in that age group. After the removal of the plaster the child continues to attend as an outpatient at regular intervals until about the age of twelve years. By this age growth is well advanced, and in most cases, significant relapse of the deformity is unlikely.

Nursing Care. As in adults, care of the limb in plaster is important (*see p.* 168–71). The main points to remember in the management of children are:

1 The child cannot always say clearly what is wrong. Crying, fretting and undue restlessness require investigation.
2 The plaster cast is much more liable to become wet, soiled and damaged. Protective waterproof adhesive strapping should therefore be applied to susceptible areas.
3 On return from theatre the position of the foot in plaster must be noted and maintained. There is a tendency sometimes for the foot to retract into a plaster cast. This must be recognised and corrected.

General care of the child is also important (*see* pp 225–7).

CONGENITAL DISLOCATION OF THE HIP

This is a condition which is of extreme importance. It occurs in about two in every thousand live births. **Females** are more commonly affected than males, and the **first born** female in particular. The condition may be **unilateral** or **bilateral.** It can be recognised at birth and if treated immediately causes little or no upset to the baby. Complete cure is almost certain. On the other hand if the diagnosis is not made until the child is walking the treatment is prolonged and arduous, and complete cure is by no means certain. It is necessary for every one dealing with babies to learn how to diagnose the condition in the newborn. It is as imperative to look for this abnormality in every newborn baby as is the routine examination for cleft palate, imperforate anus or any of the other congenital anomalies.

Diagnosis
Ortolani's test is easy to do although sometimes more difficult to interpret. The baby is laid on its back and the examiner stands facing the pelvis. The baby's knees and hips are flexed to a right angle (90 degrees). The knees are then gripped in the first web of the examiner's hands, i.e. between the thumb and index finger. The middle finger may be used in preference to the index finger as it is usually longer. The baby's left knee is held in the examiner's right hand and the right knee in the left hand. The tip of the index finger will then be on the greater trochanter. The baby's thighs are brought towards the table, i.e. abducted, and the first abnormality detected is a limitation of abduction on the involved side. When this resistance is felt, the tip of the index finger pushes the trochanter forward and the head of the femur will be felt clicking into the joint. The actual reduction may be

seen or heard. All nurses should be familiar with this test. Only experience really teaches, and like swimming and cycling, once learned it is never forgotten.

Where there is any doubt it is better to **err on the side of over-caution** than to miss the deformity, the treatment of which is more difficult in the older child and the results less certain.

Treatment

The **newborn** baby is put into a malleable divaricator **splint (Barlow's)** with hips widely abducted and externally rotated (*Fig. 8a*). The child is allowed to be taken home in this splint. The mother is given instruction in how to bath, feed and change the baby without removing the splint. It is important that the child is brought back to hospital at weekly intervals so that the doctor may check and, if

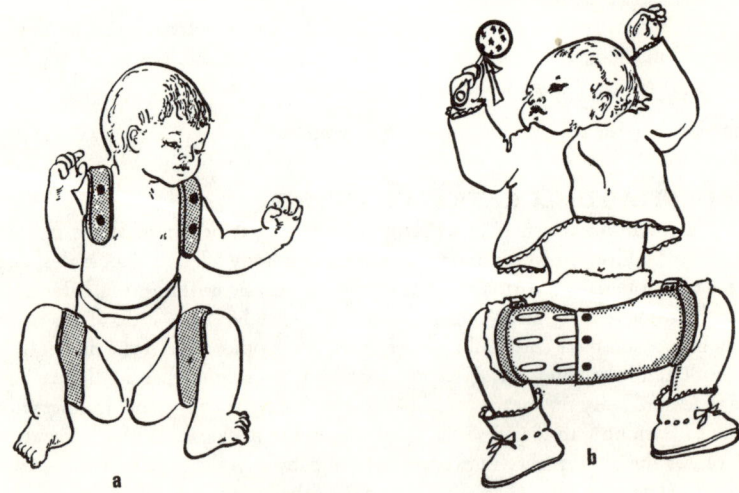

FIG. 8   (*a*) Barlow's splint
(*b*) Craig's splint

necessary, alter the position of the splint. After six weeks of treatment a **Craig splint** (*Fig. 8b*) is substituted. This is a polythene splint applied over double napkins. The mother is shown how to remove the splint for bathing and changing of the baby, and how to reapply it correctly. **Splintage** is continued in this way for a further six weeks. By this time the baby is **three months** old and splintage is discarded. The legs in the abducted, externally rotated position are allowed to descend gradually into the normal position without further treatment. The child is seen at the outpatient department at regular intervals until, on X-ray examination, the femoral head has developed and lies in the correct anatomical position in the joint. The child is often about one year old at this stage.

Late Diagnosis of Congenital Hip Dislocation

Diagnosis in the older child involves six signs which may be present in varying proportions.

1 **Shortening of the limb,** usually first noticed by the mother.
2 **Discrepancy** in the **skin creases** of the thigh, seen on inspection.
3 **Limitation** in **abduction,** found on examination.
4 **Limp.** In unilateral deformity the child tilts to the affected side on walking. In bilateral deformity there is a 'waddling' gait. The child is often late in walking, e.g. eighteen months.
5 **Telescoping** of the **femur** along the side wall of the pelvis.
6 **X-ray** appearance confirms the deformity.

Treatment

The child is admitted to hospital for one day before treatment is commenced to become familiar with her new environment. **Reduction** of the **dislocation** requires gentle manipulation under general anaesthesia. The muscles have become shortened due to the dislocation. In order to allow for complete and stable reduction, and also to prevent undue pressure on the femoral head, **adductor tenotomy** may be necessary. If reduction by this method cannot be obtained operative reduction is undertaken. As this is an extensive operation in the region of the hip joint it is avoided where possible. After reduction by either method both hips are

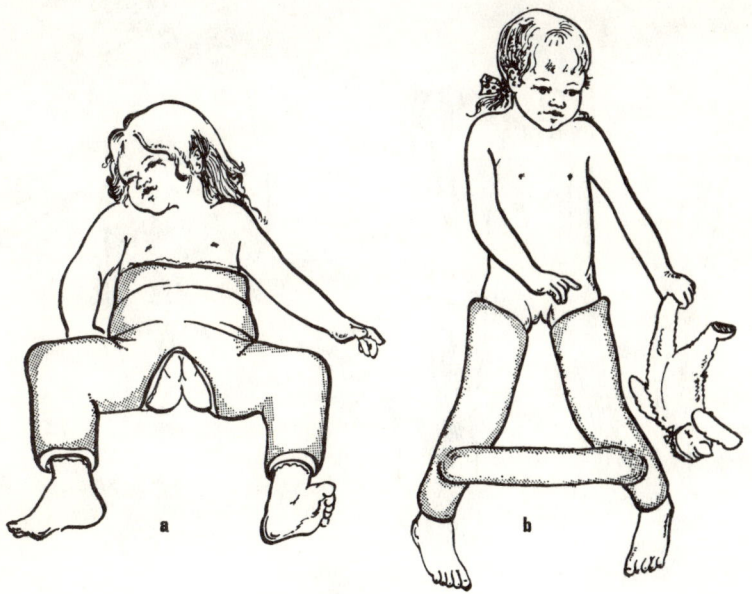

FIG. 9 (a) Frog plaster
(b) Batchelor plaster

immobilised in a **'Frog' plaster** for **six to eight weeks** (*Fig. 9a*). The child is then put into a **Batchelor plaster** which allows some function of the joints, an aid to the development of normal anatomy (*Fig. 9b*). Gradually, by the use of **serial plasters,** the limbs are brought down from wide abduction and external rotation into the neutral position and then into full internal rotation.

The child is allowed home between the changes of plaster and is actually encouraged to walk in the Batchelor plaster. The mother must, however, be aware of the necessity of returning to hospital with the child if the bar becomes loose, the plaster soft or broken. The plaster requires to be changed every two months because, in addition to becoming sodden and tight due to growth of the limb, it is necessary to alter the position of the hips in the process of treatment. In an attempt to keep the plaster firm and to avoid its digging into the skin on movement, the edges are covered by a protective waterproof strapping.

After about nine months the hips have reached the stage of full internal rotation. This is the most stable position of the hip joint. The disadvantage of this position is that the whole lower limb is also in full internal rotation. To correct this a **derotation osteotomy** is necessary. The femur is divided in the sub-trochanteric region so that the lower limb can be rotated into the neutral position with the foot facing forwards (*Fig. 10a*). This position is maintained by internal fixation. A single

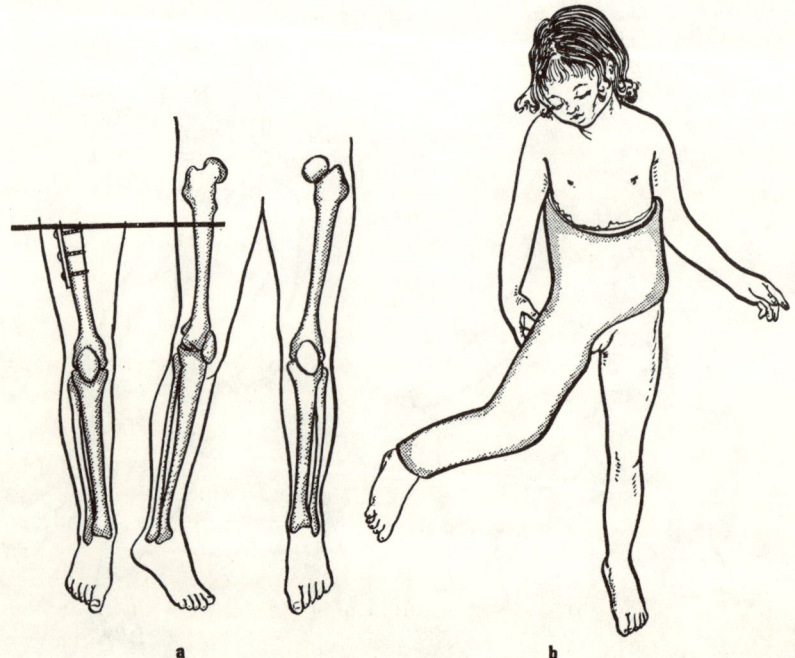

a   b

FIG. 10 (*a*) Derotation osteotomy
(*b*) Position of limb in plaster following derotation osteotomy

hip spica plaster is applied with the limb in abduction so that the relationship of the femoral head to the acetabulum is unchanged (*Fig. 10b*). The plaster is removed once the osteotomy has healed in about six weeks. The child is then allowed to mobilise freely whereby the limb adducts to the normal neutral position. Regular outpatient observation is continued for at least ten years.

In those cases showing signs of relapse, further treatment involving more complicated orthopaedic procedures is considered, e.g. **iliac osteotomy, acetabuloplasty** or even the creation of an **artificial joint.** The whole aim of treatment in this condition is to maintain a stable joint and prevent the development of painful osteoarthritis in later life.

SPINA BIFIDA CYSTICA (Myelomeningocele)

This is a condition in which there is a **defect** in the **spinal column.** The vertebral arches are absent and through this defect, the meninges with or without spinal cord tissues protrude. In an even more primitive developmental error the cord tissue may be exposed on the surface of the back. The incidence of this condition is about three per thousand live births. It may affect both sexes. As a result there is **paralysis** of those parts of the body which are supplied by nerves from the affected region. To add to the child's distress there is frequently interference with the free circulation of cerebro-spinal fluid round the brain, with resultant enlargement of the head, i.e. **hydrocephalus.** The incidence of hydrocephalus in spina bifida cystica is about 90 per cent. It is either present at birth or develops during the first few weeks of life.

In the past the majority of these children died but, with advances in anaesthetic skills and surgical techniques, many are now surviving because:

1 **Immediate closure of the spinal defect** prevents the exposed spinal cord tissues from drying and becoming infected, with resultant meningitis.

2 The **early insertion of a valve which drains the excess cerebro-spinal fluid** from the brain into the right atrium of the heart or into the peritoneum prevents the progression of the hydrocephalus.

3 The **use of antibiotics** and the **surgical techniques** available whereby the **urine by-passes the paralysed bladder** have lessened the mortality from urinary tract infection and renal failure.

Once these initial life-saving measures are completed successfully, the problem of management is centred on the limb paralysis which has now become very important. It has superseded the problem of the paralysis of poliomyelitis, now almost non-existent since vaccination against this condition has become possible.

The defect in the spinal column is found mainly in the lower thoracic, lumbar and sacral regions, so that paralysis is almost wholly confined to the lower limbs. It means that there is frequently **paralysis** of the **bladder** and **bowel,** and this adds difficulties in the total care of the patient.

The extent of paralysis of the limbs can vary considerably from a mere clawing of the toes due to paralysis of the intrinsic muscles of the foot, to complete paraplegia. To add to the difficulties of management, there may be a mixture of spastic and flaccid paralysis in the same limb, this being caused by involvement of spinal cord to one part and nerve root supply to the other.

Fortunately, in the majority of cases there is no involvement of the upper limbs although in some there is weakness, usually of the spastic type, as the result of the hydrocephalus. Thus the orthopaedic problems are confined to the lower limbs and to the spinal deformity; the upper limbs are available for the use of walking aids.

The paralysis of the nerve is total. There is not only a lack of function in the muscles but also complete **loss of sensation** in the part supplied. This area of sensory loss varies as markedly as the motor loss, which means that there may be complete lack of feeling in both limbs. The hazards of **pressure sores** are very great indeed. There is also loss of **proprioception,** i.e. muscle-joint sense. The child has no knowledge of the position of his limbs in space, unless he can actually see them.

The problem of congenital paraplegia is entirely different from that in adult life where the patient has already benefited by the experience of walking. The child may be completely unaware of the presence of lower limbs and will have to be taught, by very skilled personnel, the fundamental process of walking. The **training** of these **children to walk,** even if their muscle power will permit this, is therefore a major undertaking. The parents must be helped to understand the magnitude of the problem and to appreciate that the eventual ability of the child to walk is a major achievement. **Normal gait** is **seldom accomplished.**

The pull of the muscles which are working can often produce disabling deformities such as dislocation of the hips, club foot or calcaneous deformities of the feet. As spina bifida cystica is a congenital abnormality the paralysis is acting throughout the whole of the growth period; the deformed position can rapidly become fixed due to over-growth of bony tissue on the paralysed side.

Treatment

The aim of treatment is simple, i.e. **to give the child stable lower limbs.** This, at times, may not be easy to achieve. In order to allow anyone to stand or to walk three conditions are necessary: **stable hips, straight knees** and **plantigrade feet.** The latter term means that the heels and soles of the feet rest on the ground giving the widest possible base of weight-bearing surface. **Transplantation** of unopposed, deforming **muscles** may be required; firstly, **to stop** them pulling the foot into **deformity,** and secondly, where possible, **to use their function** in a new situation in order to prevent recurrence of the deformity. For example, an active flexor muscle group, with the opposing extensor group paralysed, may have some of its muscles transplanted to act as extensor muscles. This allows for correction of some of the deformity and some stability of the limb. In order to fulfil the third aim of providing the most adequate amount of weight-bearing surface an extensive use has to be made of **calipers.** Various operative procedures may also be necessary; these are similar to the operations used in the persistent club foot deformity, e.g. **soft tissue release** and **triple arthrodesis** (*see* Chapter 26, The Nursing of Children).

3 INFLAMMATORY CONDITIONS

Inflammation is the reaction of the body tissues to an irritant, which may be chemical, physical or organismal. The body tissues with which we are concerned are **bone** and **periosteum,** and those constituting the joint, viz. **articular cartilage** and **synovial membrane.** The inflammatory reactions which we shall discuss may be due to physical or organismal causes. Where due to a physical cause, the tissue reaction is one of a non-infective inflammation. Where organismal, on the other hand, the organism concerned invades the tissue, pus is produced and the resulting infection may be acute or chronic.

ACUTE INFLAMMATION

Physical Inflammatory Conditions
These are associated with **trauma,** e.g. a blow to the lower limb may produce a non-infective periostitis of tibia or a traumatic synovitis of the knee joint. These conditions, commonly seen in any casualty department, produce the local symptons and signs of inflammation but they **resolve quickly** and completely with **rest** and **immobilisation.**

Acute Inflammatory Conditions of Organismal Cause
The common causal organism is one of the **staphylococcal group** although others are occasionally responsible.

The mode of infection is either by (a) **direct entry** through a penetrating wound, such as in a compound fracture or through an operation wound, or (b) **via the bloodstream.** The result is inflammation of the bone or joint affected, i.e. **osteitis (osteomyelitis)** or **septic arthritis.**

Direct Wound Infection. Where a **bone** is subjected to trauma or operation the **periosteum** is **torn** or **divided** respectively; similarly in a **joint** the **capsule** is **ruptured** or **incised.** In both instances the protective coverings are no longer intact. Damage to the capillaries produces a collection of blood, haematoma, in which the invading organisms grow and multiply. Structures which are in the infected area, such as bone, periosteum, synovial membrane or cartilage are therefore exposed to invasion by the organisms. Sometimes the wound appears to have healed but, in actual fact, healing is only superficial and underneath organisms are active in the deeper structures. The body's defence mechanism resists this infection by producing an inflammatory reaction which is recognised by specific symptoms and signs.

Blood-Borne Infection. The organism is carried in the **bloodstream** from a focus in some other organ or tissue of the body. It is deposited in a **susceptible bone** or **joint** which attracts its growth and multiplication. The area affected may have suffered minor trauma at an earlier stage, often quite unknown to the patient. The infection occurs **within** the bone or joint. The **periosteum** and **joint capsule** remain **intact**. The products of inflammatory reaction, pus and abscess formation, are therefore confined within the bone or joint. Thus pus collects and as the strong fibrous nature of the periosteum and synovial membrane do not readily allow for distension there are symptoms and signs of pus formation under tension. This mode of infection is common in **infants** and **adolescents**.

Physiology of the Body's Defence Mechanism

The body reacts to any infection by an **increase** in the **heart action** thus allowing more blood to flow through the part. This results in **swelling, congestion** and **pain**. The **body temperature** is **raised** to make conditions unfavourable for the growth of the organisms. There is an **increase** in the number of **white cells** in the blood to attack the organism (phagocytosis). During this process some of the tissue cells are destroyed producing an exudate of white cells, dead tissue cells and plasma, i.e. **pus**. Where phagocytosis is efficient the pus is absorbed and resolution of the inflammatory process occurs. Significant bone damage is avoided.

Symptoms and Signs of Inflammation. The local symptoms and signs are **pain, swelling, redness, heat, tenderness** and **loss of function**. If there has been an injury or operation wound, the pain associated with this, which normally settles within three to four days, persists and increases in severity as the infection spreads within the area. In blood-borne infection the pain is dull in character at first, but becomes excruciating and intolerable as pus collects under tension in either the bone or joint affected. Swelling may be marked, the limb being tense and oedematous or the infected joint obviously distended. Redness is associated with the hyperaemia. Distended veins may be clearly seen. The skin overlying the bone or joint may be warm to touch. **Handling of the limb** or joint will produce extreme pain. In osteitis, contraction of the muscles, which have their attachment in the region of inflammation, will be painful. Muscle action is inhibited voluntarily. In septic arthritis the distension of the joint capsule with pus irritates the nerve endings. Movement stretches the capsule causing extreme pain. As a result there is guarding spasm of the muscles controlling joint movement.

The general signs and symptoms of the infection are those of a mild **anaemia,** general **malaise, headache, pyrexia, tachycardia, anorexia, oliguria, constipation** and **insomnia.**

Investigation. This includes X-ray and blood examination. The hyperaemia of the bone results in local decalcification at or around the bone ends shown on X-ray as porosis. The organism is destroyed by the white cells in the blood so that a temporary increase in the normal number is essential, i.e. leucocytosis. The toxin from the organisms damages the red cells and produces anaemia. As a result the blood is less viscous and the erythrocyte sedimentation rate is increased.

Management. Management is important. As the body reaction takes time to become manifest, a certain amount of damage to the body tissues has already occurred. Therapy, therefore, must be commenced as soon as possible to destroy the organisms. The local pain, general malaise, pyrexia and rapid pulse will demand that the patient **rests in bed. Immobilisation** of the part affected, either by pillows or sandbags, or by more adequate means, e.g. Thomas's splint and plaster cast, is important. **Elevation of the limb** will minimise swelling. The body defences now have a controlled situation in which to act.

Treatment. Treatment of the infection is by **antibiotic therapy.** In direct infection through a traumatic or operation wound there may be a discharge of pus through a sinus in the scar tissue. A **culture of the pus** should be done quickly to determine the causal organism and its sensitivity so that the correct antibiotic can be administered. In a blood-borne infection where the pus is confined within the bone or joint infected, **a blood culture** must be obtained **during a spike of fever** as well as serial blood specimens within a 24 hour period for culture and sensitivity studies. **'Blind antibiotic' therapy** is then begun. The rationale of this is to give two antibiotics selected specifically to attack all strains of the staphylococcus aureus, and as wide a range of other likely organisms as possible. If, however, the result of the blood culture later shows ineffective 'blind antibiotic' therapy the **correct antibiotic** can then be administered. **The full therapeutic dose is given.** For maximum effect the antibiotic drug may be given by injection initially. Where the patient is very ill and perhaps vomiting, the dehydration associated with this will require correction by intravenous fluid therapy which is a convenient method of effectively administering the antibiotic.

The patient's general condition, his temperature and pulse are all closely observed for the next 24–48 hours. If there is a marked improvement in the general condition and in the local symptoms and signs, early active control of the infection is usually guaranteed. Where, however, there is little improvement and the patient remains extremely ill, **aspiration of the abscess** is necessary. The procedure has several advantages: the removal of pus relieves tension under the periosteum so alleviating pain and allowing a more adequate blood supply to the bone; the presence of pus confirms the diagnosis and provides a specimen for bacteriological culture and sensitivity tests. If, after aspiration of the abscess, the condition of the patient does not considerably improve an **open drainage operation** will be necessary whereby multiple drill holes are made in the bone to allow adequate drainage from the marrow cavity. Care is taken during the procedure to avoid damage to the epiphyseal line. The instillation of a suitable antibiotic further attacks the disease locally.

It is important in the early treatment of **septic arthritis** to **aspirate the joint** when the appropriate antibiotic may also be introduced. Repetition of this procedure is often necessary during the acute phase.

Relief of pain requires the administration of potent analgesics, often by intramuscular injection initially. These are altered in accordance with the patient's relief of pain in his response to antibiotic therapy.

Prevention of deformity is important. In osteitis the patient will maintain his limb in a position of maximum comfort. There is voluntary inhibition of muscle, with the result that deformities such as drop-foot develop unless careful observation is maintained to prevent this. In septic arthritis prolonged muscle spasm will produce deformity of that joint and the articular cartilage will be damaged permanently. **Sliding skin traction** must therefore be applied to the limb to keep the joint surfaces apart until the infection subsides.

General Care of the Patient

Special Observations. A **four-hourly temperature and pulse** chart is essential initially to assess the patient's condition and his response to treatment. Where blood culture is required it is most important to record the patient's temperature frequently and to inform the doctor of the first spike of temperature. This indicates the multiplication of the organisms in the blood and gives the best chance of a positive culture.

The **limb** must be **inspected** regularly for signs of improvement or lack of response to treatment. Any unusual symptoms and signs which would suggest septic foci in other parts of the body must be noted. **Fluid balance** should be assessed until the acute phase is over, in order to prevent dehydration.

The toxic effects of an infection cause interference with normal appetite, sleep and general well-being. **Tepid sponging** initially, together with **antipyretic drugs,** e.g. Aspirin, will reduce temperature and also relieve headache. **Appetite stimulants** and an attractive **light diet,** with ample **iron** and **vitamins,** help to overcome the infection and improve the patient's general condition. **Sedation** at night will prevent insomnia. **Adequate fluids** should be given to correct oliguria and, in addition to the dietary composition, a **mild aperient** may be required to relieve constipation.

Assessment of progress is by clinical and blood examination and regular radiological review at weekly intervals.

Mobilisation of the Patient. As the general musculature is weakened by the infection it is essential, once this has settled, to build up muscle tone by means of **maintenance exercises.** Local muscle wasting of the affected limb will require more intense physiotherapy to regain normal function. These exercises are only commenced once the serological and radiological investigations confirm the clinical impression of recovery. It is at this stage that the patient can sit out of bed. Overtiredness and any attempt to stand or walk should be avoided until the muscle tone has improved. Once full muscle and physical function is restored the patient becomes ambulant.

Complications of Acute Osteitis and Septic Arthritis

Chronic Infection. Chronic infection can result and may be due to a virulent strain of organism, to poor body resistance or to incorrect or inadequate antibiotic therapy. **Abscess formation** will follow, and as more pus collects the tension increases and the abscess ruptures spontaneously bursting the skin or wound scar. A **discharging sinus** develops. In chronic osteitis (osteomyelitis) infection spreads within the bone, interfering with its blood supply resulting in local death of bone, i.e. a **sequestrum.** This may be extruded through the sinus but often requires surgical removal. As a result new bone or involucrum is allowed to form. The area is always a **site of potential infection.**

Pathological Fracture. This can occur where the bone has been weakened excessively by the infection. Any evidence of weakness or defect in the bone caused by the infection usually determines that the patient requires the support of a protective walking caliper until there are radiological signs of repair.

Septicaemia. This may be seen in association with multiple foci. Organisms may be deposited in any tissue of the body, e.g. other bones or joints, the brain, heart, lungs or abdominal viscera. This can be a fulminating type of infection producing severe toxaemia and even death. Massive doses of antibiotics to combat the infection, and as a last resort, intravenous hydrocortisone to compensate for adrenal failure are necessary to save life.

CHRONIC INFLAMMATORY DISEASE—TUBERCULOSIS

Tuberculosis is a disease characterised by its very chronic course. In the past it affected an individual in many cases for a lifetime. Hospitalisation was long term, often over many years, and recurrence not uncommon. Patients were severely debilitated due to gross tissue destruction. In those with bone and joint disease the formation of large cold abscesses and copious discharging sinuses was common. If healing eventually took place, fibrous ankylosis often with gross deformity was the end result. Where healing was delayed the loss of protein from the sinuses contributed to such conditions as amyloid disease.

Although with the introduction of anti-tuberculous drug therapy the whole pattern of the disease has been altered, there is still a significant death rate, from pulmonary tuberculosis in particular. Formerly the condition was generally more prevalent in children, in people from isolated communities or in those living in poor social conditions.

Despite an organised campaign aimed at **immunising every neonate with B.C.G.** (Bacillus Calmette—Guérin) vaccine, patients suffering from tuberculosis are still being detected in this and other highly developed countries. Mass chest radiography shows a peak prevalance in older males and young adult females. At the beginning of the century almost fifty per cent of the total number of cases notified were in the younger (0–25 years) age group. This group now comprises about twenty per cent of the total. Males over 45 years constitute around sixty per cent of the number of new cases reported.

Cause. The disease is caused by the **tubercle bacillus.** There are three main types, human, bovine and avian. All may affect human beings if in close prolonged contact with the infected creatures or following the ingestion of the milk of infected cows. The **primary lesion** is either in the **lung** and associated lymph nodes, or in the **alimentary tract** and related mesenteric lymph nodes. A small primary lung focus may not produce symptoms of lung disease. Similarly, a minor infection of the bowel may not produce significant intestinal symptoms.

Clinical Features
At the time of infection the patient is usually in a lowered state of health. Once the primary lesion is established he generally becomes further **debilitated,** often with apparent **anorexia, pallor** and **loss of weight.**

From this stage the disease may follow one of two courses. The patient's defence mechanism may halt its progress allowing **calcification** of the **lesion** with resultant **inactivity.** The organism may, however, **spread** from the lymphatic system to the **blood stream** with the development of lesions in other tissues of the body, e.g. **bone** and **joint.**

When the disease attacks bone and joint the main regions involved are the **spine, hips** and **knees,** although all other joints can be affected. Like any blood-borne infection, the tubercle bacillus is carried into the bone and deposited or trapped in an area containing, usually, a network of blood capillaries, i.e. the metaphysis of long bones as in the femur, the diaphysis or centre of short bones as in the phalanges or spine. The result is a tuberculous **osteitis.** The joint may become involved in two ways, either by direct spread from the bone through to the joint or by blood-borne infection directly to the synovial membrane, producing a **synovitis.**

Symptoms and Signs
The symptoms and signs of bone and joint disease are initially **pain** and **deformity. Swelling** results from thickening of the synovium. Joint movement is painful and is limited by protective muscle spasm. Very often a **child** suffers from '**night cries'.** During sleep the muscles tend to relax and if the child subconsciously moves the affected joints, pain is severe so wakening the child and causing it to cry. In the later stages, increasing bone or joint destruction leads to progressive deformity. This may be marked, e.g. kyphosis in a tuberculous spine. Soft tissue swellings particularly in the pharynx, back and groin indicate the presence of **cold abscess formation.**

X-ray examination confirms the nature of the lesion, demonstrates the extent of damage to bone or joint and the presence or absence of abscess formation. Blood examination may aid diagnosis. A raised erythrocyte sedimentation rate, a secondary anaemia and a rise in the number of lymphocytes may suggest the presence of the disease. The **Mantoux** (tuberculin) **test** of sensitivity to tuberculous protein is done. A positive result may be interpreted in one of three ways. Firstly, the patient may have had a minor infection by the tubercle bacillus which was resisted by th body's defence, and by this process he has acquired an immunity. Secondly, th patient may have acquired immunity from the administration of B.C.G. Thirdly, he may be suffering from active tuberculosis. With the advent of anti-tuberculous drugs it is now safe, in doubtful lesions, to establish the diagnosis by biopsy.

Treatment

Treatment is by **immediate anti-tuberculous drug therapy.** The well known group of anti-tuberculous drugs, Streptomycin, Para-amino-salicylic acid (P.A.S.) and Iso-nicotinic Acid Hydrazide (I.N.A.H.) are used.

Where one drug is used, there is a risk that the tubercle bacillus may develop resistance to it. Therefore it is essential that at least two drugs are administered and ideal if all three can be tolerated for an initial period without side effects. **Strepto-mycin** is administered by intramuscular injection. It has serious toxic **side-effects.** In particular, it produces irreversible damage to the eighth cranial nerve with result-ant **vertigo** and sometimes **deafness.** There is also the **risk** that **with defective renal function** Streptomycin will be poorly excreted and will be retained in the blood. It will soon rise to a toxic level and damage the eighth nerve. In patients with poor renal function it is preferable that an alternative drug is administered. It is, therefore, important to recognise dizziness, any defect in hearing, or an inadequate urinary output. Administration of Streptomycin is discontinued routinely after three months or immediately adverse symptoms and signs develop. P.A.S. and I.N.A.H. are administered as a combined oral preparation. These drugs are usually continued for a prolonged period, one year or longer, in order to effect a cure of the disease.

There are indications that certain strains of the human tubercle bacillus are developing a resistance to Streptomycin and possible resistance to either or both P.A.S. and I.N.A.H. Where, therefore, the patient does not show a continued response to drug therapy within the first three months, or if in fact his condition deteriorates earlier, review of the drug therapy is essential. A wide range of alternative anti-tuberculous drugs exist with which to replace one or all three drugs. If there is still no significant response to alternative treatment after a further period of three months, it is likely that the infecting organism is either an avian type or atypical mycobacterium. In the treatment of this specific form of resistant infection the group of drugs used consists of Capreomycin, Ethambutol and Rifampicin. All three drugs are administered and are available as oral prepara-tions.

If a specimen of pus becomes available even after the administration of anti-tuberculous drugs has commenced, it should be cultured, and organism sensitivity obtained in order to confirm that the patient is receiving adequate and correct drug therapy.

The aim is to attack the disease early during the synovial stage. This prevents bone destruction and retains full joint mobility. **Prolonged, complete rest** and a **nutritious diet** which were the pillars of treatment in the past are still the basis of treatment to-day. **The affected part is immobilised,** the spine in a spinal frame or plaster bed, the hip in an abduction frame or plaster spica, and the knee in a Thomas's splint. The positioning of the limbs in a functional position is important as joint stiffness may be a later result.

Once the lesion is controlled by drug therapy, and the patient is generally healthier, **surgical exploration** of the lesion may be undertaken. This is indicated by the X-ray appearance of bone or joint destruction. **Evacuation of sequestra, caseous material or pus** from the affected bone or joint accelerates the reparative process. Nowadays, this procedure may be done early, e.g. at 3–6 months. By this means, although normal joint function cannot be restored, the resultant fibrous ankylosis protects the joint against recurrence. Where the development of a strong fibrous ankylosis seems unlikely the whole joint is curetted and packed with bone chips, producing a **surgical fusion** or arthrodesis.

Immobilisation is continued until fusion is clinically and radiologically complete. Thus having treated the secondary lesion, it is important to remember that a primary focus exists and this explains why there is the need for a prolonged period of drug therapy.

Physiotherapy. This is important and initially involves **passive** movements of all unaffected joints to prevent permanent incapacity. As the patient's condition improves gentle **active exercises** of all joints distant from the lesion are encouraged, gradually involving more joints as the lesion heals. The help of the medical social worker is required, mental rest being as essential as physical immobilisation. Progress is assessed by **serial X-rays, chest, blood and urine examination.** The patient is often observed as an outpatient for several years.

Nursing management. Nursing management is important, although easier now that long-term immobilisation has been considerably reduced by drug therapy and surgery. Immobilisation is still, nevertheless, prolonged. The nurse's rôle in management is vital in augmenting with good nursing care the advantages gained by drugs and surgery. As well as understanding the disease and its effect on the patient she is required to apply and maintain the splints, appliances and plasters used in immobilisation. The complications of treatment are avoided by good anticipation. The general condition and morale of the patient is important. Verandahs afford access to fresh air and sunlight. Attention to diet is necessary to rebuild wasted body tissues. Appetite stimulants, either in the form of drugs or beverages, are useful. The patient's normal bowel habits must be maintained. Diversional therapy, encouragement with hobbies, and access to radio, library and television are all important. It may be possible to group together patients with common interests thus relieving boredom.

Splintage. The accuracy in taking measurements for spinal or hip frames will determine whether or not these fit the patient comfortably. The saddle, groin straps, pelvic and pectoral body bands must all fit correctly. The skin extension strapping of the fixed traction, used in conjunction with the hip frames and Thomas's splints, must be carefully applied. The ability to apply plaster of Paris splints and assist with plaster beds enables the nurse to do confidently, minor but necessary adjustments (*see pp.* 158, 167 on application of skin traction and plaster of Paris).

Complications can be avoided by proper use of splints and plasters, and by the knowledge and anticipation of the likely problems. Patients nursed in spinal or hip frames or plasters sometimes suffer from 'frame sickness' (a mild paralytic ileus) which usually settles if the patient's position is altered. It is important for the nurse to understand the nursing management of patients in splints or plaster casts (*see pp.* 159 168 on care of plaster and splints). The patients require to be turned regularly each day. The inclination of the frame and plaster can be altered by alternately raising the head and foot of the bed or by suspending a plaster bed or frame using a system of pulleys and weights whereby the patient can alter his position voluntarily.

Complications

A careful watch for the **development of abscesses** at all the classical sites, particularly in the lumbar and inguinal regions, is essential. **Sinus formation** following the bursting of cold abscesses is less common now since the introduction of anti-tuberculous drugs. **Repeated aspiration** of an enlarging abscess, however, may still be necessary. The nurse's warning to the doctor of the presence of a new swelling is helpful. Once a sinus has developed it is inconvenient to the patient and nursing staff as it discharges copious pus. This not only requires the frequent application of absorbent dressings, which may remain necessary for months before healing occurs, but also it is a major source of infection within the ward. Failure of a patient to improve with careful treatment often signifies poor resistance or the **development of a fresh lesion.** Continued or recurrent apathy, anorexia and general debility indicate the necessity to search for another lesion. X-ray of chest, other bony areas and abdominal or neurological examination may reveal such a lesion.

A serious complication in spinal disease (Pott's disease) is the development of **paraplegia.** This may occur during the acute stage of the disease due to pressure on the spinal cord. Pressure may result from a developing or enlarging abscess, excessive tuberculous granulation tissue or sequestra of bone or disc. The symptoms and signs of a space-occupying lesion are produced. Paraplegia may also be a late complication, months or perhaps years after apparent healing of the lesion. Tuberculous joint disease heals by a fibrous ankylosis, therefore absence of a sound bony fusion can lead to a gradual increase in the spinal deformity. Stretching of the spinal cord or nerve roots follows and this gives rise to a varying degree and type of paraplegia. A large spinal abscess causing cord or nerve root pressure may produce a similar pattern either during the acute stage of the disease or in recurrent infection. The development of flexor muscle spasms, particularly nocturnally, with associated loss of sensation and motor power suggests the onset of this complication. Treatment requires that the patient is again immobilised, if necessary for a prolonged period, in a plaster bed. If the paraplegia fails to resolve, operative spinal decompression is undertaken expeditiously.

Tuberculosis demands a high degree of co-operation amongst all members of the team caring for the patient if it is to be defeated. It offers many interesting problems in the solution of which the nurse is a very active participant.

Control and Eradication of Tuberculosis

The disease for some time remained quiescent in the community but has since become more active with the production of added resistant strains. This makes treatment more difficult, particularly if it is not established early. It is important, therefore, that there is a general awareness of the existence of the disease, of the age group it tends to affect and that it remains a notifiable disease. The following measures are necessary if the disease is to be eventually eradicated:

1 Mass chest radiography, particularly in males over 45 years and younger females.
2 The use of the tuberculin test and informed interpretation of its significance.
3 The use of B.C.G. vaccination to raise the natural resistance to the infection.
4 The search for the disease as a possible diagnosis in doubtful chest, bone, joint or kidney lesions by the family doctor and at hospital outpatient clinics.
5 Raising of the economic standards of the community, i.e. better food, improved housing and adequate recreation.

4 CHRONIC JOINT DISEASE

Of all the many diseases of a chronic nature which may affect a joint there are two which are extremely common, osteoarthritis and rheumatoid arthritis.

OSTEOARTHRITIS (OSTEOARTHROSIS)

This is a **degenerative condition** of synovial joints. Although any joint can be involved the larger **weight-bearing joints** of the lower limb are mainly affected, the hip and knee in particular. The disease may be **primary** or **secondary.** In primary cases there is no obvious cause and the condition is often generalised, affecting more than one joint. The patient is usually middle-aged or elderly. In secondary osteoarthritis the prime condition, although quiescent, has left a damaged joint in which the disease develops. Examples of such predisposing conditions are congenital dislocation of the hip, joint fractures, septic arthritis and rickets. The patient may therefore be in any age group.

The pathological changes of osteoarthritis are characterised by **degeneration** of the **articular cartilage** in the centre of the joint and the development of spurs of bone, **osteophytes** or exostoses, at the joint margins. As the disease is degenerative rather than inflammatory the term **osteoarthrosis** may be preferable to osteo-arthritis.

Osteoarthritis, whether primary or secondary, is not associated with general systemic illness. The clinical features are therefore confined to the joint or joints affected. As the disease develops the joint surfaces become rough producing **pain** on movement. **Movement** is **limited** voluntarily by the patient and also restricted by protective muscle spasm and the altered shape of the bones forming the joint, so resulting in deformity. Contracture of the joint capsule follows. Irritation of the synovial membrane gives rise to excess secretion of synovial fluid and **swelling** of the joint becomes a feature. Although pain is relieved by rest, **joint stiffness** becomes a problem. X-ray shows diminution of the joint space and the presence of the osteophytes at the joint margins.

Treatment

The three factors which determine the treatment applicable to each patient are the degree of joint damage, the number of joints affected and the age of the patient. The aim of treatment is to relieve pain, correct deformity and retain mobility.

Conservative management. Some patients are treated conservatively. Firstly, where the osteoarthritis is diagnosed at an early stage it may be possible to alter the course of the disease by **modifying known aggravating factors,** e.g.

sporting activities, overweight or physical occupational stresses. The patient may have additional therapy in the form of **short-wave diathermy** to relieve discomfort, and **exercises** to counteract deformity. Secondly, in those patients with moderate or severe generalised osteoarthritis, it is often obvious that surgical treatment of one joint, or even several joints, would still fail to relieve the patient's total disability significantly. Thirdly, the patient may be medically unfit for operation. In the latter two groups, in addition to the physiotherapy necessary to maintain joint function, **drug therapy,** e.g. Indomethacin or Phenylbutazone, is required to control pain and perhaps relieve muscle spasm. The use of these drugs is sometimes limited by the development of side-effects in some patients.

Operative management. It is in the treatment of osteoarthritis that the three classical orthopaedic operations are utilised. **Osteotomy** (*see Fig. 41*) is a surgical fracture of a long bone, usually the femur or the tibia. Where osteoarthritis affects the hip or the knee the deformity to be corrected may be coxa vara, genu valgum or genu varum. The rationale of this operation is based on the belief that an alteration in the mechanical weight-bearing function of the joint will correct deformity, relieve pain and maintain joint mobility. **Arthrodesis** (*see Fig. 39*) is a surgical fusion of a joint. By removing the diseased joint surface this operation guarantees relief of pain at the expense of joint function. **Arthroplasty** (*see Fig. 43*) is the creation of a false joint, or the partial or total replacement of a damaged joint by a prosthesis. Pain is relieved and joint mobility retained, but the continued success of the operation is dependent on the durability of the materials used and the body's reaction to them.

Each patient is assessed with regard to his fitness for operation and for the specific operation which will give him the best result to suit his particular way of life. An indication of how this decision is made may be illustrated in the following examples. A **young,** healthy adult with osteoarthritis in a **single joint,** e.g. the hip, may benefit more from the permanent relief of pain and the strength and stability of an **arthrodesis,** than from the less predictable results of osteotomy. Rather than undergo arthrodesis and risk later incapacity due to the development of stiffness in additional joints, a **middle-aged** adult with a natural tendency to stiff joints may be better advised to accept the probable relief of pain and maintenance of existent mobility offered by **osteotomy.** An **elderly** patient is nearly always a victim of some degree of joint stiffness and is exposed to all the complications of the post-operative period. An operation which necessitates a prolonged post-operative period of immobilisation is better avoided where possible. For this reason these patients are often selected for **arthroplasty.** This procedure, although a major operation, offers relief of pain, mobility and early ambulation with all its advantages. For obvious reasons the durability of the prosthesis becomes relatively less important with the advancing age of the patient.

RHEUMATOID ARTHRITIS
This is a condition affecting **synovial joints.** Although a single joint may be

affected initially the disease usually affects a group of joints. The common sites are the proximal **small joints** of the hands and feet, the wrist, knees and synovial joints of the neck. The cause of the condition is not accurately known. As it is more common in females, particularly in young adults and in women at the menopause, the disease may appear to have a hormonal source. On the other hand, research has shown that the disease may in fact be produced by a virus.

The pathological changes in rheumatoid arthritis are characterised by **thickening** of the **synovial membrane** and the growth, over the articular joint surfaces, of a **plaque of granulation tissue** which gradually erodes the articular cartilage and eventually the underlying bone. **Fibrous tissue** develops in between the bone ends forming **adhesions.** On X-ray the affected bone shows signs of **osteoporosis,** the joint space is diminished and there is erosion of the joint margins. In addition there is a generalised skeletal osteoporosis.

Rheumatoid arthritis, apart from its various joint manifestations, is also a **systemic disease.** Those mainly affected are in the middle-aged group; however, the onset may occur in childhood, Still's disease, or be first evident in old age. Although the clinical features may be related to one particular joint it is more usual to find the patient with a **polyarthritis.** The metacarpo-phalangeal and interphalangeal joints of the hand are often affected initially, and later the disease spreads to other joints. The joints affected may be involved to varying degrees, some very much more acutely than others. Damage to the articular joint surface produces **pain** which is unrelieved by rest. The thickened synovial membrane produces **swelling** of the affected joints, which further accentuates the pain. The formation of fibrous adhesions within the joint aggravates the **limitation of movement,** producing **stiffness. Deformity** becomes gradually more marked as the disease progresses. Frequently the disease extends to the synovial tendon sheaths, particularly those of the hand and wrist, although those of the foot and ankle may be similarly involved. **Cystic swellings** in the region of the wrist and ankle joints result. A cystic mass occasionally develops in the popliteal space behind the knee, i.e. a **Baker's cyst.** Rupture of this can produce symptoms and signs simulating deep venous thrombosis. Involvement of the **tendons** themselves by the rheumatoid granulation tissue leads eventually to their **dislocation** and **rupture.** This results in the development of **gross deformities,** e.g. ulnar deviation of the fingers (*Fig. 11*). The acute phase of the joint disease resembles that of an inflammatory reaction although rheumatoid arthritis is not identified as an inflammatory disease.

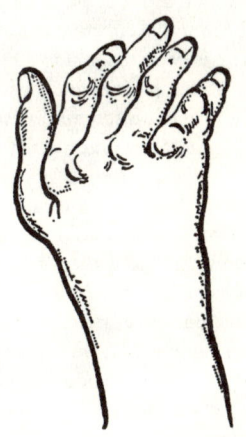

FIG. 11 Rheumatoid arthritis:
Ulnar deviation of fingers

The patient generally **loses weight,** and with her increasing muscular weakness may eventually become bed-ridden. **Wasting of muscle** is apparent on examination. **Blood changes** are many. The simplest show a **raised erythrocyte sedimentation rate,** often a secondary **anaemia,** and a **positive latex fixation test** for the presence of rheumatoid factor. Other more sophisticated serological tests may be carried out in more detailed investigation of the disease by the rheumatologist. **Biopsy of joint** tissues and examination of the synovial fluid may help in diagnosis.

Further systemic manifestation of the disease, in addition to the patient's general debility, depends on the other tissues and organs affected e.g. **dryness of the mouth** or **conjunctivitis** where the salivary or lachrymal glands are involved. **Rheumatoid nodules** are not uncommonly seen in the skin particularly over the elbows although other tissues of the body may be affected e.g. the heart or lungs. The skin nodules tend to break down and ulcerate so adding to the patient's problems.

Management

The management of this disease is essentially **medical,** organised by the physician or rheumatologist. Physiotherapy is important in maintaining and improving the range of joint movement, often with the aid of **serial plaster splints.** The place of **surgery** is to retain, or restore, joint function where increasing deformity and pain are crippling the patient. Medical treatment is aimed at relieving pain and controlling the inflammatory-like reaction. **Salicylates** are used extensively, preferably in a soluble preparation, where these can be tolerated by the patient. **Indomethacin** and **Phenylbutazone** are utilised where the response to salicylates is unsatisfactory.

The **steroid drugs,** cortisone preparations, are useful in small doses as they relieve pain and stiffness. Their use is usually restricted to the more severe type of rheumatoid arthritis where control by the drugs previously mentioned has failed. As soon as the acute manifestations are relieved, the dosage prescribed is reduced to the minimal effective maintenance level and may indeed be gradually discontinued. This is because the side-effects of these drugs are important. Salt and water retention is shown in the characteristic 'moon-face'. There is danger of adrenal failure where the drug is discontinued suddenly. This is particularly important where surgery is undertaken and a strict dosage regime must be prescribed during this period. The cortico-steroids also aggravate the degree of skeletal osteoporosis, especially where local administration (hydrocortisone) has been given by repeated intra-articular injection. Pathological fracture may result. Where it is desirable to stimulate the patient's own production of cortisone rather than give an oral preparation which depresses adreno-cortical activity, **Synacthen** (Tetracosactrin zinc phosphate) therapy is given. This is a drug substitute for A.C.T.H., the hormone which stimulates adreno-cortical function. In severe rheumatoid disease, where there is a poor response to other forms of drug therapy, the administration of either **gold salts** or **chloroquine phosphate** sometimes gives satisfactory results.

Physiotherapy. The application of gentle **heat** to affected areas is not only a comfort to the patient but it also allows for some degree of muscle relaxation. The heat treatment may be in the form of surface heat to the skin by means of **wax baths** or from an **infra-red lamp,** or deep heat which penetrates the underlying structures by means of **short-wave diathermy.** If heat treatment precedes the period of exercise, active movements are often more effectively accomplished and this gives the patient the best chance of improving his range of joint function. **Plaster splints** are made for the patient's limbs to maintain the maximum position of joint extension achieved by daytime physiotherapy. At weekly intervals the range of movement is assessed and, where improvement in extension has occurred, a new plaster splint is made to maintain the limb in this position. This regime is continued until, if possible, full joint extension is achieved. It is of vital importance that, in addition to the specific treatment of the affected joints, a programme of **maintenance exercises** for all other joints is carried out by the patient.

Surgery. This is used in an effort to preserve or restore function in the upper limbs and allow the patient to remain independent. In the lower limbs the aim is to maintain or regain mobility and stability. **Synovectomy** is an operation used in an attempt to arrest the spread of the disease in a particular joint. It may be undertaken on one joint or several joints at appropriate intervals. The aim is to remove the diseased synovial membrane and granulation tissue and to relieve the distension within the joint. As a result, pain is relieved and deformity often avoided. It is hoped that regeneration of a more normal synovial membrane will occur. The operations used in the treatment of osteoarthritis are also effective in the surgical treatment of this condition. **Osteotomy** is limited to the correction of deformity. **Arthrodesis** is particularly useful in the relief of severe pain with associated loss of function, e.g. in the wrist or knee. Its value is greatest where adjacent joints are relatively unaffected by the disease. It is because the disease is essentially polyarthritic that these two operations have a restricted use. Attention has, therefore, been concentrated on the development of satisfactory **arthro-plasties** to retain, and, where possible, increase mobility of affected joints. The development and better understanding of the use of inert metallic and plastic materials has increased the indications for this type of operation, in not only the larger joints of the lower limbs, but also the smaller joints of the hand. The combined research undertaken by the bio-engineering and medical personnel has provided the possibility of utilising total arthroplasty in a younger age group, rather than reserving it for the elderly because of the doubtful durability of materials.

Complications

In addition to the surgical measures used in the management of the joint disease surgery is often necessary to deal with the complications associated with the spread of the disease to other structures, e.g. tendon repair or transplantation is often required to correct **gross deformity.** Where the patient is unsuitable for opera-tion the application of light plastic splints helps to relieve pain, control deformity and preserve some function. In the cervical spine the joint destruction may lead to **subluxation of the joints** and may possibly interrupt the spinal cord pathway. Indeed, sudden death in rheumatoid arthritis may be due to acute atlanto-axial subluxation. The control of a developing **cervical scoliosis** may be difficult. If a light-weight collar support can be tolerated, it is provided. In more severe cases, cervical traction seems in theory the solution but is often impracticable because of the patient's general condition and the extent of the disease. Occipito-cervical fusion may seem the only means of providing stability but it is a major operation and can only be undertaken in a relatively fit patient. Other complications, such as those involving the **break-down of skin nodules,** are managed conservatively by general continuous nursing care of the patient, local application of healing agents to the affected areas, and antibiotics.

Nursing of the Rheumatoid Patient

Rheumatoid arthritis is a disease which is characterised by intermittent acute exacerbations and remissions. Various temperaments respond to the disease in different ways. Some are frustrated, others are depressed. It is yet surprising how many patients retain a cheerful, balanced outlook on life despite severe disability. As success of treatment depends so much on the maximum co-operation of the patient it is necessary to plan a programme of treatment which conveys to him the enthusiasm of all concerned. This creates an atmosphere of optimism and the patient becomes an eager participant in achieving the results. **Activity must be encouraged** if further stiffness is to be avoided, both in affected and unaffected joints. Confinement to bed should be minimal. The ward environment is therefore important. **Special low beds** fitted with patient helper devices enable him to get in and out easily, with little assistance. Lockers must be within easy reach and simple to open. Low chairs are avoided, otherwise sitting and rising become more difficult. Toilets specially adapted with the seat at a suitably high level are necessary. The provision of **good lounge accommodation** for meeting others, access to television, radio and a good library obviously add to the patient's comfort. The most important factor in preparation for operation is the supervision of **drug therapy,** particularly where a patient is on steroids. It may be necessary to give these drugs intramuscularly, or even intravenously, over this period.

In view of the tendency to stiffness, post-operative immobilisation should be minimal. Where possible, internal fixation is used in preference to plaster cast immobilisation in operations such as osteotomy and arthrodesis. Synovectomy requires only a supporting bandage until wound healing has occurred. Total arthroplasty, being less dependent on regeneration of tissues, does not necessitate rigid fixation. As soon as the patient feels well enough, he is encouraged to get out of bed in order that general body function will be interrupted for as short a period as possible.

During the early convalescent period the patient is helped and instructed by the physiotherapist in a course of graduated exercises designed not only to restore muscle tone affected by operation, but also to enhance the functional results of the p ocedure. Where patients cannot benefit from surgery the aim is to keep them mobile and independent. Patients who are severely crippled will require more intensive nursing care. Assistance on to bed-pans, into wheelchairs and on to examination plinths will be necessary. The nurse's help is vitally important to those patients who can neither feed themselves nor attend to their personal hygiene because of their joint disability.

On discharge from hospital it is possible for patients to obtain **helpful devices** designed to overcome certain difficult situations met within the course of living independently at home, e.g. gadgets to help put on socks and shoes and to facilitate cooking and feeding, and appliances for use in general housework. These are obtained from the *Arthritis and Rheumatism Council*, Faraday House, 8–10 Charing Cross Road, London WC2.

5 AFFECTIONS OF THE NERVOUS SYSTEM

The nervous system is exposed to many diseases. The two which require more intensive orthopaedic management are anterior poliomyelitis and cerebral palsy.

ANTERIOR POLIOMYELITIS (INFANTILE PARALYSIS)

Although once a common infectious disease, poliomyelitis is now a rarity in this country. The victims who contracted the disease before it was controlled effectively still require orthopaedic supervision and treatment of its life-long effects. Before the development of a vaccine this was a dreaded disease. If the patient, often a child, survived the initial illness, the possibility remained that he would have been crippled to an extent which destroyed all hope of his future career; he would have had to be dependent on assistance from others, only able to get around with difficulty wearing calipers, a spinal brace or confined to a wheelchair. This disease presented in sporadic cases and as epidemics. How it spread was not clear as there did not seem to be a pattern, as there is for example in the spread of influenza. Nowadays as the vaccine is widely used and administered in the first year of life it is only the sporadic case that is seen.

It has been shown to be a **virus** which gains entry through the upper respiratory air passages. It then follows the olfactory nerves through the base of the skull into the cerebro-spinal fluid bathing the brain and spinal cord, so causing **infection** and **inflammation** in the **brain, brain stem** and **spinal cord.** The virus is excreted from the gastro-intestinal tract in the faeces, thus the chain of reinfection begins again with the next unprotected victim. The disease is more commonly contracted in midsummer, particularly in July and August. Infection of the brain stem may result in a fatal respiratory paralysis. The more usual picture is of a stage of infection, a stage of paralysis and a stage of recovery.

The **stage of infection** results in an illness mistaken for influenza or gastro-enteritis and can be so **mild** that it is unrecognised. After three to four days, the **stage of paralysis** is established which varies from **mild** to **severe,** and can even result in death due to brain stem infection. The severity of paralysis is always greater if **physical activity** is carried out during the period of incubation. The patient complains of general **malaise,** mild **fever** and marked **pain** in the affected **muscle,** the handling of which causes discomfort. The paralysis is maximal to begin with and is due to damage to the motor cells in the anterior horns of grey matter or brain-like tissue in the spinal cord. There is, therefore, **flaccid motor paralysis** without sensory involvement, a **lower motor neurone lesion** (*Fig. 12*).

Patterns of paralysis are produced which depend on the level and extent of the cord affected. For example, if cervical segments five and six are affected, there is partial or total involvement of the muscles supplied from that level resulting in the loss of some or all the movement in the shoulders and arms. The **stage of recovery** follows, during which **maximum improvement** occurs in the **first six months** but may not be **complete** for **two years.** Even then there may still be **residual paralysis.**

Treatment

The stage of infection is treated in an **infectious diseases hospital.** Here the patient is visited by the orthopaedic surgeon, and an assessment made of the severity of the condition. The **limbs** are **splinted** in the **neutral position** using

Normal brain interpretation

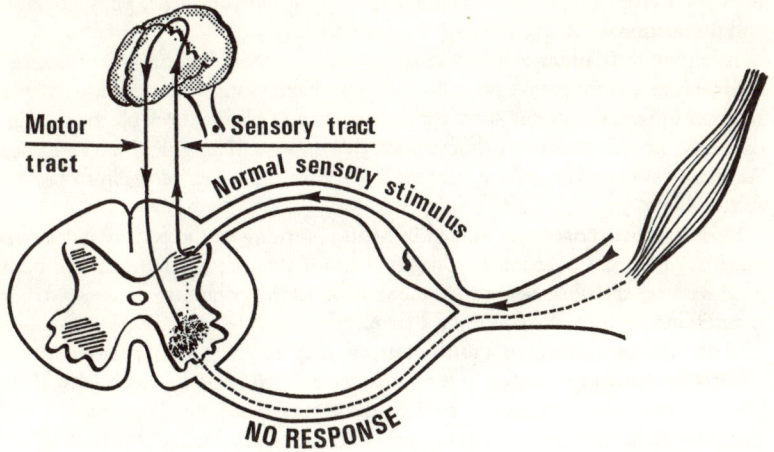

FIG. 12   Anterior poliomyelitis: Lower motor neurone lesion

supporting pillows. After three or four days, when the stage of paralysis is apparent, a more specific picture of the extent of the palsy is seen. The surgeon and physiotherapist chart the degree of paralysis which is then reviewed weekly. Initially the muscles are tender to touch and passive exercises are not possible. Active exercises also increase the severity of the palsy and are therefore avoided. Where there is balanced muscle weakness, the trunk and limbs are splinted in a neutral position while paralysis exists. When one group of muscles is paralysed, e.g. the extensor muscles of a limb, the opposing active group will pull the limb into flexion deformity and over-stretch the paralysed muscles. This is avoided by splintage in a slightly over-corrected position. It involves the making of **special plaster splints** which must be **carefully padded** and **well-fitting** to avoid pressure on the paralysed limbs. Sometimes where adequate support can be achieved by the use of **pillows** and **sorbo rubber pads** plaster casts are avoided.

Pain during the stage of paralysis must be relieved by **analgesics.** Once it has settled, and the patient can tolerate handling of the trunk and limbs, physiotherapy starts with **passive** joint **movements.** Any evidence of developing muscle contracture is prevented by passive stretching and splintage in the corrected position. As each group of paralysed muscles shows signs of recovery, the patient is encouraged to use them. **Gentle active exercises** are therefore commenced graduating to more intensive physiotherapy as recovery becomes more complete. This can involve long months of effort on the part of the patient.

Management

Nursing management can only be carried out successfully by a nurse who has sympathy and understanding, great patience, unfailing enthusiasm and the ability to work well as a member of a team consisting of doctor, nurse, physiotherapist and occupational therapist.

Attention to **bladder** and **bowel** is important. Although there is no neurogenic lesion present constipation can often be a problem, sometimes requiring digital removal of faeces. Extreme constipation can produce bladder neck obstruction and difficulty in micturition with retention of urine and overflow incontinence. Regular aperients with intermittent enemata in certain cases will help to prevent this problem.

Skin pressure sores are avoided by regular turning of the patient and movement of the skin. Inspection of splinted areas for pressure is important. All bony prominences, the ulnar nerve area, the sacrum, lateral popliteal nerve area, tendo Achillis and heels must be examined frequently.

When the patient becomes **ambulant,** he may be able to walk only with the aid of a **spinal support** such as the Milwaukee brace, if he has a scoliosis. If the hip muscles are weak he may require a **walking caliper** jointed to a pelvic band. The joint at the hip level is made to lock and so stabilise him while standing and to unlock in order to allow flexion on movement. He can walk with both hip joints locked, using crutches, in a tripod or three point type of gait, or else with one locked and the other unlocked. Similarly where the main weakness is in the muscular control of the knee joint a long leg caliper jointed at the knee is used. Over a period, as muscles recover, the amount of splintage can be reduced until only below knee calipers and a drop foot appliance are required. Eventually these are discarded altogether.

Some patients, however, are destined to wear calipers all their lives, unless surgery can successfully stabilise the joints controlled by the weakened muscles. For instance drop foot appliances can be discarded after a **triple arthrodesis** (*see p.* 11), a long leg caliper removed following an **arthrodesis of knee** (*see Fig. 39a*), or a Milwaukee brace discarded after a **spinal fusion** (*see p.* 197). In the upper limb, **tendon transplantation** is helpful (*see p.* 46), e.g. for stabilising a drop wrist or weakness of extension. For the less fortunate, unable to benefit from surgery, it is important that calipers and supports should be not only strong and durable, but also light-weight to allow weakened muscles to cope with them. In this field the science of biomechanics is concentrating on the reduction in the bulk of these calipers and the introduction of durable light-weight modern materials. The patient benefits not only from the increased functional efficiency of these appliances but also from their less conspicuous, more aesthetic appearance.

Throughout this illness the **morale** of the patient must be upheld. He will often despair and wonder whether or not he will be able to use the paralysed parts again and, if the legs are involved, whether or not he will walk again. The nurse plays an important part in encouraging him to keep trying. At apparent or real setbacks he needs support. Later, as the final result becomes more or less established, a period in a **rehabilitation** unit may help him to resettle and realize his limitations. The resettlement officer will take a personal interest in his particular problem and see the patient employed in the job which he will be able to do satisfactorily, despite his disability. For badly disabled patients, a **wheelchair** for indoors and motorised **invalid car** for outdoors provide some enjoyment in life. They can at least meet other victims of the disease at the various organisations which provide facilities and interests for those in a severely crippled condition. Very often they acquire a determination to overcome their handicap and, with the use of the available facilities, can earn a living so that they become less dependent on society.

CEREBRAL PALSY (SPASTIC PARESIS)

The causes of cerebral palsy may be classified into three groups; **pre-natal, natal** and **post-natal.** The post-natal group may be further subdivided under three headings; **traumatic, inflammatory** and **degenerative** causes, e.g. head injury, meningitis or cerebro-vascular disease. In this chapter, we discuss the problems of cerebral palsy arising in the pre-natal and natal periods. It is a condition in which the **primary lesion** is in the **brain.** The specific area of the brain damaged determines the pattern of functional impairment in the area of the body it controls. The pre-natal causes include developmental anomalies and disease. The natal causes are those occurring during the process of childbirth.

The motor or pyramidal tracts of the cortex of the brain are not fully developed until about the eighth month of foetal growth. Any interference with this process during the early months of pregnancy may predispose to congenital defects in the nervous system with spastic paresis. The basal ganglia, the centre of origin of the extra-pyramidal tracts, may be damaged, e.g. in a condition known as erythro-blastosis foetalis which gives rise to haemolytic jaundice in the newborn. Pigmentation of the cells of the basal ganglia, i.e. kernicterus, causes the athetoid type of cerebral palsy. During prolonged or difficult childbirth these centres, or their tracts in the spinal cord, can also be damaged by cerebral anoxaemia or trauma. The effect may be spastic paresis, athetosis or a mixed pattern of these two types. Both **spastic paresis** and **athetosis** are **upper motor neurone lesions.** The former arises in the cerebral cortex and its related **pyramidal system**; the latter is centred in the basal ganglia and its associated **extra-pyramidal system.** The **paralysis** produced is **spastic** in type.

Clinical Features

The clinical picture varies according to the degree of cerebral damage. In severe cases, spasticity or athetosis will be obvious at birth. In mild cases the child may appear perfectly normal. His failure to advance at the same rate as a normal child may be the first indication of any abnormality. Delay or difficulty in the child's ability to lift his head, sit, and later to crawl, stand or walk may be noticed.

The child may be generally clumsy in performing simple movements. Development of bowel and bladder control may be delayed and toilet training difficult or unsuccessful. While the child's **mentality** is often quite unaffected, all degrees of mental retardation including idiocy may be detected as the child grows. Varying degrees of **blindness** or **deafness** may also become apparent and further delay progress. Sometimes **speech** is affected. This may be mechanical, due to weakness of the facial muscles, or related to the degree of mental retardation. In some instances the child may be completely aphasic. **Epilepsy** is not uncommon in spastic hemiparesis.

Examination of the child shows the pattern and extent of muscle involvement. The **muscles,** deprived of control by the damage to the higher centres, overact or are **hypertonic.** They produce an exaggerated reflex response to a sensory stimulus. Passive movements of joints result in almost rigid resistance by the hypertonic muscles in contraction, i.e. spasticity. This resistance is overcome by continuous, steady, passive opposition which counteracts the muscle spasm. When the muscles relax it is then possible to complete the range of movement of the joint. There is no true paralysis of the opposing group of muscles, but they are relatively weak in comparison to those in the spastic group. The distribution of muscle impairment varies. **Monoparesis** is the term used to describe weakness of one limb. Where the arm and leg on the same side are affected the condition is known as **hemiparesis.** Spastic **paraparesis** refers to the involvement of both lower limbs and if all four limbs are affected the term **tetraparesis** or **quadriparesis** may be used.

Deformity is produced by the imbalance of muscle action. The characteristic appearances in the upper limb are of a flexion deformity of the elbow, pronation of the forearm, palmar flexion and ulnar deviation of the hand and wrist. In the lower limb, there are flexion deformities of the hip and knee and an equinovarus deformity of the foot with hyperextension of the toes. The flexion deformity of the hip is associated with the development of a secondary lumbar lordosis. Adductor spasm may lead also to crossing of the lower limbs or a **'scissors-gait'** in walking. The gait is distinctive. The hypertonicity of the spastic muscles produces exaggeration of the normal 'springy' gait often with an associated **jerking arm action.**

In **athetosis,** there is **impairment of the control of voluntary movement.** Any attempt to perform even a simple movement may be interfered with by the action of other muscle groups, e.g. an exaggerated intention tremor on volunteering to use the arm. Slow rhythmic movements of the head and neck, with peculiar **grimacing** movements of the facial muscles, occur. Emotion often exaggerates such involuntary movements inhibiting further the patient's attempts to perform the required action. This consequently reduces the patient to a helpless demoralised state. In a purely athetoid type of cerebral palsy the mentality is normal.

In the mixed type of cerebral palsy there is athetosis superimposed on the spastic paresis, the **athetoid spastic.** There is therefore, in addition to the spasticity of muscle, uncontrolled involuntary movement.

Management of Cerebral Palsy

As the **primary lesion** in the brain **cannot be cured,** the management of this condition depends on the mental and physical disability it has produced. In the severely mentally and physically handicapped child the need for **institutional care** is usually obvious. Some parents, however, feel it is imperative for them to care for their child. It is a major undertaking on their part, but this can be relieved by occasional admission to an institution when special circumstances arise, e.g. illness or to enable the parents to benefit from a holiday.

Nursing of the severely handicapped child with spastic **flexion contractures** and the problems of **immobility** and **incontinence** requires endless patience and constant complete general nursing care.

Where the child is less severely affected, the management is by the combined effort of a team consisting of physiotherapist, orthopaedic surgeon, neurosurgeon and speech therapist. Management is best conducted through a special **cerebral palsy unit** attached to a hospital or, in some cases, within a special **school for handicapped children,** e.g. a school for the deaf. These children are taught by teachers specially trained in the education of the handicapped. The situation related to the child's prognosis is assessed. A programme of treatment is organised starting in childhood and continuing throughout the growth period into adult life. The principles of treatment are muscle relaxation and re-education, splintage, surgery and speech therapy. **Muscle relaxation** and **re-education** are initially in the form of **passive** exercises. Their function is to relax spastic muscle contraction, improve the tone of weak muscles, retain full joint mobility and correct deformity. **Hydrotherapy** is of particular value in the treatment of this condition as it provides the maximum muscle relaxation.

Physiotherapy. It is important that physiotherapy is continuous. The exercises are basically simple and can be done by the parents thus enabling the child to live at home. Instruction in manipulation of the limbs is given to the parents by the physiotherapist. The child is brought to hospital for review by the physiotherapist and doctor at regular intervals and progress is assessed.

Splintage. Where deformity is increasing in spite of adequate physiotherapy the utilisation of splints will be necessary. The aim is to get the child who is mentally normal sufficiently mobile to attend school so that he may be educated according to his age, aptitude and ability. These splints may be in the form of **below-knee calipers** with **drop foot appliances** or, when there is excessive instability of the knees, **long leg calipers** may be worn. Where there is a marked scissors gait, the long leg calipers are jointed together by a pelvic band, or in some cases by a corset brace. **Footwear** will require **regular servicing** and **replacement,** particularly where there is equinovarus deformity. Two pairs of surgical shoes or boots are provided, due to the high rate of wear.

Surgery. Operation is often necessary to correct deformity of the limbs. In the upper limb the aim is to improve function of the hand. In the lower limb, the object is to achieve stability. Operation is only undertaken after careful assessment of each patient. There are several problems to be considered. Firstly, if the child is still growing, interference by surgery may further add to his problem if the growth pattern is affected. Secondly, although severely physically handicapped, many patients compensate for their deformities extremely well and are fully mobile despite their peculiar gait. Operation in these patients may only alter their equilibrium and indeed, as a result, they may be further crippled. Correction of marked deformity and improved function of the hand are in some cases achieved by **arthrodesis** of the wrist. If the patient experiences difficulty in walking, **lengthening of the tendo Achillis** may be beneficial. **Tendon transplantation** is sometimes a means of stabilising a joint, e.g. transplanting the tendon of the spastic hamstring muscles into the anterior aspect of the femur or quadriceps expansion. This will improve the function of the quadriceps and perhaps at the same time reduce the flexion deformity of the knee. Where there is adductor spasm, e.g. in the scissor type of gait, **adductor tenotomy** or **obturator neurectomy** are undertaken to reduce spasm. In the foot, **triple arthrodesis** may give stability in some selected cases.

Neurosurgery. In the athetoid spastic, neurosurgery may be indicated occasionally in the form of **injection** of a **sclerosing agent** into the **basal nuclei** in an attempt to control the involuntary movements.

Speech Therapy. For those with difficulty in speech, an important part of the treatment is speech therapy. This includes exercises for **breathing** and the development of **lip** and **tongue control.** The use of such accessories as mirrors and tape-recorders is of added value in speech training. These training sessions are usually conducted in a special room free from any distracting influence.

Drug Therapy. Where epilepsy exists, it is controlled by mysolin and phenobarbitone. Valium is used as a general tranquillizer in patients with cerebral palsy. It is also a useful muscle relaxant.

The Problems in Nursing Management
Nursing of patients with cerebral palsy requires considerable understanding. Many patients are **emotionally unstable** while others are, indeed, **mentally subnormal.** Athetoids in particular are very dependent on the family unit and the members of the cerebral palsy team. When they have to come into hospital they are often very emotionally upset. This is aggravated by the fact that many have **difficulty in communication** because of some degree of speech defect, and

difficulty in speech co-ordination. **Incontinence** of bladder and bowel may be a problem. Muscle spasm and **deformities** of the limbs will tend to make the patient appear clumsy. He has **difficulty in feeding, dressing** and **toilet.** In bed, the patient with flexion contracture of the hips lies with one hip abducted and externally rotated. The other limb rests on top, with the hip adducted and internally rotated. This hip is very liable to **'silent' dislocation** in this 'wind-swept' position. Pillows between the legs and regular passive movements are essential, as well as regular changing of position, to avoid this complication.

Post-operatively, where **plaster immobilisation** has been utilised, it must be remembered that recurrent spasticity following recovery from anaesthesia may lead to pressure on the skin, blood vessels and nerves. Observation of the **circulation** and **peripheral nerve function** must be carried out with particular care.

6 METABOLIC BONE DISEASE

Although bone is the hardest of all the body tissues, it is nevertheless a living tissue and has its own metabolism. Bone metabolism is the process by which selected materials from the bloodstream are utilised by the bone tissue cells in the growth and maintenance of the skeleton. There are various factors necessary for **normal bone metabolism:**

1 **Osteoid tissue** is the ground proteinous structure which is the basis of bone formation.
2 The bone cells, **osteocytes,** are of two types, the osteoblasts which are bone-forming cells, and the osteoclasts, which are bone-destroying cells.
3 **Ossification** is the term which describes the hardening of the bone. The osteoblasts require the deposition of calcium salts in the osteoid tissue, i.e. calcification, to enable them to complete this process of ossification.
4 **Calcium** is taken into the body in foodstuffs and absorbed from the small intestine. Absorption can only take place in the presence of vitamin D.
5 **Vitamin D** is found in foodstuffs, e.g. fishliver oils, and is also obtainable from the ergosterol produced by the sun's action on the skin. It can also be synthesised and taken in the form of capsules.
6 Calcification of bone is controlled by an enzyme, **alkaline phosphatase,** which is a biochemical product of osteoblastic activity.
7 **Parathyroid hormones.** There are two known hormones influencing bone metabolism. Parathormone controls the ratio of calcium to organic phosphate in the blood. It also stimulates osteoclastic activity. Calcitonin, the other hormone, inhibits the action of the osteoclasts. These hormones regulate the amount of bone resorption taking place.
8 As a result of metabolism, **waste products** are produced and excreted by the kidneys and bowel. These include urea, creatinine and unused calcium salts.

In the growing child the osteoblasts are particularly active, to allow for the growth of bone in length and girth. There is a more balanced action of osteoblasts and osteoclasts in the adult, where bone tissue is being continually renewed but actual growth has ceased. In the ageing person there is a generalised lessening of bone activity.

METABOLIC BONE DISEASE

In this condition **normal metabolism is upset.** This may be due to a fault in the bone structure, bone cells, the supply and utilisation of calcium, or a hormonal upset. The effect of such changes produces a wide variety of symptoms, and it is for this reason that patients are seen and referred from many different departments. A patient may, for example, be admitted to a medical ward with symptoms of general rheumatism or renal failure, to a urological ward with renal calculi, to a psychiatric ward with mental disturbance or to an orthopaedic ward with back-ache, muscle weakness or generalised pain.

Osteoporosis

Although in this condition the bone is normal in composition and structure, there is an insufficiency of it. It is seen mainly after the menopause in women but affects both sexes in the elderly age group. Only when the **structural weakness** gives rise to fracture after minor stress is the presence of the disease recognised. Otherwise it is usually quite **symptomless.** Fractures of the spine, causing low back pain and kyphotic deformity, Colles' fracture and fracture of the neck of the femur, are among the more common **pathological fractures.** X-ray shows a decrease in bone density.

Blood biochemical examination is normal except where there is a pathological fracture in which case the alkaline phosphatase will be raised. A loss of calcium from the body may be evident on urine examination. **Bone biopsy** from the iliac crest will show **decreased amount of bone.**

Treatment. The treatment is to relieve the pain produced by the fracture and to prevent deformity. In the wrist and neck of femur, the **principles of fracture treatment** are applied. To prevent the development or worsening of the kyphotic deformity of the spine, a **supporting corset** is fitted. Occasionally, in a younger patient gentle **back extension exercises** will help provided she can tolerate them. Diet is important. As the elderly are mainly affected and are often less diet conscious, they should be instructed in the importance of a **balanced diet,** with a daily intake of at least half a pint of **milk.** Small doses of **vitamin D** weekly and **calcium** daily produce good results although there is no real evidence of their deficiency. Sometimes hormones are given to post-menopausal patients, but such drugs usually have unpleasant side effects.

Osteomalacia

In this condition there is **vitamin D deficiency** and consequently, calcium depletion. It is essentially a **dietary deficiency,** as seen in poor social conditions with malnutrition, but it may be related to a **malabsorption syndrome,** e.g. coeliac disease in the child and idiopathic steatorrhoea and post-gastrectomy syndrome in the adult. Premature babies and infants under eighteen months are susceptible to the juvenile form called **rickets,** while adults with poor dietary intake of vitamin D and calcium develop osteomalacia. The lack of calcium produces **softening of the bones.** This is further aggravated by a compensatory function of the hormones of the parathyroid glands which, in their effort to regulate the blood calcium level, stimulate the mobilisation of existent calcium from the bones. Where the response of these glands is poor, however, the patient will develop a low blood calcium, **hypocalcaemia,** which gives rise to the additional signs and symptoms of **tetany.**

Symptoms and Signs. The symptoms and signs associated with osteomalacia vary considerably. The patient may complain of **severe aching pain,** often in the back and thighs. Physical examination of the patient may reveal generalised **tenderness over the bones. Pathological fractures** may occur, e.g. of the metatarsal bones. The softness of the bones leads to the development of **deformities** of the spine, pelvis and lower limbs. **Coxa vara** deformity produces a waddling gait. There is usually an associated iron deficiency **anaemia,** and, if the condition is not diagnosed until it is well advanced, the patient can become generally **debilitated** and **confined to bed.** There is then a marked tendency to the development of bed sores. The additional symptoms and signs of **tetany** may be apparent. These include **paraesthesia, muscle weakness** and **twitching,** and sometimes autonomic nervous system upset, e.g. biliary colic.

Investigation is by means of X-ray, blood examination and urine analysis. X-ray shows decreased bone density, blood examination reveals the lack of calcium, and urine analysis confirms the raised level of calcium and phosphate excretion.

Treatment. Treatment is firstly by the administration of **vitamin D** orally to improve the absorption of calcium, and secondly by the administration of **calcium.** All children under eighteen months should have a daily intake of 400 units of vitamin D to prevent rickets. Where a **malabsorption syndrome** is the primary feature, it will require treatment, either by **special diet** or **surgery.** Treatment of secondary complications, e.g. anaemia and pathological fracture, will also be necessary.

Hyperparathyroidism

This condition is associated with **overactivity** of **parathyroid** tissue. It can be due to a general overgrowth, **hyperplasia,** of the tissue of all four glands, or a **tumour** or adenoma of one of them. A **secondary hyperplasia** of the four glands can be a **compensatory** reaction to an existing low blood calcium.

The raised blood calcium predisposes to the formation of **renal calculi** as the kidneys attempt to excrete the excess calcium. **Thirst, polyuria,** general **weakness, anorexia,** and **mental disturbance** are symptoms of a raised blood calcium level. **Renal infection, colic** and **haematuria** indicate the presence of renal calculi. **Loss of height** and **deformity** occur in the bone manifestation of the disease. The deformities include kyphosis, alteration in the shape of the pelvis, stubbing of the fingers and swelling of the lower limbs, due to tumour-like formations. **X-ray changes** occur in the **bones** particularly of the skull, round the teeth and in the fingers. **Tumour-like cysts** are also seen in the long bones. A **barium swallow** shows a defect where there is enlargement of the parathyroid glands. **Blood examination** results show a raised calcium and a correspondingly low phosphate level. **Urine analysis** is necessary to estimate the level of calcium and phosphate excretion. **Bone biopsy** confirms the loss of calcium from the bone.

Radio-isotope studies are sometimes done to investigate the utilisation of minerals, calcium in particular, by the body.

Treatment. This is essentially **surgical,** by removal of excess parathyroid tissue. Dehydration must be corrected prior to operation, and any signs of tetany post-operatively must be immediately noted and treated by calcium therapy.

NURSING MANAGEMENT

The nursing management of metabolic bone disease is important. The investigation includes many **special tests** and **analyses.** X-ray examination shows a picture similar to that of many non-metabolic diseases and does not establish the diagnosis. The ability of the body to utilise various elements can be tested by giving the patient a known quantity of any one of them, thereafter estimating the amount cleared from the blood and excreted in the urine and faeces. The preparation of the various **diets** is usually the responsibility of the dietician, but the nurse must make sure that the patient receives his portions of diet required in the particular test, and that the whole portion is taken. Any remnant should be carefully preserved to be taken into consideration in the final analysis.

Preparation of the patient and equipment for the removal of venous blood for electrolytes and **special biochemistry** is also necessary. Accurate **urine and faecal collections** are important. A five day faecal fat collection involves conservation of the whole specimen each time, and the total for the five days is despatched in a container to the laboratory. Special containers for this specific purpose are usually available. Urine collections must be commenced at the exact time stated and over the required number of days. For example, in a twenty-four hour urine collection commencing on Monday the patient would empty his bladder at 8.00 am and the urine would be discarded. All further urine passed would be kept in a special bottle until 8.00 am on Tuesday morning. The patient would then empty his bladder and the urine would be added to complete the collection. Good communication is necessary so that the patient and all the nurses on day and night duty appreciate the reason for the test. The biochemist is dependent on the co-operation between patient and nurse to provide reliable results.

Specific nursing care will vary according to the way in which the disease presents. Pain can be relieved by adequate **analgesics.** Total bed rest is better avoided as these patients are generally in the older age group and prone to the complications associated with immobilisation. In addition, it has been shown that complete immobilisation can produce osteoporosis which would merely aggravate the problem. **Care of the skin** and the **prevention of joint contractures** are important. **Breathing exercises** will help lung expansion and help prevent infection. **Adequate fluid intake** keeps the kidneys functioning and less liable to renal infection and stone formation. **Mild aperients** may be required to relieve constipation. Pathological fractures associated with metabolic bone disease are managed by observing the **principles of fracture treatment** (*see p.* 94). Normal union of the fracture usually occurs although in some instances the process of healing is delayed.

7 BONE TUMOURS

A tumour or neoplasm is a **collection of cells** or tissue in the body which develops a metabolism and **growth pattern independent** of the rest of the body. There are two types, **benign** and **malignant.** The nature of the tumour depends on the type of cell from which it originates. There are many different types. Benign tumours do not endanger life because they do not spread; malignant do, by spreading all over the body. A bone tumour is a tumour, benign or malignant, which involves bone. A malignant bone tumour is either a **primary** tumour arising in bone or a secondary, or **metastatic,** deposit in bone from a primary tumour in a tissue situated elsewhere in the body. Initially, the clinical picture may not reveal the true nature of the lesion which could be benign, malignant, or even a non-neoplastic condition simulating a tumour. The doctor must decide whether the lesion is neoplastic or non-neoplastic; if neoplastic, whether it is benign or malignant; if malignant, whether it is primary or secondary. Only then is he in a position to decide on treatment.

Primary bone tumours may arise from any tissue in the body, e.g. **cartilage, bone, fibrous tissue, nerve, marrow** or **blood vessels.** For most tissues there is a benign and malignant tumour counterpart. The malignant one is called a sarcoma, i.e. of endothelial origin. From cartilage, for example, there is a benign chondroma and a malignant chondrosarcoma. Some of these tumours are very rare and only the commoner ones will be discussed.

Classification

Tissue or Cell of Origin	Benign	Malignant
Cartilage (cartilage cell)	Osteochondroma Chondroma	Chondrosarcoma
Bone (osteoblast)	Osteoid osteoma	Osteosarcoma
Fibrous tissue (fibroblast)	Fibroma (rare) Giant cell tumour	Fibrosarcoma Giant cell tumour
Bone marrow (connective tissue) (blood forming tissue)	— —	Ewing's sarcoma Multiple myeloma
Nerve tissue (nerve cell)	Neurofibroma	—

Tissue or Cell of Origin	Benign	Malignant
Blood vessels (endothelial cell)	Angioma	—
	Aneurysmal bone cyst	—

Sites. Primary bone tumours develop mainly in the **metaphysis** of a long bone. The lower end of the femur, upper end of tibia, upper end of humerus and lower end of radius are common sites.

BENIGN TUMOURS
These may be **single** or **multiple.** They are **localised,** do not invade surrounding tissues and would only endanger life from their bulk in an enclosed space, e.g. in a cavity such as the skull. They may cause swelling and so pressure on blood vessels, nerves and the skin. Pathological fracture of a bone may occur due to weakening of its structure.

Clinical Picture of Benign Tumours
Some tumours may remain entirely within the bone, e.g. chondroma, and therefore be unsuspected unless a **pathological fracture** occurs, or they may draw attention to themselves because of **pain,** e.g. osteoid osteoma. Others may protrude from the bone and be palpable as painless **swellings** unassociated with any invasive change in the soft tissues, e.g. osteochondroma. Finally, others may expand the bone and produce **local tenderness** and an **increase in skin temperature,** e.g. giant cell tumour.

Treatment
Osteochondroma need only be removed surgically if pressure symptoms and signs occur, or enlargement suggests malignant change. Chondromata are often seen as incidental findings on X-ray examination for some other reason. Once identified they are usually ignored. Where pathological fracture has occurred, curettage and bone grafting is necessary. An **osteoid osteoma** produces pain which is relieved by the administration of salicylates. Diagnosis is sometimes obscure because of the difficulty in demonstrating the lesion radiologically. Once it is localised it is surgically removed. A **giant cell tumour,** once diagnosed histologically after biopsy is treated by curettage and bone grafting when in an accessible site. If in an inaccessible site it may be treated by radiotherapy.

PRIMARY MALIGNANT BONE TUMOURS
These are most often seen in **childhood** or **adolescence.** However, young adults and the elderly with an underlying Paget's disease may be affected. Such tumours arise usually in the **medulla of a long bone,** but soon show their local **invasive reaction** by spreading through and in turn destroying the cortex and periosteum. Once the tumour penetrates the periosteum, muscle is involved and eventually it ulcerates on the surface of the skin. The bone is weakened by the local destruction

and may develop a **pathological fracture.** The tumour **spreads** by the **blood stream** to the **lungs** and destruction of lung tissue eventually causes death.

Clinical Picture of Primary Malignant Bone Tumours

The onset is characterised by the **gradual** development of **pain** in a limb often following some minor trauma. The pain becomes rapidly more **severe,** particularly at night time. Function is interfered with and a lump or tumour develops in the limb. Local indurated **swelling** occurs towards one or other end of a long bone. It is **tender** to touch and the **skin temperature** is **raised. Blood vessels** are **distended** and are seen clearly in the skin. Pathological fracture may occur. **Anorexia, loss of weight** and a dry unproductive **cough** follow due to development of metastases in the lungs. Death usually occurs inside five years. **Diagnosis** is by X-ray, blood examination and biopsy. X-ray shows loss of bone density and later destruction of bone. It may be difficult to differentiate amongst the main types of sarcomata radiologically, although there are characteristic features which tend to suggest an individual diagnosis. The lungs may be clear or they may show tumour tissue. Blood examination shows **anaemia, raised E.S.R.** and possibly **hypercalcaemia.** Biopsy demonstrates the type of tumour and indicates the degree of malignancy. Whilst these are all virulent tumours the most aggressive is the osteosarcoma.

Treatment

This varies slightly with each particuar tumour. Initially, **osteosarcoma** is treated by **high dosage X-ray irradiation** which really withers the limb. A **protective walking caliper** is worn where the tumour affects the lower limb, and the upper limb may require the support of a **sling.** If after six months the lungs are still uninvolved and the consent of the patient or, in the case of a child, the guardian has been given, the limb is **amputated** proximal to the tumour and a prosthesis supplied. Regular yearly assessments are carried out thereafter. In **chondrosarcoma,** the tumour is less malignant and in certain sites it may be completely **excised** and the area **bone grafted.** However, this is not always possible and usually **amputation** of the limb or even the limb plus half the pelvis or scapula, as the case may be, is carried out. In **fibrosarcoma,** arising from the periosteum, **local excision** with **bone grafting** is sometimes possible. If impracticable, or where the tumour is very malignant, **amputation** is again the only method of treatment.

SECONDARY MALIGNANT BONE TUMOURS

These are very much **commoner** than primary bone tumours.

Site. Any bone may be affected. They arise mainly in the **spine,** in the cancellous bone in the centre of the vertebral bodies, and in the centre or the upper ends of the shafts, or diaphyses, of the long bones. The **femur, humerus, ribs** and **skull** are common sites in addition to the spine. Death is caused by destruction of bone marrow, blood cells and lung tissue. Locally the tumour weakens the bone and pathological fracture is common.

Origin. These secondaries originate from primary soft tissue malignant tumours elsewhere in the body. They are **carcinomas,** i.e. of epithelial origin. The **breast** in females and the **lung** in males give the commonest secondary tumours. **Thyroid** carcinoma, when it occurs, gives the highest percentage of secondaries. **Prostatic** carcinoma is fairly common in the male. **Renal** tumours often have only a solitary metastasis for a long time, which gives some scope for treating both it and the primary.

Spread. The spread of primary soft tissue malignant tumours is by the **lymphatics** to the lymph nodes and by the **blood** to the lungs and bones.

Clinical Picture of Secondary Malignant Bone Tumours
This is very similar to that of primary tumours as far as the limbs are concerned except that the site differs. It tends to be more towards the centre of the shaft of the bone. Initially there may be one site only, but after a varying period other similar sites may be involved. In addition to involvement of the limbs, the spine and other tissues such as the lungs, liver and central nervous system may be affected. The patient's general condition deteriorates, as shown by **anaemia, anorexia** and **loss of weight.** His pain increases and he requires more and more sedation. **Pathological fracture** may occur, either in the spine or in the long bones and is revealed by sudden increase in pain, local tenderness and deformity. This is associated with an increase in the soft tissue swelling, due to tumour tissue. **Secondaries** in the **brain** produce personality changes, and in the lung, **haemoptysis.** An X-ray of the affected bone or bones shows destruction with little evidence of effective healing. A **skeletal X-ray** survey shows the extent of the lesions. Blood examination shows **anaemia, raised E.S.R.** and often **hypercalcaemia.**

Treatment
Pain requires **sedation** starting with the weaker analgesics, e.g. salicylates, and progressing through the newer, more powerful drugs, to morphine derivatives eventually. The **lesion** is **biopsied** to determine its nature. With the knowledge that the lesion is a secondary, and of its nature, a search for the **primary** is carried out. Having found it in one of the sites mentioned the next decision is on its treatment. This may be **surgical removal, radiotherapy** or by **radio–isotope.** The treatment of the **secondary** may be discussed with a radiotherapist. He can give advice on such measures as the use of **radiotherapy, hormone therapy** or **cytotoxic drugs,** or a combination of hormone therapy and cytotoxic drugs. **Combined therapy** is more successful in relieving pain. Side effects from these methods may include skin damage, e.g. erythema and alopaecia, or blood damage, e.g. anaemia and agranulocytosis resulting in septicaemia. The organisms enter, e.g. via a catheter and, as the blood is low in white cells, infection spreads.

Treatment of a pathological fracture is influenced by the tumour and the fracture. Surgery, treating the fracture on conventional lines, will not prevent the tumour from growing. Therefore, while immobilisation is necessary to allow even pathological callus to form, treatment of the tumour causing the fracture is also a necessity. Immobilisation in the case of an arm would be by a collar and cuff sling and posterior plaster shell to allow of expansion, inspection and therapy. In the lower limb, traction in a Thomas's splint is useful. In some cases, internal fixation by a nail and plate, or by intramedullary nail, gives stability to the fracture, with sufficient comfort to the patient. For the spine only bed rest will help, as paraplegia, ascending renal infection or liver failure will inevitably cause death.

NURSING MANAGEMENT

Benign tumours require hospital care should pain or pathological fracture occur. Either plaster immobilisation or bone grafting may be required, so that the nurse is involved in **care of plaster** and in the post-operative management of bone grafting. Malignant tumours, either primary or secondary require relief of pain, **correction of anaemia,** general nursing care, plaster or splint care, and the pre-operative and post-operative **management of amputation.** Reassuring and comforting the patient who often suspects the diagnosis become extremely important. Naturally, the doctor must discuss the matter fully with relatives, and as fully as is possible, or wise, with the patient. The nurse, however, is closer to the patient emotionally and can often answer questions that would not be put to the doctor, either by the patient or the relatives. The emotional factor is at its severest in young children with primary bone tumours and limbs destined for amputation. **Care of the skin, bladder, bowel** and **chest** are of vital importance. Pressure sores, urinary infection, constipation and hypostatic pneumonia only add to the patient's burdens in this distressing set of circumstances. **Careful, continuous nursing** should prevent these. The use of **antibiotics** in the prevention and treatment of infection is not striving to maintain life needlessly. On the contrary, it is a kindness which it is charitable to afford someone in this most unfortunate state. The **adequate relief of pain** is vital. Weak analgesics are more to be abhorred than worrying about the dangers of addiction to morphine or other such drugs in a dying patient. To ensure the patient's comfortable demise, the steady progression from weaker to stronger drugs requires good judgement by the doctor, who is usually guided by the nurse's careful and compassionate interpretation of the patient's daily condition (*see p.* 200, Amputation).

PART I

SECTION II

REGIONAL ORTHOPAEDICS

8 COMMON AFFECTIONS OF THE SPINE

BACKACHE

Many people at some time in life complain of backache. The majority suffer a minor form such as a mild strain which although painful is transient, and rapidly and completely disappears. A smaller number, however, suffer from chronic or recurrent backache, and a few indeed experience an acute incident.

Causes. The causes of backache are many. They include **poor posture, congenital anomalies, injury, inflammatory conditions** of pyogenic or tuberculous origin, **degenerative processes** e.g. osteoarthritis, rheumatoid arthritis, **metabolic bone disorders** e.g. osteoporosis or osteomalacia and **secondary neoplasms.** In a generalised condition the spine is only one of the areas affected. Any one of the constituents of the spine may be mainly affected disrupting either its structural or protective function. Osteoporosis, for example, will affect the vertebral bodies while osteoarthritis involves the synovial interarticular joints. Inflammatory lesions and tumours may not only cause destruction in the vertebral bodies but also implicate the contents of the neural arch by compression from abscess or tumour formation. Although these various conditions are all important they constitute only about ten per cent of the total causes of backache. In the large majority of patients with backache the cause is more specifically related to the spine itself. These include chronic lumbo-sacral and sacro-iliac strain, spondylosis, intervertebral disc lesions, spondylolisthesis and ankylosing spondylitis.

Chronic Lumbo-sacral and Sacro-iliac Strain

Chronic strain of the strong ligaments in the lumbo-sacral and sacro-iliac regions of the spine is thought to be the pre-disposing factor in the development of a particular type of low back pain. The patient is often female and usually in the twenty to forty age group. There are often **known aggravating factors** present such as pregnancy or the postural attitudes involved in the care of young children. **Pain** is the main feature, particularly on standing and bending. It **radiates into the buttocks** and **back of the thighs.** Clinical examination reveals **local tenderness** in the lumbo-sacral and surrounding area together with **restriction** of flexion and extension **movement** of the spine. There are no other signs and X-ray examination is negative.

Treatment. Discussion with the patient often discloses an aggravating factor. It is usually a faulty postural habit. Advice is given in the conservative regime for backache which relieves the present attack and avoids recurrence.

Conservative regime for backache. If the patient is to avoid aggravating his lesion either gradually or suddenly it is essential for him to understand which movements produce pain and therefore how to avoid making them. He should make a **conscious effort to keep his back straight** which will avoid undue stress on the discs and ligaments. If he neglects this rule and flexes his spine his backache will increase or recur.

When trying to pick up or lift objects off the floor, while washing at a sink or when sitting in a chair, the back should be kept extended and the head held erect. The body is lowered by **bending at the hips, knees and ankles.** Low or 'easy' chairs should be avoided during an acute phase and stools or high (dining room) chairs used instead. The patient's back should rest against the back of the chair so that it will be kept straight. The importance of a **firm bed** which does not sag like a hammock cannot be overstressed. It is preferable that the mattress should be firmly sprung and should rest on a firm base. Where this is not so, it should be supported by placing beneath it a wooden platform which is made to cover the whole spring or base of the bed. Sufferers from backache should **learn to get out of bed by first rolling on to the prone position,** and to extend the back by pushing upwards with the arms. The patient can then gradually slide his legs over the side of the bed until they reach the floor. In this position the hips, knees and ankles should be flexed. In order to stand erect, the patient uses the thrust of his arms on the side of the bed to push his trunk upwards and at the same time he extends his back, hips and knees.

Coughing, sneezing and **laughing** can all cause further damage to the back and should therefore be controlled if possible. When this is not possible, the back should be protected by arching or extending it. A full bowel often aggravates backache by pressing on the lumbo-sacral plexus on the posterior wall of the abdomen and pelvis. **Constipation and straining at stool** should be avoided and a gentle laxative is recommended if necessary.

When backache is acute, prolonged and uninterrupted, bed rest is usually necessary. The patient lies supine, on his side or prone, whichever is the more comfortable, as long as his trunk and limbs are in the same straight line. The patient usually finds difficulty in using a bed-pan and it is often wiser to compromise and allow him to get up to use a commode or to go to the toilet. Bathing should be discouraged because of difficulty in getting in and out of the bath. After a minimum of three weeks, or once the pain has settled, **gentle physiotherapy** is commenced. This constitutes gentle back extension exercises perhaps augmented by backward extension of each leg in turn off the bed. Such exercise may indeed further ease the pain. These movements might almost be described better as 'self-manipulations' rather than exercises for they are not vigorous. **If the pain fails to settle, sliding traction** may be implemented. Its effect can be tested by first applying manual traction to each leg in turn and then to both. Sometimes the patient experiences lessening of the pain during one of these manoeuvres. It is then possible to determine to which leg or legs the traction should be applied. Intermittent traction in the physiotherapy department may suffice and is usually carried out as part of outpatient treatment. Occasionally the pain and stiffness of backache may be relieved by **manipulation** either with or without anaesthesia but this is a treatment which must be prescribed rarely and carried out only in experienced hands as there is the **danger of leaving the patient with a permanent handicap.**

Finally where the patient's back tires markedly as the day progresses causing a 'postural slump' he may feel the need of a **support.** A short, light plaster jacket worn for a minimum period of six weeks may give considerable relief. A less rigid support, e.g. a lumbo-sacral corset (*see* Appendix, *Fig. 51c*) should be substituted at this stage. It is worn during the day. Once the pain has remained settled for several months it can be discarded and held in reserve for use in any further recurrence.

Spondylosis

This is a **degenerative condition** of the **cartilaginous joints of the spine,** as opposed to osteoarthritis which affects the synovial joints. Often the two conditions co-exist. It is more common in people over forty years of age. Both sexes are affected although men are perhaps more susceptible because of their manual activity. Sometimes the condition is symptomless, revealed only on X-ray examination for some other reason. The whole spine may be involved, but more particularly the mobile cervical and lumbar areas. **Pain** and **stiffness** are the characteristic features. The pain is initially localised to the spine. Later as the degenerative changes advance there may be involvement of the nerve roots and the pain then radiates into the upper or lower limbs. The **neurological signs** vary considerably and do not conform to any particular pattern. X-ray examination of the spine shows the degenerative changes. Blood examination excludes other causes, e.g. secondary neoplasm or tuberculosis.

Treatment. The patient must avoid any activities which aggravate the condition, e.g. lifting heavy weights. He is instructed in the **conservative regime for backache.** Gentle **neck and shoulder bracing exercises** are often of some value in the treatment of cervical spondylosis, and **back extension exercises** in spondylosis of the lumbar region. Where the degeneration is more marked and produces **severe symptoms,** a period of **bed rest** on a firm bed with the cervical and lumbar curves supported will allow the pain to settle. The patient is then fitted with a **cervical collar** or **lumbo-sacral support.** When pain settles completely, gentle exercise helps to relieve muscle spasm and reduce stiffness.

Intervertebral Disc Lesions

The **disc** is composed of **two types of tissue** and has **two functions.** The outer strong fibro-elastic cartilaginous ring of each disc binds the vertebra above to the one below, thus forming one continuous spinal unit; the inner gelatinous mucoid substance has the function of absorbing shocks and distributing stress throughout the vertebral bodies. The superior and inferior borders of each disc unit are

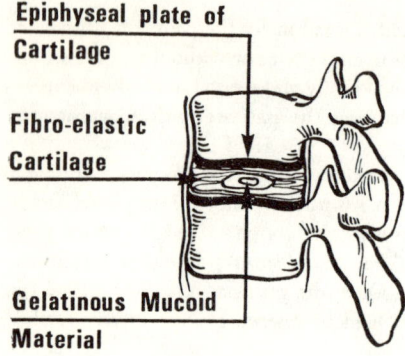

Epiphyseal plate of Cartilage

Fibro-elastic Cartilage

Gelatinous Mucoid Material

FIG. 13   Intervertebral disc

provided by the epiphyseal plate of cartilage of the two adjacent vertebral bodies (*Fig. 13*).

Disease or damage to an intervertebral disc causes disruption of that part of the spine as a functioning unit. Shocks and traumatic forces being neither absorbed nor distributed throughout the spine are concentrated locally, so aggravating the condition. Degeneration of intervertebral discs starts early in life, in adolescence. Changes occurring in the outer disc ring make it thinner and weaker. When undue stress is applied to the area the inner mucoid material bulges through the weakness consequently causing pressure on the nerve roots.

Discs may be damaged by disease, e.g. inflammatory lesions such as tuberculosis, or by injury from forces causing flexion of the spine, e.g. a fall on the buttocks, repetitive flexion of the spine or unexpected stress on the spine in the flexed position. Disc lesions may occur at any level of the spine but the lumbar region is the most common site.

The **symptoms and signs** of a **lumbar disc lesion** vary from those of vague backache to those constituting a neurosurgical emergency. In the **non-acute lesion** intermittent low backache, aggravated by poor posture and activity, is relieved by good posture and rest. There may be some muscle spasm restricting movement. X-ray examination sometimes reveals a **narrowing of a disc space.** This condition is referred to as a **recurrent lumbago.**

In an **acute lesion** the patient is often a young healthy adult with a marked **limp.** The pain is severe. It is centred in a specific area of the spine and radiates into the thigh and leg, i.e. **sciatica.** Coughing, sneezing and bending cause sudden exacerbations of the pain. Examination of the patient shows a **scoliosis,** marked lumbar muscle spasm and inability to touch the toes. When the patient lies supine he is **unable** to **lift his leg straight off the bed.** Any attempt to turn in bed is associated with a sudden increase in the pain. There are definite signs of **nerve root irritation, motor weakness** and **sensory loss** in the part of the limb supplied by the nerves affected by the lesion.

The spinal reflex arc is also inhibited and the **knee** or **ankle jerk** responses may be **sluggish or absent. Drop foot** is another significant feature of nerve root pressure. Where the lesion compresses the cauda equina, i.e. in a **central disc lesion,** both limbs are affected and in addition there is **paralysis of bladder and bowel.** These cases are **neurosurgical emergencies.**

Treatment. The treatment of **lumbago** is **conservative.** Initially the patient may have two or three weeks **bed rest,** only being allowed up to the toilet. The bed must have a firm mattress with a fracture board beneath it. This is followed by physiotherapy, consisting of gentle back extension and postural exercises designed to keep the back straight. Where it is obvious that maintenance of posture is difficult the patient is put into a **plaster jacket** for a minimum of six weeks. Thereafter he is fitted with a **lumbo-sacral corset support** which need only be worn when he suffers minor recurrence.

The **acute disc lesion** demands a different approach. **Bed rest** is essential. Where manual traction to one or both legs relieves discomfort, **continuous skin traction** is assembled. After a minimum of three weeks, where improvement has been maintained, **gentle back extension exercises** for periods of ten minutes, three times a day, can be commenced. The patient can then sit up with his legs over the side of the bed, and eventually stand. At this stage, his spine is immobilised in a **plaster jacket** for at least six weeks after which he is fitted with a **lumbo-sacral corset support.**

Where bed rest and limb traction do not relieve pain, a **myelogram** is indicated. Once disc protrusion is diagnosed and located, or if significant features like drop foot persist, operation is indicated. Excision of one or more laminae, i.e. **laminectomy,** exposes the affected nerve root stretched over the protruded disc, the removal of which relieves the pressure.

Post-operative management is simple. The patient's pain is relieved almost immediately. He is nursed on his back or side. Stitches are removed in 7–10 days. As soon as he feels fit he is allowed to sit in a chair, and when the pain settles gentle back extension exercises are given. He may be discharged wearing a lumbo-sacral support. Later, some patients develop a recurrence of backache due to osteo-arthritis and may then require a local spinal fusion.

Spondylolisthesis

This is a **slipping,** or **subluxation,** forwards of the body of one vertebra on that of the one below. Although it may occur at other levels it is usually seen in the **lower lumbar spine.** The interlocking structure of the posterior articular joints of the spine provides the stability which normally prevents forwards subluxation. **Defects** in these, which are either **congenital** or **acquired,** allow movement to occur.

The **displacement** is **gradual** over a number of years before becoming complete. It is commonest in adolescents and young adults. It leads to stretching of ligaments, disruption of the intervertebral disc and muscular strain. The symptoms are of **low back pain,** often with **sciatica,** depending on whether or not the damage to the intervertebral disc causes nerve root pressure. Examination shows forward displacement of the spine above the level of the affected vertebral spinous process (*Fig. 14*). There is **local tenderness** and, where there is nerve root pressure **neurological symptoms** and **signs** are present. X-ray examination demonstrates the defect and confirms the diagnosis.

Treatment. This varies with the type and severity of the lesion, the age and the

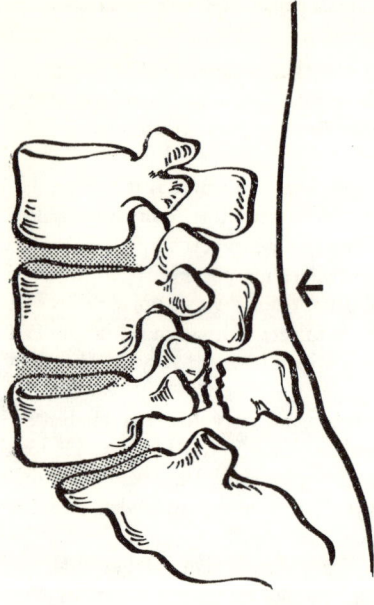

FIG. 14 Spondylolisthesis

physical condition of the patient. In a young fit person it is desirable to stabilise the spine by local fusion. Conservative regime is that of chronic lumbo-sacral strain (*see p.* 60).

Ankylosing Spondylitis

This disease results in loss of mobility of the spine converting it from a strong, resilient structure to a rigid, rod-like structure i.e. 'bamboo spine'. It usually commences in the sacro-iliac joints and spreads upwards throughout the whole spine to the occiput resulting in obliteration of all the synovial and cartilaginous joints and their replacement by bone. **Flexion deformity of the spine** results. Although the spinal cord is uninvolved, the intercostal nerve roots may be irritated and produce pain radiating round into the chest. Fixation of the ribs by involvement of the costovertebral joints and costal cartilages results in a **'fixed chest'** and respiratory impairment. The disease afflicts **young adults,** usually **males.** The cause is unknown. The pathological changes involve all the soft tissues related to joints, i.e. synovium, capsular ligament, intervertebral discs and muscles. The symptoms and signs are initially those of **lumbago** and low back pain without sciatica and have to be differentiated from the many causes of backache. As the disease progresses the patient's posture deteriorates. An increasing **kyphosis,** which later results in a fixed 'C' shaped deformity of the spine in severe cases, makes it difficult for the patient to see ahead. This is further aggravated by stiffness of the hips, and the patient develops a **shuffling gait.** A few patients develop an **iritis.** X-ray examination reveals the joint changes. Blood examination shows a **raised E.S.R.**

Treatment. The aim is to relieve pain and retain mobility. **Radiotherapy** is most effective in relieving pain and may appear to halt progress of the disease in some patients. Its disadvantage is in its side-effects. **Cortisone drug therapy** is also used but the subsequent development of osteoporosis is a complicating factor. When the pain settles **physiotherapy** is important to redevelop muscle tone, maintain posture and chest expansion. The patient must realise the importance of sleeping on a **firm bed** with only one pillow under the head so limiting the tendency to further deformity. These patients are also advised on how to maintain **good posture** and the conservative regime necessary to prevent recurrent backache.

Where the hips are affected it is now possible that **total hip replacement** will be used frequently to restore mobility. The kyphotic deformity in an otherwise fit patient with some chest excursion may be corrected by spinal osteotomy but this is rarely possible.

NURSING MANAGEMENT OF BACKACHE

Patients with backache should always be **nursed on a firm bed,** i.e. one with a special orthopaedic mattress or, alternatively, a flock mattress on top of a fracture board. The majority of patients are more comfortable lying supine with one pillow underneath the head. Those who have a high disc lesion, however, much prefer to sit up supported by pillows as the pain is aggravated in the supine position. In an acute lesion movement is restricted because of pain. The **patient's position** should be **changed frequently** as he is reluctant to move and pressure on the skin may soon become a problem. He is turned in bed in the same way as the patient with a fractured spine. The head, neck, spine, pelvis and lower limbs are treated as one unit. Pain is relieved by the regular administration of **analgesic drugs** which are gradually reduced as the condition settles. Application and care of **sliding traction** is often part of the initial nursing management (*see* Part II, *pp.* 158–63). The pain associated with severe backache and the supine position of the patient sometimes interfere with normal **bladder and bowel function.** This is quite distinct from the paresis of bladder and bowel which results from pressure on the cauda equina in central disc lesions. A daily estimation of fluid balance indicates whether or not the bladder is being emptied satisfactorily. Distension of the bladder further aggravates pain and the patient may require to be catheterised if he finds difficulty in micturition. Where constipation is a problem the collection of faeces in the rectum may produce bladder neck obstruction. The administration of rectal suppositories, or even an enema, may be required initially and a regular bowel evacuation thereafter controlled by the oral administration of mild aperients. It is better to allow the patient to sit on a **commode chair** in order to empty his bladder and bowel than to seat him on a bed pan, which is often painful and unsuccessful. The patient gets out of bed by turning into the prone position, pressing up with his arms to keep his back extended, gradually allowing his legs to slide over the side of the bed until they reach the floor. In this way the erect position can be attained without flexing the spine. The conservative management of acute backache sometimes demands that the patient lies flat and immobile for several weeks. As the relief from pain is a gradual process, some patients tend to become frustrated and somewhat depressed. Continual encouragement and re-assurance help to give them a more balanced outlook over this period. (*See pp.* 196–7, nursing management of patients after spinal surgery.)

9 COMMON AFFECTIONS OF THE SHOULDER AND UPPER LIMB

THE SHOULDER

The shoulder girdle consists of the scapula, humerus and clavicle. Functionally it is capable of circumduction or movement in any direction. The other joints in the upper limb have a more restricted range of movement. Stiffness of the shoulder restricts the usefulness of the movements of these other joints. The shoulder joint is a synovial ball and socket joint between the scapula and the humerus. The three muscles arising from the back of the scapula form the **rotator cuff,** or tendinous hood (aponeurosis), covering the shoulder joint. This is necessary to allow the deltoid muscle to act efficiently in abduction of the shoulder. In addition, the long tendon of the biceps muscle assists in maintaining the head of the humerus in close apposition to the glenoid cavity of the scapula. The capsule of the shoulder joint is slack and 'sac-like'. The glenoid labrum deepens the socket. (*Fig. 15.*)

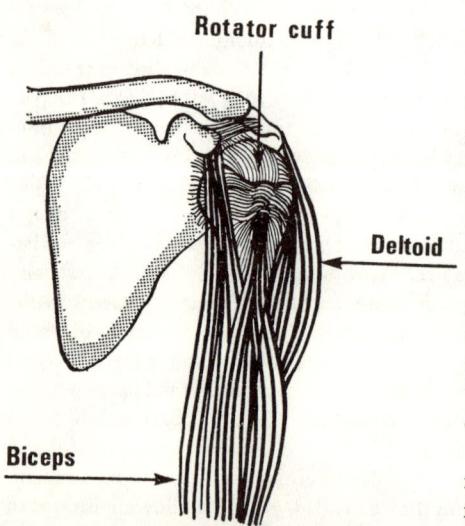

FIG. 15   The rotator cuff mechanism

Pain in the shoulder region may arise locally or be referred from the neck (cervical spondylosis), chest (lung or cardiac lesion) and abdomen (visceral injury, e.g. spleen). Pain localised to the shoulder may arise from the shoulder joint itself, or the acromio-clavicular joint which lies above it. The lesion can be any one of the diseases of synovial joints, such as acute or chronic inflammation or one of the rheumatic diseases. The conditions more commonly associated with the shoulder region, apart from fractures and dislocations, are traumatic or degenerative in origin and all affect the gleno-humeral joint.

Supraspinatus or Rotator Cuff Tendinitis

As this structure initiates abduction of the arm it may be damaged by repetitive activities or by direct contusion in falls on the upper limb or shoulder. The patient complains of an aching pain in the shoulder, aggravated by movement and often present nocturnally. On examination there is local tenderness and a **'painful arc'** through which the shoulder moves.

Treatment. Treatment is by the injection of **local anaesthetic** to deaden the pain, and **hydrocortisone** to minimise the inflammatory reaction. The treatment of tendon lesions by hydrocortisone is somewhat restricted by the side effects produced. Healing may be delayed and the structure weakened to the extent that tendon rupture can occur. This complication is more likely where such injections have been repeated. If the pain is more diffuse, **short wave diathermy** may be effective.

Degenerative Tendinitis

Degenerative changes may occur anywhere in the rotator cuff tendon producing partial or complete rupture. **Partial rupture** of the **tendon** resembles the clinical picture of rotator cuff tendinitis. A **complete rupture** is, however, a more serious condition. The onset is sudden and there is always a history of indirect injury to the shoulder. Pain is severe and there may be some localised shoulder swelling. Abduction of the shoulder is impossible as the deltoid can no longer function efficiently. X-ray examination confirms upward displacement of the head of the humerus.

Treatment. This is usually **conservative.** Surgical repair of the torn tendon usually fails because of the degeneration already present in the tendon. A **simple inside collar and cuff sling** is fitted until the pain settles after which an **outside support** is substituted (*see* Appendix, *Fig. 48a and b*). **Physiotherapy** is then commenced to develop the remaining shoulder girdle musculature. The end result is a limitation in abduction of the shoulder, a disability which the patient is usually willing to accept.

Calcification of the Rotator Cuff Tendon

Repeated stress causes gradual degenerative change and the formation of a small plaque of calcium (not unlike toothpaste) in the substance of the rotator cuff tendon. The calcium plaque may rupture through the tendon into the subdeltoid space (bursa) where it is gradually absorbed. It is a very painful condition which is aggravated by the slightest movement of the shoulder and also disturbs sleep. Clinically the condition is not unlike a septic arthritis but the patient does not have the symptoms and signs of inflammation and the calcification is seen on X-ray examination.

Treatment. The pain may be alleviated by a course of **short-wave diathermy** combined with rest. Where this fails, or if indeed the condition is aggravated, an injection of local anaesthetic may be given into the painful spot and an attempt made to **aspirate the calcium.** If the symptoms persist, operative removal of the calcium deposits is necessary.

Recurrent Dislocation of the Shoulder (cf. Dislocation of the Shoulder, *p.* 119). The original injury is produced by **indirect violence** to the shoulder due to a fall on the out-stretched arm. This is associated with pain and marked muscle spasm which holds the head of the humerus in the dislocated position. The act of dislocation ruptures the joint capsule. After reduction the torn capsule may fail to heal adequately. This may be due either to the nature of the lesion itself or to an insufficient period of immobilisation. Subsequently the shoulder may dislocate during the course of a simple movement, for example putting the arm into a coat sleeve, producing similar, but less severe, symptoms and signs to those of the original injury.

Treatment. Many patients learn to live with their disability which need not inconvenience them greatly, provided they are not involved in manual or sporting activities. Where discomfort is significant operation is necessary. This may involve re-attachment of the detached capsule to the scapula as in **Bankhart's repair** or strengthening of the rupture as in **Putti-Platt operation.** Post-operatively, the shoulder is immobilised in a collar and cuff sling with the arm bandaged firmly to the body using a crêpe bandage reinforced by strips of elastoplast. Although the sutures are removed in 10–14 days, the immobilisation is maintained for a further 3 weeks. Thereafter, treatment is by outpatient **physiotherapy.** Both operations give good results enabling the patient to pursue previous activities.

THE ELBOW
The elbow is a synovial joint formed by the lower end of the humerus articulating with the upper ends of the ulna and radius. The true joint is that between the humerus and ulna. It is a hinge joint and has two movements, flexion and extension. The joint between the humerus and radius is a ball and socket joint which, in addition to flexion and extension, allows rotation. This is a particularly important joint as, together with the inferior radio-ulnar joint at the wrist, it controls the pronation and supination of the hand. With the elbow fully extended and the hand in full supination, the forearm is normally deviated laterally from the line of the humerus by 5–10 degrees. This is known as the **'carrying angle.'**

The elbow is a joint exposed to trauma at all ages. It can also be affected by any of the diseases associated with synovial joints, e.g. rheumatoid arthritis. Stiffness or deformity of the joint is a serious complication, not only because of the local restriction of movement but also because of the effect it has on the function of the hand.

Valgus and Varus Deformities
Valgus and varus deformities respectively increase or decrease the carrying angle of the forearm and are usually the result of **malunion of supracondylar fractures.** Valgus deformity produces a traction lesion of the ulnar nerve which gradually occurs over a period of months leading to a typical ulnar nerve palsy. Varus deformity is important because of its unsightly appearance. Both are seen

in children and often require operative correction by **supracondylar osteotomy.**
Internal fixation is used and in most cases the child regains a normal elbow.

Osteochondritis Dissecans

This is a condition in which a portion of the lateral condyle of the humerus
becomes detached, forming a loose body in the elbow joint. Intermittent locking
of the joint occurs. There is pain and swelling due to synovial effusion. Treatment
is by **removal of the loose body.** Where degeneration is marked the cartilage is
trimmed but, in severe cases, **excision of the head of radius** may be necessary.

Tennis Elbow

This is the name given to a condition in which there is pain localised to the **lateral
side of the elbow.** It is seen not only in tennis players but also in anyone whose
job demands repetitive strong gripping movements of the hand. To grip requires
fixation of the hand by the wrist extensors whose common origin is from the
lateral epicondyle. Chronic muscular strain or partial rupture of these fibres gives
rise to this condition. Tennis elbow is recognised by a dull aching discomfort of a
commanding nature which is aggravated by activity and by localised pressure.
Full extension is painful and eventually becomes limited. X-ray examination is
negative.

Treatment. Local anaesthetic, hyalase to disperse it, and **hydrocortisone** to
combat formation of excessive scar tissue are injected into the most tender spot.
If this fails a course of **short wave diathermy** and massage may help. Complete
muscular **rest** is most important. Should the symptoms persist they may be
alleviated by complete **immobilisation in plaster** for 3-4 weeks. **Operative**
division of the common extensor muscle origin may be required in extreme cases.

Olecranon Bursitis

This may result from direct trauma to the point of the elbow or chronic pressure
from repeated leaning on the elbow (student's elbow). The olecranon bursa is a
synovial sac which overlies the point of the elbow lessening friction on the olecranon. Inflammation of the bursa leads to a synovial effusion which distends it
producing a bulbous, soft deformity over the olecranon. Pain is minimal and many
patients only seek reassurance that the swelling is not a tumour. In the absence of
further trauma most cases will subside. In persistent cases aspiration or even
surgical excision may be required. Occasionally olecranon bursitis may be due to
pyogenic infection or gout.

THE WRIST, HAND AND FINGERS

The wrist consists of eight small bones arranged in two rows of four. These bones
articulate with each other. The scaphoid and lunate in the proximal row articulate
with the radius. Each of those of the distal row articulates with one metacarpal
except the most medial one, which articulates with two, the 4th and 5th. All the

joints of the wrist are synovial. Although each individual joint does not have a wide range of movement, the wrist itself is an extremely mobile unit. Rotation of the radius round the ulna, at the upper and lower forearm joints, permits pronation and supination of the hand. The **triangular fibro-cartilage** is an intra-articular disc binding the lower end of the radius and ulna together, and separating the ulna from the proximal bones of the wrist. Disease or injury of bone or joint in this region interferes with strength and mobility, which can be a serious handicap particularly in a manual worker.

Ganglion

The wrist is the commonest site of ganglion formation. A ganglion is a cyst, variable in size, which has an outer capsule, an inner synovial lining and contains a gelatinous material. It is found in either a joint capsule or fibrous tendon sheath and the swelling appears usually on the back of the hand, either centrally or to the radial side. As the tense swelling enlarges, pain becomes a feature and function of the hand is restricted. The ganglion may disappear spontaneously but can persist indefinitely. The cyst can be **ruptured** by **digital pressure** or **aspirated** under local anaesthesia, both of which are temporary measures. **Surgical excision** is usually curative although the condition occasionally recurs.

Kienboch's Disease

Post-traumatic avascular necrosis of the **lunate** is commonly seen after dislocation of the bone. The nutrient vessels are torn with the capsule. Collapse of the bone and degeneration of the articular cartilage predispose to osteoarthritis of the wrist. **Arthrodesis** may be necessary to provide a strong painfree wrist.

Triangular Fibro-Cartilage Syndrome

Although the triangular fibro-cartilage is a powerful structure it may rupture in a fall on to the outstretched hand, either as an isolated injury or commonly in association with a **Colles' fracture.** The lesion produces an aching discomfort on the ulnar side of the wrist, local tenderness on palpation and a painful clicking in the wrist on movement. As X-ray examination is negative the lesion is sometimes undiagnosed. Function of the hand is limited in the supinated position and this can severely incapacitate the manual worker. **Excision of the lower end of the ulna and triangular fibro-cartilage** removes the annoying 'click' and relieves pain. Although the wrist is weakened function is not unduly impaired.

Carpal Tunnel Syndrome

The carpal tunnel is the space surrounded by the concave aspect of the carpal bones posteriorly and the carpal ligament anteriorly. The contents of the tunnel are the median nerve, the flexor tendons and tendon sheaths to the fingers.

Compression of the median nerve occurs due to swelling of the tendon sheaths in the water retention of pregnancy, hypertrophy of the synovial membrane in rheumatoid arthritis, or projection of osteophytes in osteoarthritis or trauma. Apart from injury and osteoarthritis the condition is often bilateral, occurs in women and is worse nocturnally. The patient complains of pain and a burning sensation in the fingers. Clumsiness in the finer movements of the fingers, e.g. fastening a belt, and burns of the fingers while cooking are not uncommon complaints. The classical signs of median nerve palsy, hypoaesthesia, atrophic skin changes in the radial $3\frac{1}{2}$ fingers and weakness of the short abductor muscle of the thumb are present. **Treatment** is simple and effective. **Division of the carpal ligament** anteriorly under general anaesthesia decompresses the median nerve and produces dramatic improvement.

Trigger Finger (Stenosing Tenovaginitis)

This condition affects the fibrous tendon sheaths of the fingers. Thickening of a sheath occurs without obvious cause, perhaps due to trauma. This produces an area of constriction in the tunnel of the sheath which hinders the smooth gliding of the tendon it contains. The tendon develops a constriction in relation to the thickened sheath with a bulbous swelling proximal to it. (*Fig. 16.*) When the swollen part of the tendon is forced through the obstruction during flexion and extension of the finger, a 'click' is produced. Eventually the finger may be fixed in flexion and require passive extension by the patient himself. Extension is then associated with a painful click, i.e. trigger finger. It is an annoying condition.

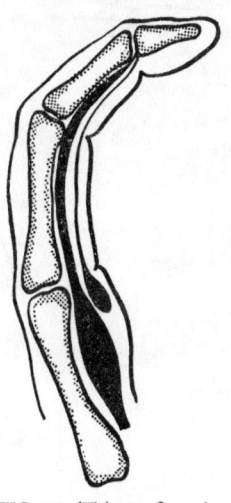

Treatment. Treatment is simple and curative by **surgical division of the fibrous tendon sheath** under general anaesthesia with excision of a small portion of the sheath to avoid recurrence. **Local injection of hydrocortisone** occasionally cures mild cases. The

FIG. 16 'Trigger finger' (stenosing tenovaginitis)

condition is also seen in infants, the thumb being most commonly affected, and it is sometimes bilateral. The thumbs are fixed or 'locked' in the flexed position. Surgery is necessary to free the tendon and in order to allow the thumb to be extended.

Mallet Finger

This deformity occurs due to rupture of the extensor tendon insertion into the terminal phalanx. It occurs when excessive stress is applied to the fingertip while the tendon is contracted during extension of the finger, e.g. catching the finger in a sheet while bed-making, or catching a cricket ball. The tendon itself may be torn or, if it remains intact, a piece of bone is pulled off the terminal phalanx. The tip of the finger cannot be extended and droops (*Fig. 17*). Pain, swelling and immediate loss of function are obvious.

Treatment. Where a piece of bone is avulsed it can be replaced and sutured successfully. Splintage is by a **mallet finger splint** until the wound has healed. Where it is the tendon that is ruptured, treatment is sometimes less successful, because it is technically difficult to approximate the torn ends. The patient may well have to accept the deformity which does not interfere greatly with function of the hand.

Site of rupture

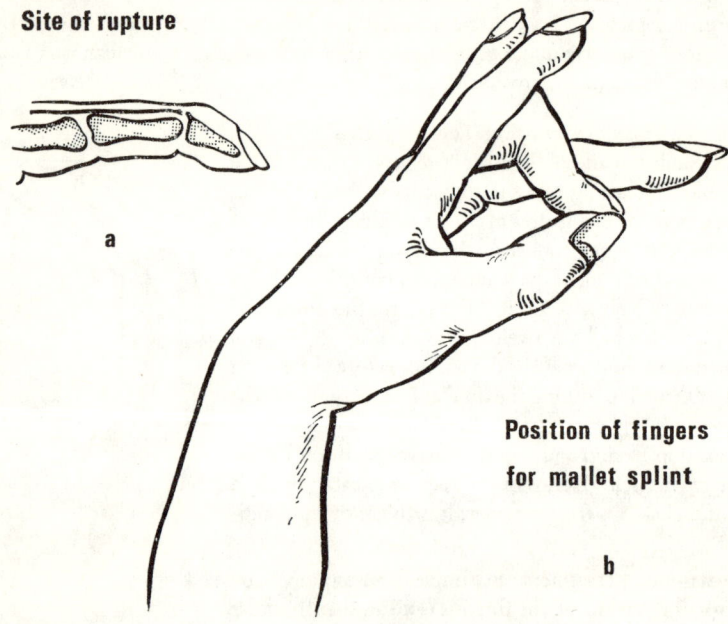

a

Position of fingers

for mallet splint

b

FIG. 17   (a) Mallet finger deformity
(b) Position of fingers for splintage

Dupuytren's Contracture

This condition is more commonly associated with the palms of the hands but the soles of the feet can also be involved. It appears to be an inherited disease and is often bilateral. Gradual thickening of the skin occurs in the palms of the hands, usually opposite the ring and little fingers. The thickening is in the palmar fascia which has extensions into the base of each finger. Contracture occurs and the fingers are pulled down into the palm at the metacarpophalangeal joints. This interferes with the grip. Dupuytren's contracture can sometimes be painful.

Treatment. This is conservative in mild cases. **Passive manipulation** is carried out several times daily by the patient. In progressive, severe cases **surgical excision of the contracting palmar fascia** prevents the fingers from being pulled down into the palm of the hand and becoming functionless. With the **open palm technique,** the wound is allowed to heal by secondary intention without skin grafting. The patient must attend the outpatient department for several weeks for wound dressings. Where the patient comes for advice late, and the fingers are flexed functionless into the palm, the condition cannot be relieved. Amputation of the affected fingers may be considered.

Volkmann's Ischaemic Contracture

This is a **crippling deformity** involving the forearm, wrist and hand. There is wasting of the flexor muscles of the forearm and flexion deformities of the wrist and fingers. Although specifically a complication of **supracondylar and forearm fractures,** particularly in children, a similar picture is occasionally seen in the muscles of the lower limb, in fractures of the tibia. Pressure on the brachial artery interferes with circulation to the structures of the forearm and hand. The degree of tissue damage will depend on whether or not the vessel is partially or completely occluded. Complete occlusion will produce total death of tissue, i.e. gangrene. This is uncommon as the collateral circulation usually compensates partially for the obstruction. The blood supply is, however, diminished and ischaemia of the tissues results. The main structures affected are the flexor muscles in the forearm. Some of the muscle fibres die and are replaced by scar or fibrous tissue. This contracts, later producing the flexion deformities of the wrist and fingers. The nerves can be damaged either by the ischaemia itself or by constriction due to the fibrous contracture within the muscles. Volkmann's ischaemia **develops insidiously over a period of several hours.**

Cause. Anything which obstructs the circulation to the limb can produce this lesion. **Pressure on the brachial artery** may result from **displaced bone fragments,** a **tight plaster cast** or **bandage,** or **swelling of the soft tissues.**

Clinical Features. Painful clawing of the fingers is a classical sign of a developing lesion. The pain is aggravated on gentle passive extension of the fingers. The patient often complains of a burning sensation or **paraesthesia** in the forearm and hand. There may be a patchy loss of sensation. The **radial pulse** may be **weak, present intermittently** or **absent** altogether. The fingers are cold with a bluish mottled appearance because of the **sluggish circulation.** As time progresses, there is increasing **weakness of flexion of the fingers.** Once the true deformity has developed, the shortened flexor muscles hold the fingers and wrist in a position of flexion, making extension of the fingers impossible.

Treatment. This is essentially **preventative.** Observation of the circulation and the **careful supervision of plaster splintage** is vitally important (*see pp.* 168–71). Where there is a defective circulation, which persists despite the removal of the plaster splintage, the limb is **X-rayed** as a bony fragment of a displaced fracture may be the cause of pressure. If the X-ray is negative, **exploration of the artery** is the only alternative. Sometimes there is arterial spasm and this may be relieved by the **local infusion** of a **smooth muscle relaxant.** If, however, the patency of the vessel is questionable, a **replacement graft,** e.g. a piece taken from the long saphenous vein, is used to replace the damaged segment. **Passive movements** of the fingers are performed post-operatively to overcome the tendency to deformity.

Where the **true deformity** has developed, the ischaemia cannot be rectified and treatment is aimed at correcting the deformity. Sometimes **passive correction,** by physiotherapy or splintage, helps to reduce the degree of contracture but surgery is required in most cases. A **muscle slide operation** is undertaken. The common origin of the flexor muscles is detached from the medial epicondyle of the humerus. Extension of the wrist and fingers, i.e. correction of the deformity, causes the muscle origin to slide further down the forearm. The limb is immobilised in a special splint which, although intended to keep the fingers extended, allows gentle active flexion movements in order to prevent stiffness. Splintage is maintained until the muscle origin forms a new attachment in the soft tissues of the forearm. Thereafter, correction is maintained by physiotherapy.

THE HIP

The hip is a ball and socket joint. It allows movement in all directions. The lever acting on it, the femur, is the longest bone in the body. All the weight of the trunk passes through the sacro-iliac joints to the pelvis and hip. The long femoral lever transmits and magnifies any force it experiences to the hip joint. The ability to extend the hips is necessary to allow one to stand erect. A child who cannot extend his hips will not learn to walk. The ability to flex the hips allows one to sit. The combination of movements occurring at the hip allow normal walking. Disease of the hip joint leads to difficulty in sitting, standing and walking. As most cases have flexion deformities walking is the main problem. In ankylosing spondylitis, however, the hip is stiff in extension and sitting is difficult. The commonest hip diseases vary with age. Congenital and infective lesions are commonly seen in infancy and early childhood (*see pp.* 17, 23), Perthes' disease in children from 5–9 years, slipped upper femoral epiphysis in adolescence, rheumatoid arthritis mainly in adult life and osteoarthritis and secondary bone tumours in advancing age (*see pp.* 33, 34, 54).

Disease or injury in the region of the joint may result in a deformity of the hip, in which there is a diminution in the femoral neck/shaft angle with an accompanying limp. This deformity is known as **coxa vara.** Coxa vara produces mechanical dysfunction of the short gluteal muscles which control the tilt of the pelvis while walking. For example, while standing on one leg and lifting the other as if to make a step, the contraction of the gluteal muscles on the weight-bearing side tilts the pelvis towards that side. This gives room to swing the non-weight-bearing leg through to complete the step. Where the short gluteal muscles are inefficient a reverse tilt is produced. This is the basis of the medical term known as the **Trendelenburg's sign** which, in this case, is positive (*Fig. 18*).

Perthes' Disease

The disease affects a **child** classically between 5–9 years of age, although appearances resembling Perthes' disease may be seen earlier. The cause is not established but it may be traumatic. Appearances similar to those of avascular necrosis are shown in the femoral head. This causes it to collapse and become mushroom-shaped. The disease process is slow, over eighteen months to two years. Although pain is not significant the child develops a **limp.** Examination of the hip shows some **limitation of movement.** X-ray confirms the presence of **avascular necrosis** and **deformity of the femoral head.**

Treatment. The child is treated by the avoidance of weight bearing on that side for up to two years. This is achieved in various ways, e.g. by **bed rest in traction,** by a **pelvic sling** suspending the leg, or by a **weight-relieving walking caliper** with a patten on the opposite shoe to equalise the leg lengths. The results of these different methods seem comparable. As it is desirable to avoid prolonged bed rest,

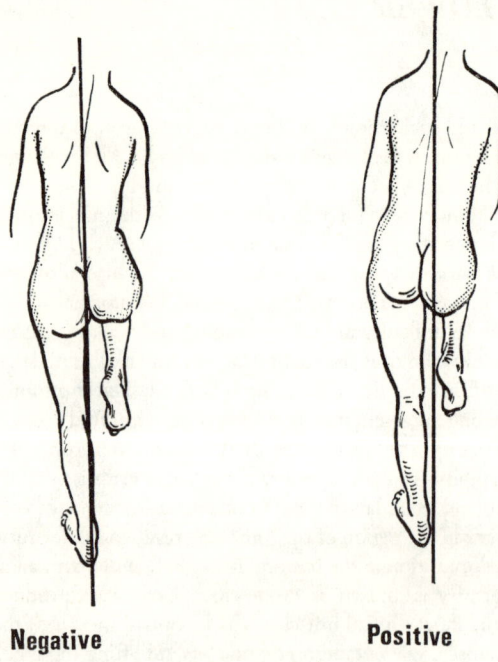

Negative   Positive

FIG. 18   Trendelenburg's sign

either of the latter two methods is now preferred particularly in the later stages of the condition when the head of the femur has reached the healing stage (*see* Appendix, *Fig. 50a and b*). Once X-ray shows that the femoral head has revascular-ised, weight bearing can commence. The patient remains trouble free until middle life when some patients develop a secondary osteoarthritis.

Coxa Vara

In the adult the normal angle between the neck and shaft of the femur is between 120° and 140°. Where it is less, i.e. nearer a right angle, the deformity is called coxa vara. Less commonly the angle may be increased, and the deformity is termed **coxa valga.** Coxa vara may be caused by damage at different sites at the upper end of the femur, viz. the head, the epiphysis, the neck or the trochanters. The nature of the damage varies. It may be congenital, traumatic, inflammatory (pyogenic, tuberculous), degenerative (osteoarthritis, rheumatoid arthritis), metabolic (osteoporosis, osteomalacia), neoplastic (secondary tumour) or idiopathic, i.e. of unknown origin. Common conditions resulting in coxa vara are Perthes' disease, slipped upper femoral epiphysis and femoral neck and trochanteric fractures.

Adolescent Coxa Vara

Slipped upper femoral epiphysis is seen between the ages of 12–16 years. In the young child the upper femoral epiphysis sits horizontally on top of the neck and is less liable to slip. In the adolescent the epiphysis is in the 'cocked-hat' position and under certain circumstances has the tendency to shift (*Fig. 19*). The predisposing

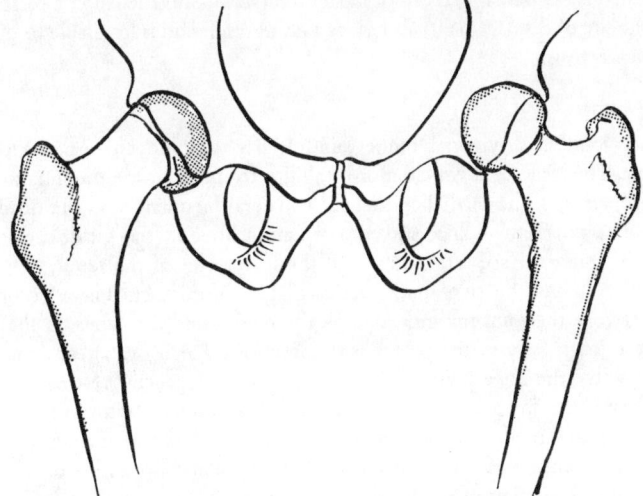

FIG. 19 Coxa vara: Slipped upper femoral epiphysis (Right side)

factor is an **endocrine upset** where there is imbalance between the growth and sex hormones. There are two physical types, the **long lean** individual and the **short Dickensian 'fat boy'.** The other epiphyses are not affected probably because they are more horizontally placed. The **slip** occurs **gradually** and may be **partial** or **complete.** Trauma, however, can produce an acute slipping of the epiphysis. The symptoms and signs are classical, in that the subject is a boy of one of the two types described; he usually complains of **referred pain** in the **knee** and has a **limp.** It may be some weeks before pain is felt in the hip. There is difficulty in rotating the foot inwards and a tendency to walk with it externally rotated. Occasionally the condition is bilateral. There is usually no significant tenderness on palpation of the hip although extremes of movement may be painful. There is an **external rotational deformity** and a **coxa vara** with a **positive Trendelenburg** sign. X-ray shows the degree of displacement of the femoral epiphysis. No endocrine defect is evident.

Treatment. This is either conservative or surgical. Complete **bed rest** for a year, or perhaps longer, would allow early fusion of the epiphysis in a partial slip. This long period of immobilisation can be shortened by surgery. **Internal fixation** (e.g. Austin Moore pins) not only prevents further slipping but also stimulates fusion of the epiphysis, usually within three months. Where an acute total slip of the epiphysis has occurred, gentle **manipulative reduction by traction** prior to internal fixation is necessary. When the displacement is gradual a severe degree of slipped epiphysis with marked deformity may develop before the condition is diagnosed. The deformity may be corrected by **osteotomy.** Transcervical osteotomy, at the site of the displacement, gives excellent correction but may be complicated by avascular necrosis of the femoral head. Subtrochanteric osteotomy, below the site of displacement, also gives a good result and is less liable to produce avascular necrosis.

THE KNEE

The knee joint is a synovial hinge joint. It has two movements, flexion and extension. The structures which afford stability to the joint are the intercondylar cruciate ligaments, the medial and lateral collateral ligaments and the quadriceps muscle. The **patella**, or knee cap, is a sesamoid bone in the quadriceps muscle tendon. Its inner surface articulates with the lower end of the femur. The knee joint also contains the two semilunar cartilages or menisci. These occupy the spaces between the joint margins, one on the medial and the other on the lateral side of the joint. Any of the generalised conditions which can affect joints commonly involve the knee joint, e.g. inflammatory or degenerative diseases. Apart from disease, the knee is particularly exposed to trauma, with damage to the joint structures. The degree of flexion of the knee at the time of injury, together with the mechanism of injury, determine the particular structure or structures involved and the extent of resultant damage.

Tears of the Menisci

A **meniscus** is composed of **fibrocartilage.** Such structures are found in the interior of the wrist, knee and temporo-mandibular joints. Of the two menisci in the knee joint, one is situated at the inner (**medial**) side and the other lies at the outer (**lateral**) margin. They are **crescent-shaped** and occupy the triangular space between the opposing condyles of the femur and tibia, being attached to both by ligaments. They have a limited degree of mobility within the joint, the outer or lateral meniscus being more mobile than the medial. In stresses and strains on the joint the menisci, along with the articular cartilage, absorb some of the shocks or pressures on the joint. A meniscus may be torn in one of several ways. When part of the torn meniscus is displaced it can restrict extension of the joint.

Clinical Features. There is a history of either a **violent injury,** often at sport, e.g. in a footballer, or of a **repetitive** or **awkward movement** at work, e.g. in a miner. **Pain** is the most significant feature. Traction on the synovial membrane gives rise to a **synovial effusion** which produces **swelling** of the joint. The swelling causes inhibition of the quadriceps muscle function and the patient feels a sensation of **instability** in the joint. **'Clicking'**, or even intermittent **'locking'** of the joint is a common feature, caused by the intervention of a part of the torn meniscus between the joint surfaces. Where the joint is 'locked' the pain is severe and the patient is unable to extend his knee. Either he may be unable to bear weight on the affected limb, or he may do so with a marked **limp**. Severe instability of the knee is always associated with further structural damage, e.g. rupture of the anterior cruciate ligament.

Examination. Swelling of the knee joint is obvious. **Wasting** of the **quadriceps muscle** is apparent and is due to inactivity of the knee particularly where there has been recurrent locking. In a 'locked' knee there will be an obvious **flexion deformity**. **Tenderness** is elicited on pressure over the damaged meniscus.

If the knee is manipulated by the doctor through the range of flexion, rotation and extension, a loud painful 'click' may be produced (**McMurray's test**). This will confirm the presence of a tear in the meniscus and its location in either the medial or lateral side of the joint. The integrity of the cruciate ligaments and the stability of the joint are also tested at this stage. An X-ray of the knee joint usually appears normal.

Treatment. The meniscus cannot be repaired because it is composed of fibro-cartilaginous tissue which lacks its own blood supply and will not heal. Removal of the meniscus is called **meniscectomy** (see p. 177). If this operation is undertaken early enough, and there are no other complicating factors such as tears of the cruciate ligaments, the knee should subsequently function normally. Sometimes the patient does not present with his problem until after several incidents of joint 'locking'. The constant locking and unlocking process damages the articular cartilage which predisposes to degenerative osteoarthritis in later life.

Recurrent Dislocation of the Patella

The shortest distance between two points is a straight line. Where the quadriceps muscle, the patella and the patellar tendon are in one straight line, a direct pull on the patella results and stability is maintained. Where the patella lies medial to the straight line joining the quadriceps muscle and the patellar tendon, a triangle is formed. Contraction of the muscle produces subluxation or dislocation of the patella into the straight line between the muscle and tendon. This situation commonly arises in girls with a broad pelvis and a tendency to knock knees. Other anatomical factors which interfere with the normal quadriceps extensor mechanism may produce this condition. The symptoms are of **pain,** a feeling of **instability** in the knee and the impression of **'locking'**, symptoms not unlike those of a torn cartilage. The continued instability can in fact cause intra-articular damage such as a torn cartilage, chondromalacia patellae and eventually osteoarthritis. The condition is **recurrent** although, occasionally, it may be **chronic**.

Treatment. Treatment is surgical by **transplantation of the tibial tuberosity.** The tibial tuberosity is raised from its bed by osteotomy leaving the tendon attached to it. A fresh bed is made for it more medially so as to convert the triangle into a straight line thus correcting the tendency to lateral displacement. After wound closure a **plaster cylinder** is applied. One week later a graduated course of exercises is instituted and after a further week the plaster is removed.

Loose Bodies

A loose body is found in a synovial joint either as the result of injury or disease. The knee is the commonest site of loose body formation. Loose bodies can originate from any of the structures forming the joint, i.e. articular cartilage, meniscus, bone or synovium, or from the results of haemarthrosis or septic arthritis, i.e. fibrinous loose bodies. There may be one single loose body in the joint or many, depending on the predisposing condition. The fragment may be existent for some time and is only apparent when it interferes with joint function giving rise to specific symptoms and signs. When the loose body lodges in between the joint surfaces it produces sudden **pain** and **'locking'** of the joint. **Dislodgement** is usually **spontaneous** and freedom of joint movement is restored. At varying intervals the situation **recurs.** Eventually the affected joint **swells,** there is **instability** of the knee and the patient walks with a **limp.** The repetitive incidents cause local damage to the articular cartilage.

Treatment. Where the loose body is of bony origin it can be located on X-ray examination and removed surgically. Where the diagnosis cannot be confirmed by X-ray, e.g. in cartilaginous or fibrinous loose body formation, exploration of the joint is necessary in order to identify the presence of one or more fragments. Surgical removal cures the locking but the prognosis is dependent on the underlying cause and the extent of damage already present in the joint. Secondary osteoarthritis is a common complication.

Chondromalacia Patellae

This is probably one of the more common causes of loose body formation. The predisposing factor in this condition appears to be **trauma** to the kneecap and indeed there is often evidence of a scar from an old injury in the region of the knee. There is a characteristic softening, roughening and actual **breaking-up** of the previously smooth **articular cartilage** of the opposing surfaces of the patella and femur. Pieces of cartilage form a semi-detached 'seaweed-like' appearance within the joint. Eventually pieces actually become detached forming **loose bodies.**

Clinical Features. There is vague discomfort present in the knee which is followed by an ill-defined **ache** behind the patella. A painless **'cracking'** of the knee develops. Often after the knee 'cracks' there is temporary relief of the discomfort. Exercise, kneeling and climbing all contribute to exaggeration of the symptoms. **Crepitus,** a grating sensation, may be experienced later on pressing the kneecap against the femur. When the separation of pieces of cartilage form loose bodies within the knee joint, the knee **'locks',** the **joint swells** and the patient develops **a limp.**

Treatment. The early treatment, before loose body formation occurs, consists of **rest** and the **avoidance** of all possible **aggravating factors. Weight reduction** where necessary, is advised to relieve the mechanical 'load' on the joint and often a change of occupation is indicated. Sometimes a course of **short wave diathermy** is beneficial but physiotherapy is avoided as it makes the condition worse.

Operation involves **removal of the loose bodies** and trimming of the articular cartilage thus partly reconstituting the smooth surface. Occasionally when the condition is far advanced it may be necessary to remove the patella. This relieves the acute symptoms. Although function is improved by **patellectomy** it may remain somewhat inferior to that of a normal knee.

Osteochondritis Dissecans
This is a condition in which a fragment of bone and cartilage gradually separates from what usually appears to be a normal part of a joint leaving a saucer-like depression. The condition is more commonly seen in the knee, particularly in the medial femoral condyle, but it may be found in the elbow, hip or ankle joints. The cause is thought to be either **traumatic** or part of an **inherent defect.** In some instances it has been shown to be **familial.** The loose body gives rise to sudden **pain** and **locking, swelling** and **instability** of the joint. An X-ray shows the loose body and the site of origin in the condyle. At **operation,** if the loose **fragment** is relatively undamaged it is **replaced** and internally fixed using a **Smillie pin.** Weight bearing is avoided on the affected limb for about twelve weeks until the fragment appears to have united to its base. The joint is then exposed and the pin removed. Osteoarthritis is a common complication, often occurring in the younger age group.

THE ANKLE
Although the ankle joint is perhaps more commonly involved in injury, it is, nevertheless, liable to any of the diseases affecting synovial joints. Two common causes of chronic weakness in the ankle are recurrent dislocation of the joint and rupture of the Achilles tendon.

Recurrent Subluxation or Dislocation of the Ankle Joint
Where total rupture of the lateral ligament is inadequately treated recurring instability results. There is **pain** and **swelling** of the ankle joint after each incident. Eventually the patient dreads walking on uneven surfaces because of the tendency for the foot to invert. Sometimes the patient actually falls to the ground. The **instability** of the ankle joint can be demonstrated by X-ray comparison of both ankles under stress.

Treatment. In **subluxation** without true dislocation, **physiotherapy** strengthens the peroneal or evertor muscles of the foot. The stability of the ankle joint is increased if the patient is willing to wear a **solid low-heeled shoe,** the heel being further broadened by flaring it laterally. These measures may be sufficient to resist the tendency of the foot to invert when the patient walks on uneven ground.

Where, however, inversion and instability persist, a **below-knee caliper** will prevent inversion of the foot and give stability to the ankle joint.

In severe cases where transient **dislocation** occurs treatment is by **operation.** The **damaged ligament** is **repaired** using the tendon of one of the less important peroneal muscles. After immobilisation in a plaster cast for 3–6 weeks, mobilising ankle and foot exercises are carried out. A supporting shoe with lateral flaring of the heel is again necessary.

Rupture of the Achilles Tendon (tendo calcaneus)
The tendo Achillis is the strong tendon of the powerful calf muscles on the posterior aspect of the lower leg. It is inserted into the os calcis. The function of the calf muscles with their common tendon is to plantar flex the foot in the 'push-off' phase of walking, running and dancing. In middle life degenerative changes occur in the tendon. If physical activity is suddenly increased at this stage the degenerate tendon is liable to rupture.

Clinical Features. The clinical picture is of sudden **localised pain** in the calf of the leg. There is **swelling** behind the ankle as a result of haematoma formation. As muscle function is impaired, the patient is **unable to stand on tiptoe** and so walks with a **limping gait** which is described as 'duck-like'. On palpation of the back of the leg a **hollow** is felt, denoting absence of the firm, tendinous, cord-like structure.

Treatment. If the injury is untreated, healing by fibrosis with lengthening of the structure occurs and, although pain disappears and swelling diminishes, the limp persists. **Surgical repair** of the tendon is undertaken early. Post-operatively the foot and ankle are immobilised in a long leg **plaster** with the knee bent and the foot in equinus. After two weeks the sutures are removed and a below-knee plaster, with the foot still in equinus, is applied.

In subsequent plaster applications the foot is gradually dorsiflexed from the position of equinus until, by about six weeks, it is at right angles to the tibia. The patient is allowed to walk on the affected limb at about the fourth week of treatment. The plaster is usually discarded after six weeks and physiotherapy is commenced. The ultimate aim is to regain full mobility in the foot and ankle.

THE FOOT AND TOES
Pain in the sole of the foot may be due to any of the diseases which affect bones or synovial joints. In addition there are certain mechanical ailments peculiar to the feet. These include metatarsalgia, chronic foot strain, plantar fasciitis and march fracture.

Metatarsalgia
Pain in the transverse metatarsal arch (ball of the foot) is referred to as metatarsalgia. This arch resembles a shallow dome and weight is taken on the heads of the 1st and 5th metatarsal bones. The other metatarsal heads are 'cushioned' by a pad of fat. The arch is maintained in this position by the small muscles of the foot and

the supporting ligaments. Pain is produced where this dome is flattened, resulting in **strain on the joints, muscles and ligaments.** This may be due to long hours of **standing, obesity,** or a debilitating illness. **Trauma** to the arch or a **badly moulded plaster cast** predisposes also to metatarsalgia.

The condition is usually of a chronic nature. It is **often bilateral** but one foot is predominantly affected. As pain becomes marked the patient develops a **limp.** **Local tenderness** is present over the heads of the metatarsals. There may be a slight **swelling** of the dorsum of the foot.

Treatment. Treatment is **conservative** reconstruction of the metatarsal arch. This can be achieved immediately by the temporary insertion of a **dome pad** into the shoe (*see* Appendix, *Fig. 50e*). The predisposing cause must, however, be treated where possible, e.g. **weight reduction.** Physiotherapy aims at redeveloping the weakened muscles by active exercise, and electrical stimulation of the muscles is necessary to begin with in severe cases. In fracture treatment the plaster must be carefully moulded to conform with the arch in order to avoid deformity.

Morton's Metatarsalgia

This resembles metatarsalgia in the situation of the pain. The character of the pain is different. It is intermittent, acute and radiates into the adjacent sides of the 3rd and 4th, or 4th and 5th toes, and is associated with **tingling** or **'numbness'** in these areas of the toes. **Localised tenderness** exists between the heads of the metatarsals. Examination also confirms loss of sensation to light touch and pin prick in the numb areas. The cause of this condition is interference with the blood supply to the interdigital nerve between the 3rd and 4th or 4th and 5th metatarsals. Nerve degeneration occurs and a **neuroma** is formed. When the patient walks the neuroma is squeezed by the metatarsal heads so producing painful symptoms. Treatment is by **surgical excision of the neuroma.** This relieves the pain completely, but the division of the digital nerves leaves permanent numbness of these toes.

Chronic Foot Strain

This is mainly related to the longitudinal arch of the foot. This arch is maintained by the shape of the bones, the tone of the muscles and the strength of the ligaments. It is usually the 'spring' ligament at the apex of the arch which is strained. The arch may not be flat but there is an obvious tendency for it to flatten. **Fatigue** and **obesity** contribute to weakening of the muscles and straining of the ligaments. If these factors can be relieved before the foot becomes stiff the condition is correctable by means of physiotherapy to redevelop the muscles of the foot.

Plantar Fasciitis

Where chronic foot strain persists plantar fasciitis develops and the arch flattens. The plantar fascia is a thick, strong band of fibrous tissue which lies under the skin of the sole of the foot covering the short muscles. It is attached to the heel posteriorly and the deep surfaces of the skin of the toes anteriorly. When the longitudinal arch flattens the plantar fascia is stretched, producing a severe aching pain, particularly on **weight-bearing** and on **pressure.** The pain is more exaggerated nearer the heel, at the attachment of the fascia to the bone. The patient can barely tolerate his shoe and begins to **limp.** The condition is usually primary but may be seen secondary to a more generalised disease, e.g. ankylosing spondylitis.

Treatment. Treatment is by injection of **local anaesthetic** and **hydrocortisone** initially to relieve symptoms. The injection may be repeated at fortnightly intervals. A **tarsal pad** is fitted into the shoe of the affected foot. Physiotherapy is necessary to re-educate the small muscles of the foot, sometimes with additional electrical stimulation. Aggravating features such as obesity and excessive standing must be relieved in order to effect a cure.

March Fracture

This is a stress fracture commonly associated with the.second metatarsal bone although other metatarsals may be affected. It is seen where a long period of **unaccustomed weight-bearing** has occurred, e.g. new recruits in the army. There is no history of trauma. It is occasionally seen in metabolic bone disease, e.g. osteomalacia. Clinically it results in a painful **swelling of the forefoot,** producing a marked **limp.** Initially the fracture is difficult to detect radiologically, but after a fortnight, callus formation can be demonstrated.

Treatment. This is by immobilisation in a **below-knee walking plaster** until the foot is painfree in about 4–6 weeks. Thereafter a temporary **metatarsal arch support** is inserted into the shoe until physiotherapy completely restores the function of the foot.

Pes Cavus

This is a deformity of the foot in which the longitudinal arch is exaggerated. It may be **congenital** or **acquired.** In both instances there is an underlying **neurological disorder** which produces the muscular weakness responsible for the development of the deformity. In the congenital type, the pes cavus may be part of a generalised neurological disorder or it may be associated with traction on the cauda equina as in spina bifida occulta. It is usually bilateral. In the acquired type, it may be secondary to disease of the nervous system, e.g. poliomyelitis. In some cases, the cause is unknown.

Clinical Features. The fitting of suitable, comfortable shoes is difficult because of the degree of **deformity** of the feet. In addition the shoes quickly become distorted and worn out. The patient complains of pain in the toes and soles of the feet and walks with an **awkward gait.** On examination the longitudinal arch in each foot is high, there is weakness in dorsi-flexion with dropping of the forefoot and a clawing of the toes due to loss of function and contracture of the small muscles of the foot (*Fig. 20*). **Corns** and **callosities** are usually seen overlying the prominent parts of the foot, i.e. the heel, the metatarsal heads or ball of the foot, and the dorsal aspect of the clawed toes.

Treatment. In mild cases **conservative** measures suffice. Footwear must be roomy with strong soles and therefore has to be made specially for the patient. As callosities develop chiropody becomes necessary. In severe pes cavus **surgery** may be required in an effort to correct the deformities. Operation involves a **soft tissue release procedure** combined with **manipulation of the foot** in order to lessen the height of the arch and improve muscle function of the toes. A **below-knee walking plaster** is applied in which the plaster does not conform to the longitudinal arch but is constructed in the 'flat-foot' position. The purpose of this plaster is to encourage the arch to settle with weight-bearing before the muscle tendons become re-attached to their new

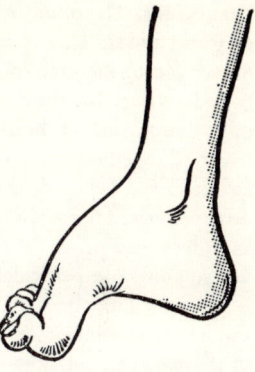

FIG. 20 Pes cavus

situation. The function of the toes may be further improved by **tendon transplantation.**

Where there is a fixed bony deformity, e.g. as seen in the **adult pes cavus,** the function of the foot may be improved simply by correction of the claw-toe deformity. The interphalangeal joints in each toe are excised and the bones fused, i.e. **Lambrinudi's arthrodesis.** Interphalangeal pins or wires are used to fix the bones internally until fusion is complete (*see Fig. 39c*). A below-knee plaster is applied with the toes and pin projections encased in a **'hood' extension.** Weight-bearing is not permitted until the pins are removed when fusion is complete in about six weeks. Physiotherapy to re-educate the foot muscles is important.

When this procedure fails to improve function adequately additional correction of the arch deformity is necessary; the operation involves a combination of **triple arthrodesis** and **fusion of some of the tarso-metatarsal joints.** Plaster immobilisation is maintained for 10–12 weeks but weight-bearing is allowed at about 3–6 weeks. It will remain important after operation for footwear to be made specially for the patient and for regular treatment to be given by the chiropodist.

Hallus Valgus

This is a deformity of the big toe in which it is deviated laterally towards the other toes. The deformity occurs at the metatarso-phalangeal joint, resulting in prominence of the metatarsal head. The second, and in severe cases, the third toe are displaced and overlap the big toe. The function of the foot is therefore impaired. Metatarsalgia of the undisplaced toes may result.

The cause may be congenital but it is usally acquired. Females are more commonly affected. Badly-designed shoes restricting free movements of the toes may be a predisposing factor. The overlying soft tissues are subject to pressure by footwear. They become indurated and thickened with the formation of a bursa between the skin and the metatarsal head. Infection of the bursa may be a complication.

Treatment. The ultimate success of any procedure is enhanced by the **wearing of good shoes.** These give sufficient length, breadth and depth to allow of free movement of the toes. In addition when the patient is obliged to stand for long periods, reasonably thick soled shoes will ease the strain on the feet. The simplest operation is that of **bunionectomy** in which the inflamed bursa (bunion) is removed together with the protuberant part of the metatarsal head. This not only facilitates the fitting of shoes but improves the appearance of the affected foot. **Arthrodesis** of the metatarso-phalangeal joint corrects the deformity, relieves pain and gives strength to the foot. The main disadvantage is that the angle of fusion will suit only one particular height of heel. Immobilisation in plaster for 6–8 weeks is necessary for sound fusion. **Arthroplasty** (Keller's) relieves pressure and pain, and leaves a mobile joint. It involves removal of the base of the proximal phalanx of the big toe, and although the toe is shorter it retains its mobility. The post-operative period is less than in arthrodesis. Weight-bearing is possible at the end of two weeks after which a short period of physiotherapy is necessary. It is contra-indicated where there is metatarsalgia and better avoided when deformity is severe.

Hallux Rigidus
In this condition there is stiffening of the big toe at the metatarso-phalangeal joint. Although the disturbance occurs at this joint, in children the predisposing cause is pressure, acute or chronic, on the tip of the great toe. In the acute form the patient has sustained a direct blow as in 'stubbing' the toe; in the chronic type the pressure is produced by hosiery and footwear of inadequate length. In the adult the joint shows osteoarthritic changes, either as part of a general osteoarthritis or following disease or injury.

As a result of the associated muscle spasm the big toe is held in a plantar flexed position. Dorsi-flexion is limited by pain and spasm or by capsular contracture. The pain and stiffness produce a limp.

Treatment. In the **child** temporary rest from sport and a change to **longer socks and shoes** relieves pressure on the big toe and allows the condition to settle. In the **adult, roomy, thick, rocker-soled shoes** may relieve milder cases. **Surgery,** where indicated, may involve only the simple removal of the exostosis on the dorso-lateral aspect of the joint. If this fails, pain can be relieved either by **Keller's arthroplasty** or, where the interphalangeal joint is mobile, by **arthrodesis** of the metatarso-phalangeal joint.

Other Deformities of the Toes
Control of the movements of the small joints of the toes arises from the balanced action of three groups of muscle tendons inserted into them. Should the function of any one of them be deficient, deformity arises. The commoner deformity is **hammer toe** in which there is undue prominence of the proximal interphalangeal joint. Direct pressure on the dorsal aspect of this joint by footwear results in a corn which often becomes infected. One or more toes may be affected. Less common is

mallet toe in which the terminal phalanx is flexed downwards. There is pressure on the tip of the toe and this is often the site of a painful corn.

Treatment of Hammer and Mallet Toe Deformities. The provision of special roomy footwear with supporting insoles as well as attention to corns by the chiropodist may be an effective method of conservative treatment, particularly in the elderly. In the younger patient, hammer toe deformity is perhaps more successfully treated by operative **fusion of the proximal interphalangeal joint.** Mallet toe is treated by surgical **fusion of the distal interphalangeal joint.** Intramedullary wires are often used to maintain satisfactory alignment until fusion is complete in 6 weeks. Where the deformities are established and the toe is completely functionless but painful, **partial amputation in mallet toe** and **total amputation in hammer toe** may be a quick and effective procedure.

If there is infection of the corns, however, operation is withheld until this has been treated successfully.

Ingrown Toenail. This occurs where the nail of the big toe grows into the skin on the dorsum of the toe. The skin breaks down and becomes infected with the development of granulation tissue. Treatment is by removal of the nail and instruction in the correct manner of cutting the big toenail (*Fig. 21*). Roomy footwear should be worn. If this fails radical excision of the nail bed prevents recurrence.

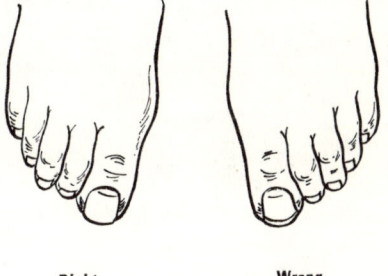

Right   Wrong

Subungual Exostosis. This is a bony outgrowth beneath the distal end of the toenail. The resultant tension produces acute, throbbing pain. Treatment is by removal of the nail allowing excision of the exostosis with complete cure.

FIG. 21   Method of cutting toenails

Onychogryposis. This is enlargement of a toenail which becomes thickened and claw-like. Although the big toenail is most often affected all toes may be involved. It is commonly seen where the hygiene of feet is poor and also in the elderly. Treatment by chiropody is necessary, as cutting of the nails becomes more difficult. In extreme cases, removal of the toenail with radical excision of the nailbed cures the condition.

PART I

SECTION III

TRAUMA

_11_ INTRODUCTION TO FRACTURES

To fracture means to break. A fractured bone is therefore a broken bone. The injury **damages** not only the **bony skeleton** but also the **surrounding soft tissues.**

Damage to the soft tissues can vary from a minor bruise to an open wound. The soft tissues support important structures such as **nerves** and **blood vessels** which are also liable to damage.

In long bones, e.g. the femur, and short long bones e.g. a phalanx, the fracture may be either in the shaft or epiphyseal area where it may extend to include a joint. In small bones the fracture is through the body of the bone and usually involves a joint, e.g. fracture of the scaphoid. In fracture of the shaft of the **long bones** the main problems are **shortening** and **deformity**, whereas in **joint fractures** the problems are **deformity** and **stiffness.**

Where possible, treatment is immediate in an effort to restore normal anatomical position, a necessity if full function is to be achieved. The principles of treatment are **good early reduction, adequate splintage** to avoid deformity and a sufficient period of **immobilisation** to allow union to occur.

Conservative management achieves and maintains good reduction in the majority of fractures. Where this is not possible **open reduction and internal fixation** is carried out. Whether the treatment be conservative or operative, after the patient leaves theatre, the early ward management during the first three weeks is vital to the patient and to the success of the particular procedure. It is during this period that the nursing principles matter most. Ischaemia, nerve palsy, pressure sores, wound infection and deformity are complications which develop rapidly, but these can be anticipated and so avoided. Once they exist, new and perhaps more difficult problems of management are created. Lack of knowledge in the use of appliances and plaster casts and in the relevant nursing care of the patient can produce any or all of these complications. Good liaison between all medical and nursing staff will contribute greatly to the well-being of the patient and the standard of treatment.

Causes of Fractures

1 Trauma. _Direct Violence:_ The **point of application** of the force is usually the **point of fracture,** e.g. a blow on the shin fracturing the tibia. The soft tissues are damaged from without by the blow causing the fracture.

Indirect Violence: The **point of application** of the force is **remote from the point of fracture,** e.g. a fall on the outstretched hand may produce a fracture of both bones of the forearm or a fracture of the humerus. The damage to the soft tissues is caused by the broken bone ends rather than by the external force.

2 Stress. A fracture of the neck of the 2nd or 3rd metatarsal, referred to as a march fracture, is an example of where persistent strain from an excessive force results in a fatigue fracture of a bone at a weak point. This particular fracture was seen classically among recruits training in the Army, hence the term 'march fracture'.

3 Pathological. A disease process weakens the bone and fracture will occur even without any abnormal stresses or strains being applied to it, e.g. a pathological fracture of a vertebral body due to a bone metastasis.

Classification of Fractures

A **simple** or **closed** fracture is one in which the bone is broken; there is some degree of soft tissue damage but the skin is intact. There is no communication between the fracture and the exterior.

A **compound** or **open** fracture is one in which the bone is broken; the overlying soft tissues and skin are torn allowing direct communication between the fracture and the exterior.

Types of Fracture

The different types of incomplete and complete fracture are illustrated in Figure 22.

Stability of Fractures

A fracture may be classified as **stable** or **unstable.** In a stable fracture either the bone ends are undisplaced and reduction is unnecessary or, despite initial displacement, the bone ends are easily maintained in position after reduction. In an unstable fracture the bone ends are displaced and there is a tendency after reduction to redisplacement, unless some method is used to maintain their position.

Clinical Features

Where the fracture has been caused by trauma there will be a **history** of **direct** or **indirect violence.** In stress fractures the patient can relate his injury to some repeated or continued stress or strain. If the cause is pathological the patient may not have had any preliminary symptoms or signs e.g. osteoporosis. Some patients may have suffered minor trauma; others may have experienced pain or discomfort in the bone particularly at night-time. Sometimes the patient gives a history of several months general debility and complains of lack of appetite and loss of weight. These, together with the patient's present symptoms and signs of fracture may suggest the presence of a neoplastic lesion e.g. a chest, breast, genito-urinary or other primary tumour. **Pain** may be throbbing in character and localised to the site of injury. It is aggravated by any attempt at active or passive movement. **Loss of function** results because of pain and the instability of the broken bone. A patient with a fracture of the tibia for example, would be unable to stand on that leg as it would collapse under him. **Swelling** due to oedema and the effusion of blood, haematoma, will vary according to the extent of the soft tissue damage. **Deformity** occurs in two ways. There is an **angular** deformity of the limb produced by the displacement of the bones; **shortening** of the limb occurs due to overriding of the bone ends, except in an impacted fracture.

INCOMPLETE

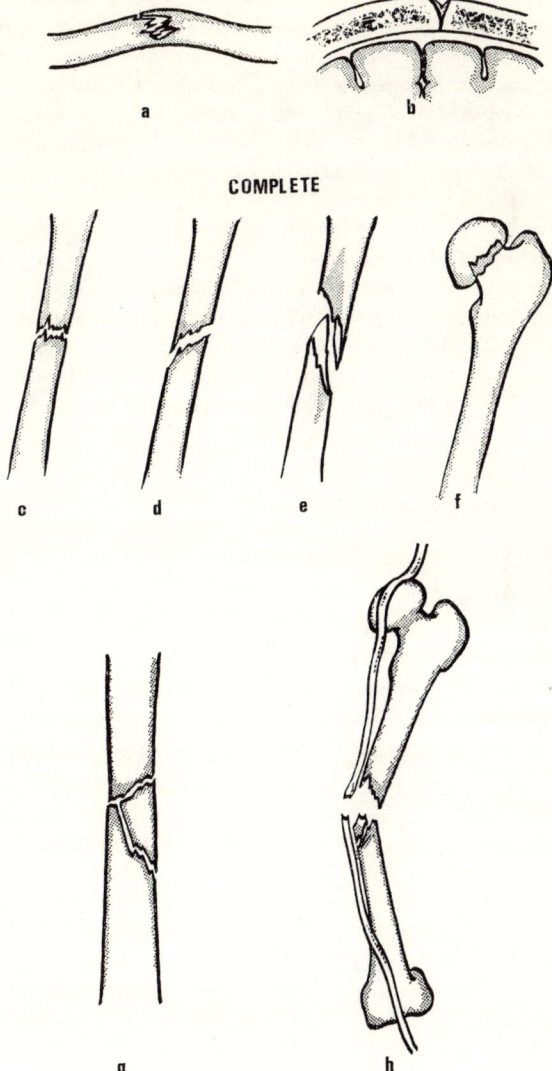

COMPLETE

FIG. 22 Types of fracture

Incomplete: (*a*) Greenstick; (*b*) Fissure

Complete: (*c*) Transverse; (*d*) Oblique; (*e*) Spiral; (*f*) Impacted;
(*g*) Comminuted; (*h*) Complicated

Unnatural mobility of the limb can be demonstrated under an anaesthetic. The distal fragment can be put through an unnatural range of movements at a site other than a joint, again with the exception of the impacted fracture. **Tenderness** of both the soft tissues and the bone can be elicited at the level of the fracture. Where the bone is more superficial the tenderness will be more clearly localised to the line of fracture. **Crepitus** is the grating sensation heard and felt when the broken surfaces of the bones are allowed to rub against each other. This feature should not be produced deliberately as it is painful to the patient. Where the bones are fixed, as in an impacted fracture, crepitus is absent.

Investigations

X-ray examination confirms the diagnosis. Two views at least are taken at right angles to each other, as the fracture may be masked in one view where there is overlap of the bone ends. These are referred to as **antero-posterior** and **lateral** X-ray views. When a long bone is being examined the joint above and below is included in the X-ray, and where small bones are involved the whole region is examined, e.g. in the wrist or foot. Oblique or strain views are special X-rays used in an attempt to reveal an obscure fracture.

Treatment of a Patient with a Fracture

There are five main aims (the five R's):

1 **Resuscitation** of the patient
2 **Reduction** of the fracture
3 **Restriction** of movement, i.e. immobilisation
4 **Restoration** or maintenance of function
5 **Rehabilitation** (*see* Chapters 27 and 29)

Resuscitation. Where a patient has sustained an injury, whether minor or major, he is liable to suffer from **shock.** This is a term used to explain the body's reaction to many different circumstances; in this chapter it is specifically related to the response to **blood loss** and to **pain** resulting from injuries producing fractures and associated soft tissue damage. A similar clinical picture may be seen although usually to a lesser degree, following orthopaedic surgery.

Symptoms and signs of shock. The patient is **anxious** and often **distressed.** He looks **pale** or **ashen,** his **skin** is **cold** and usually **moist** with perspiration, i.e. 'a cold sweat'. The **features** are **pinched,** the **eyes sunken** and the tip of the nose appears prominent. The **pulse** is **rapid and feeble,** the **temperature** is **subnormal** and **breathing** is **shallow** at first. If the patient is losing fluid from the body, **thirst** and **oliguria** become additional features. Either the patient remains **semi-conscious** (faints) or lapses into **unconsciousness** when breathing becomes deeper and more irregular.

In the large majority of minor casualties the degree of shock is minimal and the question of resuscitation only occasionally arises. It is important in each case to make a quick assessment to establish whether or not a serious state of shock is present by:

1 The general appearance of the patient
2 The patient's pulse and respiration rates and the blood pressure level
3 The degree of swelling of the limb in a simple fracture
4 The assessment of the blood loss in a compound fracture
5 The appreciation of the patient's excessive pain

Shock can be relieved or limited by early simple resuscitative means. **Careful handling** of the injured part is important. Relief of pain may be achieved by **temporary immobilisation** where feasible, e.g. in a splint. The patient should be kept **warm** in an effort to maintain the body temperature. Overheating should, nevertheless, be avoided as it dilates the blood vessels and causes further oedema or bleeding. Where the pain is severe **analgesia** is required. If the blood pressure is low and the pulse weak preparations must be made for **temporary circulatory fluid replacement therapy**, e.g. Macrodex. When the blood loss is significant replacement **blood transfusion** is necessary before any operative treatment can be carried out.

Reduction of the Fracture. A fracture of a bone, e.g. in a skeleton, would not present any problem. It is because of the interpretation of the pain stimulus that the muscles contract causing distortion or displacement of the bone ends. **Reduction is the method by which these displaced bone fragments are brought back into their anatomical position.** This involves overcoming the muscle contraction, or as it is often referred to, 'protective muscle spasm'. Reduction of a fracture is usually better achieved if the patient is given a general anaesthetic but in some instances of minor fracture, or where a patient is generally unfit, local anaesthesia may suffice. Complete reduction has four main requirements:

1 **Good apposition** which means there must not be anything between the bone ends
2 **Good alignment** which means that there is no angulation at the site of reduction
3 **Full length of the limb**
4 **Normal rotation**

If in a lower limb a fracture were to be reduced and allowed to heal with good apposition but bad alignment there would be a weakness through which the body weight would be directed when the patient stood on the limb, and refracture would possibly occur (*Fig. 23a*). Good alignment with poor apposition does not create quite the same problem. If even only one-third of the diameter of the distal fragment of the broken bone is in apposition with its proximal fragment, bony union can still take place. The remodelling process takes care of the deformity (*Fig. 23b*). If, however, good apposition can be achieved it will ensure full limb length (*Fig. 23c*). Where a fracture is unstable and there is a tendency for the bone ends to displace, the muscle spasm causes them to overlap and shortening occurs which of course is undesirable (*Fig. 23d*).

To avoid rotational deformity the limb is placed in its normal anatomical position, e.g. in reduction of a fracture of the tibia the patella and the toes must point forwards in the same direction and in the same straight line. This type of deformity is not clearly seen on X-ray but is more obvious on clinical inspection of the limb.

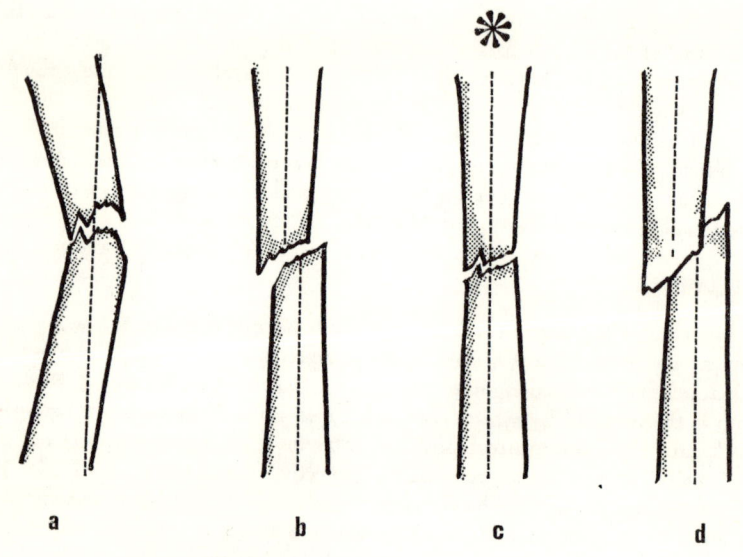

FIG. 23   Reduction of fractures
   (*a*) Bad alignment
   (*b*) Good alignment with poor apposition
   (*c*) *Good reduction in alignment and apposition
   (*d*) Displacement of fragments with shortening of limb

Restriction of Movement or Immobilisation. This is the method by which a fracture, after its reduction, is maintained in position until bony union takes place. The method used depends on the site and type of the fracture. It may involve the application of splints or traction, plaster of Paris or the use of internal fixation. Good immobilisation necessitates the effective control of movement by incorporating the joint above and below the injury in the splint or plaster. Adequate maintenance of splintage is essential until healing is complete.

Restoration or Maintenance of Function. During the course of immobilisation of a fracture there is a tendency for other muscles in the body to weaken and uninvolved joints to stiffen. In a fracture of the wrist, for example, which is usually immobilised in a plaster cast, there is a tendency for the shoulder joint and the finger joints to stiffen. It is imperative during the course of treatment of any fracture to maintain the function of all joints with the exception of those directly involved in the immobilisation. This can be done by the physiotherapist or, if the patient is given adequate instruction, he will be able to practise the exercises in his own time. Exercises of the muscles and joints closely related to the fracture are commenced whenever possible. Such exercises are gentle at first and are graduated so that the limb returns to full functional mobility.

Healing of Fractures (*Fig. 24*)

In a fracture the bleeding from the bone ends is produced by the ruptured branches of the nutrient artery carrying blood to the bone. There is also bleeding from the vascular layer of the damaged periosteum and from the torn muscle attachments to the bone. Further bleeding may occur from other sources if there is extensive soft tissue damage.

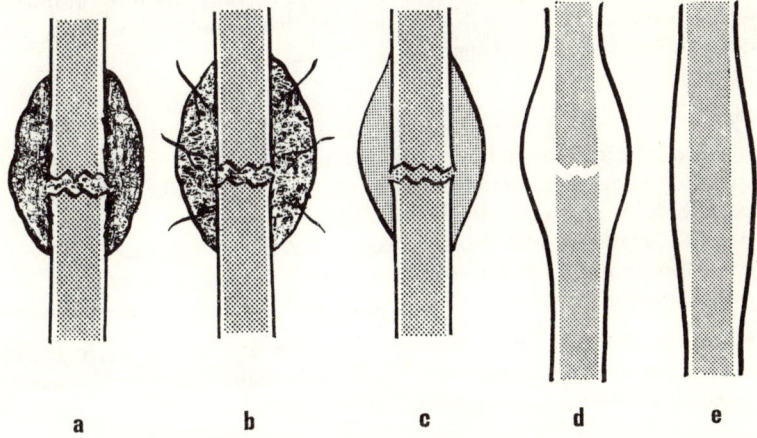

| a | b | c | d | e |

FIG. 24 Healing of a fracture
     (*a*) Blood clot formation at fracture site
     (*b*) Growth of blood vessels in fibrinous framework
     (*c*) Osteoid tissue formation
     (*d*) Ossification
     (*e*) Remodelling and recanalisation of the bone

The clotting mechanism of the blood causes the **formation of a clot** between and around the bone ends which organises into a loose fibrinous framework (*Fig. 24a*). Blood vessels grow into this clot thus providing an adequate blood supply (*Fig. 24b*). **Calcium** from the bone ends is **deposited** in the fibrinous clot forming osteoid tissue resembling bone, but soft, opaque and pliable (*Fig. 24c*). Bone cells (osteocytes), mainly **osteoblasts,** the bone builders, are active in this framework and so **ossification** takes place. The process continues until the gap between the bone ends is full of new bone. This **'callus formation'** can be seen clearly on

X-ray and also palpated on clinical examination indicating that bony union of the fracture is taking place (*Fig. 24d*).

The **altered shape** of the bone as a result of the 'callus' mass is **remodelled** by the removal of unnecessary material, a process brought about by the function of the **osteoclasts,** the bone destroyers. They also **recanalise the medullary canal** so completing the programme of reconstruction (*Fig. 24e*). This may take 6–9 months in a child and 12–18 months in an adult, although the patient can walk on the affected leg before the process is altogether complete. After the appropriate period of immobilisation for the particular fracture, clinical and X-ray examination out of splintage is important. A plaster is bivalved and the limb is cradled in the posterior half; traction apparatus is dismantled and the limb rests freely in the splint. As the doctor lifts the patient's limb, the nurse removes the remaining plaster or splint, inserting a pillow on to which the limb is gently placed. The doctor then tests it for clinical union. **Freedom from local tenderness on palpation** and **stability on the application of stress suggest that union is complete.** X-ray examination out of splintage **confirms that sound callus exists.** The fracture is then judged to be united.

Complications of Fractures

Infection. Where a wound exists there is always a risk of infection. This is particularly so in a **compound fracture** where there is often some damaged or devitalised tissue as a result of the injury. Where the wound is surgical as in the **operative treatment** of a simple fracture this risk, although greatly reduced, nevertheless remains. The danger in both these cases is that the infection may spread beyond the soft tissues and infect the underlying bone, i.e. **osteomyelitis.**

Mal-union. This means union of a fracture in the wrong position. It may be due to an **unsuccessful reduction,** to **inadequate immobilisation** or to the tendency to deformity inherent in an **unstable fracture.**

Delayed union. Although union occurs it is delayed beyond the average period for that particular fracture. This may be due to a relatively **poor blood supply** to one of the fragments, e.g. in fracture of the lower end of tibia, or to **interference with the formation of callus,** e.g. by repeated manipulative reductions in unstable fractures, by distraction or by inadequate immobilisation.

Non-union. There are various reasons why a fracture may fail to unite. Those which lead to delayed union if exaggerated will produce non-union. Sometimes **soft tissue** gets **interposed between the bone ends,** e.g. a flap of periosteum, a piece of muscle or tendon. In the presence of **infection,** unhealthy granulation tissue may form between the bone ends which eventually leads to the formation of an avascular fibrous tissue (scar tissue) and local bone necrosis. The normal healing of a fracture, which depends on an adequate blood supply to the bone ends, cannot therefore take place. Where non-union of a fracture occurs, a **bone graft** is usually necessary to stimulate new bone formation to fill the gap.

Fat Embolism. This is a plug composed of fatty matter which occludes a blood vessel. The actual cause is unknown although there are two common theories: the source of the fat deposits may be from the bone marrow at the site of fracture or from some alteration in the physical state of the fat in the blood. The manifestations of this obscure disease and its effects vary from minor to major degree. The degree appears to depend on the size of the embolus or emboli, the location of the blood vessel or vessels involved and the importance of the territory supplied by these vessels, e.g. skin, lung, kidney or brain.

The condition is usually recognised by the appearance of **petechial** (freckle-like) **haemorrhages** particularly in the loose folds of the **skin** in the axilla, neck and conjunctiva. If the condition is more severe the whole of the upper trunk may be covered in these petechiae. The rash usually appears within the first 72 hours of fracture, and in many cases is limited to skin alone. It rapidly fades within 24–36 hours. Where other important regions are affected, e.g. **brain, lung** or **kidney,** the patient may show dramatic changes in his general condition with or without signs of haemorrhages in the skin, e.g. cerebral irritability or loss of consciousness, pneumonic symptoms and signs such as breathlessness, or renal failure where the kidneys are involved.

The diagnosis is established by recognising petechial haemorrhages in the retina by means of an ophthalmoscope and by finding fat deposits in the sputum or urine on pathological examination. **Chest X-ray** may show the characteristic 'snow storm' appearance in positive cases. E.C.G. changes may be evident. The **blood platelet count** is **diminished. Blood gases** are **monitored** since successful therapy depends on their measurement. The administration of a **high concentration of oxygen** is required if hypoxia has to be reversed and mechanical ventilation will often be necessary. In severe cases 100 per cent oxygen may be used together with intermittent positive pressure respiration. If the patient's condition is serious, intravenous **hydrocortisone** may be given to combat inflammatory oedema in the lungs. Some success has been achieved in the treatment of fat embolism by the use of low molecular Dextran and Trasylol in certain cases. Antiobiotic therapy is necessary where there is lung involvement. Renal dialysis may be required in cases of renal failure.

Damage to Other Important Structures. In complicated fractures there will be involvement of other structures such as **nerves** or **blood vessels** and the resultant palsy or ischaemia may present many problems in management.

Complications of Immobilisation. These include **chest** and **urinary** infection, **stiffness of joints,** circulatory disturbances, e.g. **deep venous thrombosis,** and the development of **bed sores.**

12 METHODS OF IMMOBILISATION OF FRACTURES

TRACTION

Traction is used in orthopaedic practice to exert a force, either a direct or indirect pull to a particular part of the skeleton. It may be used in the **reduction of fractures, fracture dislocations** or in the **conservative treatment of other conditions,** e.g. prolapsed intervertebral disc. It is, however, most frequently utilised in the treatment of **fractures of the shaft of the femur.** The pull is exerted on the distal fragment. The traction force necessary for the fracture reduction is that which equalises the pull of the muscles in the opposite direction. Where the fracture is successfully reduced by manual traction and is stable, all that is required is a mechanical substitute which will maintain this reduction until union occurs. This is called **fixed traction.** Where the fracture is unstable, even after manual reduction, and the bone ends tend to displace producing shortening of the limb, a mechanical system is necessary which can be adjusted readily and which exerts a sufficient continuous pull on the distal fragment in order to obtain a satisfactory reduction. This is called **sliding, balanced or continuous traction.** It is usually a temporary measure; once reaction has settled, reduction has been achieved satisfactorily and the fracture appears stable a maintenance traction i.e. fixed traction is substituted.

Simple Traction Mechanics

Fixed Traction. In fixed traction (*Fig. 25*) the forces act within **one unit.** This unit consists of the splint, the leg and the extension mechanism, either skin strapping or a skeletal pin. **Anything outside this unit has no part in its mechanical function,** e.g. suspension of the splint, elevation of the bed, etc. The splint must be of the **correct size in ring circumference and length.** The fracture is reduced by manual traction which is maintained until its replacement by mechanical traction is complete. The Thomas's splint with supporting slings is slipped carefully on to the limb, and the ring is held firmly in position in the groin providing the first of the **two fixed points.** The fixing of the second point is the replacement of the manual traction by the tension on the extension cords from either the skin or skeletal appliance, as they are tied to the U-piece of the splint.

Sliding Traction. Sliding traction (*Fig. 26*) is a means of applying a pull on one fragment of a fracture against a counter force in the opposite direction. It is based on the principles of balance and there are **no fixed points.** It is easily understood if one is aware of the forces involved.

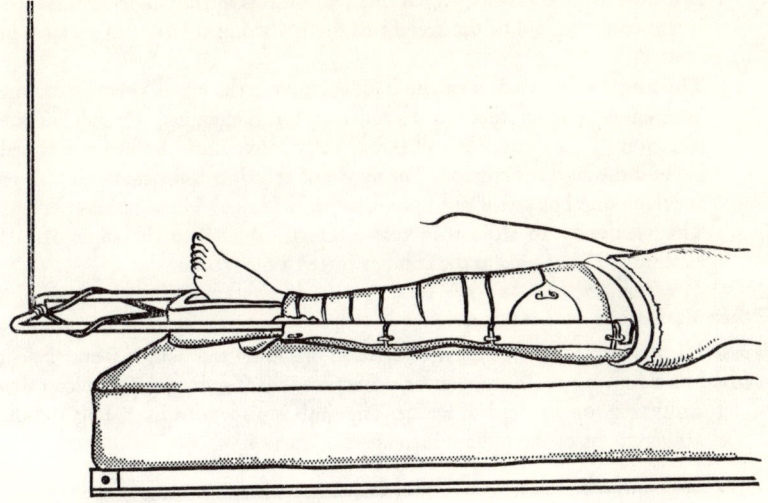

FIG. 25   Fixed traction

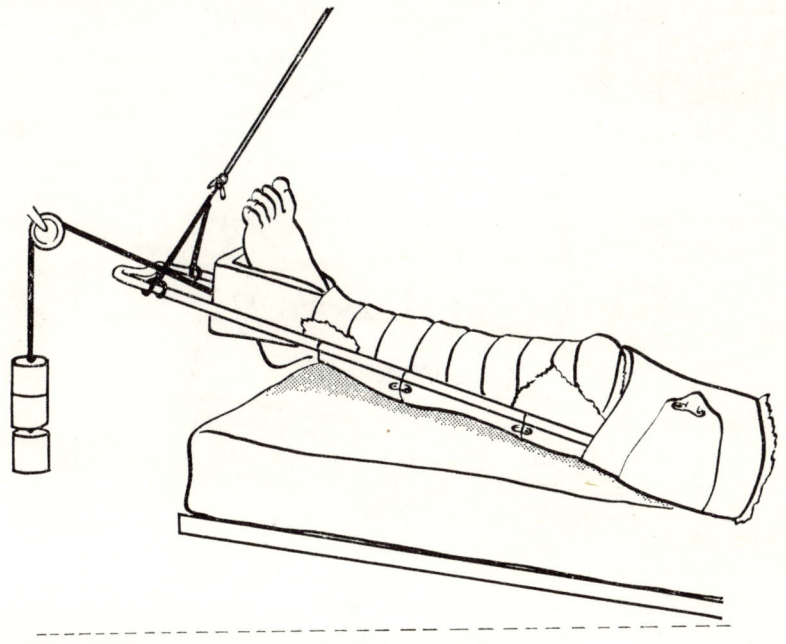

FIG. 26   Sliding traction

1 **Friction** is the resistance which one body meets in moving over another. It is directly related to the weight of the body and the type of surfaces in contact.

2 **The angle of elevation of the bed.** As soon as the bed is altered from the horizontal position there is a tendency for the patient to slide in the direction of the slope. He will not actually move until the bed is elevated beyond the angle of friction. The **angle of friction** is the maximum slope at which one body will rest upon another without sliding down.

3 **The tendency to slide** is therefore directly related to the angle of bed elevation. This is used as the counter force to the traction.

Other Variations of Traction

Russell Traction (*Fig. 27*). This is a variation of sliding traction. It is an efficient method of achieving more traction on a fracture where reduction is difficult due to deformity, e.g. upper third of femur. The limb is suspended by a sling and the special arrangement of the pulleys increases the traction.

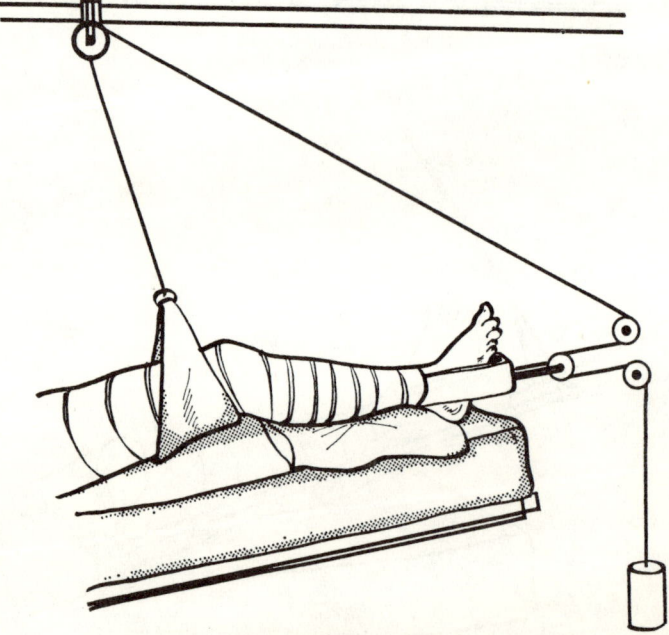

FIG. 27 Russell traction

Gallows Traction. Gallows traction (*Fig. 28*) is a useful form of weight traction used in smaller children with fractures of the femur. It utilises gravity as its basic mechanism of function. Skin traction is applied to both limbs and the extension cords are led over pulleys on a frame to weights so that the legs are suspended at right angles to the body. The weights are the traction force and the weight of the body and limbs are the counter traction force. It is important that the **child's buttocks are clear of the bed** (usually sufficient to allow a hand to slip between

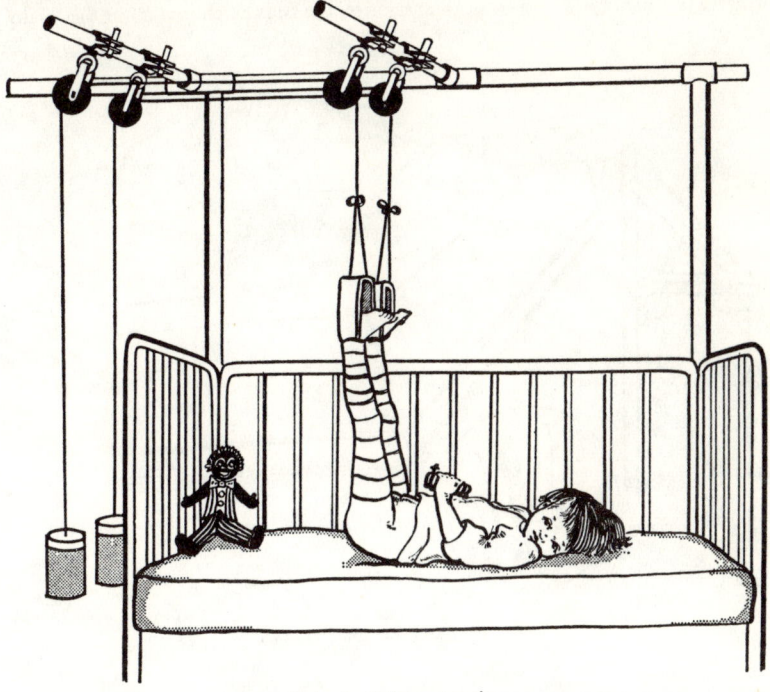

FIG. 28 Gallows traction

the buttocks and the bed) otherwise the counter-traction or gravitational force is absent. The **circulation of both limbs** must be carefully checked as **ischaemia** is a complication due to arterial spasm.

Skull Traction (cervical traction). Skull calipers are introduced into the thick part of the skull about 2 inches (5 cm) above and in line with the external auditory meatus. An extension cord is attached to the caliper, led over a pulley at the head of the bed and weights are suspended (*Fig. 29*). The head of the bed is raised. The mechanical principle is similar to that of sliding traction. This type of traction is used in **the reduction of cervical dislocation.** Alternatively, sometimes preferably in order to prevent chest complications, this traction is assembled with the patient in the sitting position supported by a back-rest and pillows. The pull must be exerted in the same axis as the cervical spine. An extension piece to the head of the bed will be necessary to which is attached a pulley over which the extension cord passes to be attached to the weights. The bed remains level if this method is used.

'Halo Traction'. This is a type of fixed traction used to maintain the position of reduced fractures or dislocations in both **cranio-facial and cervical spine injuries** (*see Fig. 33*). In cervical spine fixation the rods extending from the 'Halo'

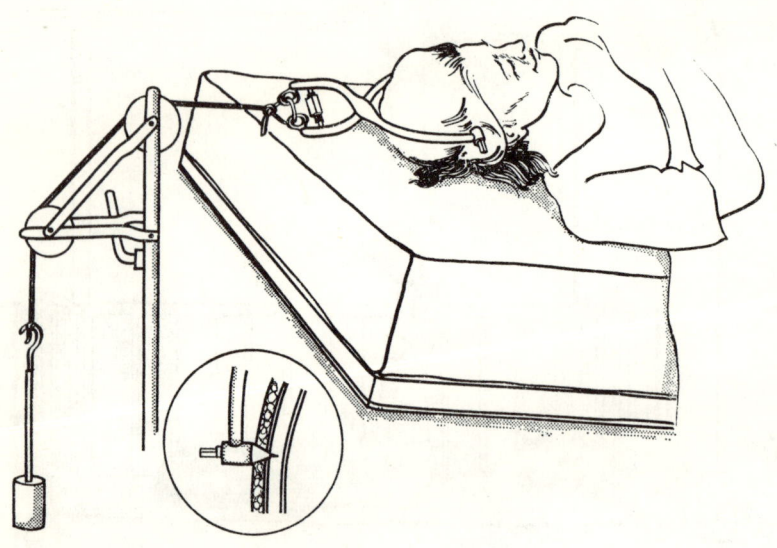

FIG. 29   Skull traction (cervical)

frame are fixed into either a body frame or into a plaster jacket in order to produce stability. This method of traction allows patients with such injuries to become ambulant earlier in their period of treatment.

PLASTER OF PARIS

Plaster of Paris is made from gypsum or calcium sulphate. The calcium sulphate crystals have been heated and dehydrated into an anhydrous state. This powder is incorporated in a firm muslin bandage (produced in varying widths, e.g. 3 in., 4 in., 6 in. and 8 in. (7.5 cm, 10 cm, 15 cm and 20 cm). When the bandages are immersed in tepid water the chemical process whereby the crystals take up moisture produces heat as the plaster sets or hardens. The higher the temperature of the water, the quicker the plaster sets. **This is the commonest type of conservative and post-operative immobilisation used in any orthopaedic and accident unit.**

INTERNAL FIXATION

This is the procedure used in the operative treatment of fractures. **Where a**

fracture is irreducible by any other means, and in particular where a joint is involved, operative reduction and fixation is necessary, e.g. in fracture of the capitellum in the elbow joint. In **potentially unstable fractures** where conservative treatment is usually unsuccessful, stabilisation by internal fixation is indicated, e.g. in a trimalleolar fracture in the ankle joint. Where the nature of the fracture is such that **other important structures are liable to damage,** e.g. in an unstable fracture of the femur, internal fixation may have to be used in preference to conservative management. In the **management of multiple fractures,** those more effectively treated by internal fixation are thus stabilised in order to facilitate the treatment of others more suited to conservative management. Often, as a result, the problem of nursing the patient successfully is eased considerably. In the elderly where early mobilisation is essential, it is often more practicable to stabilise the fracture by internal fixation so that early weight-bearing is possible.

Methods of Internal Fixation
Four common methods of internal fixation are shown in Figure 30.

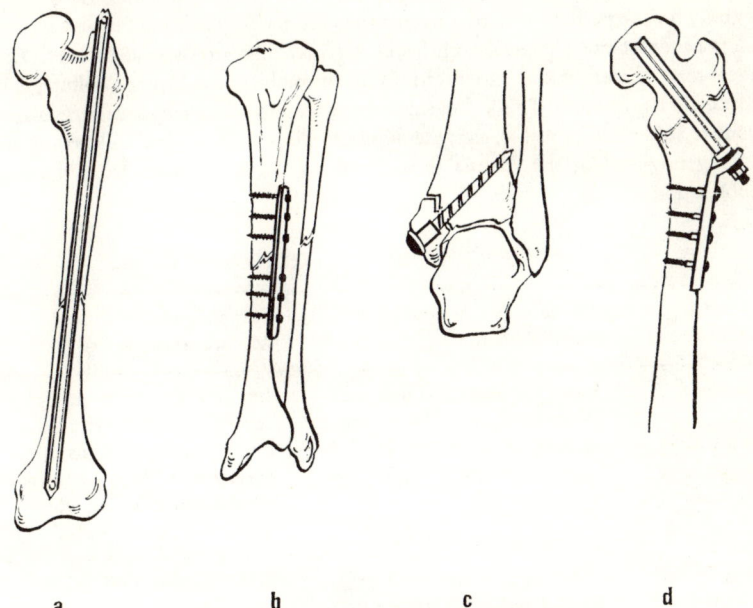

a   b   c   d

FIG. 30   Methods of internal fixation (common types)
      (*a*) Intramedullary nail (Küntscher)
      (*b*) Bone plate
      (*c*) Screw
      (*d*) Nail and plate

13 COMMON FRACTURES AND THEIR MANAGEMENT

The following tables show the more common fractures and indicate any characteristic deformity. They outline the usual method of treatment, the average length of immobilisation and the special points in nursing management. The tables will serve only as a reference guide to the nurse in the management of individual fractures. Obviously there are many variations in treatment and these can be found in any complete textbook on the management of fractures.

Upper Limb Fractures

To immobilise a fracture adequately, the joints above and below it require to be included in the splintage. Full mobility in the joints of the upper limb is essential, not only for the performance of movements necessary for one's job but also for the maintenance of one's general well-being, e.g., feeding, dressing and toilet. The nurse may therefore see modifications of immobilisation where splintage is reduced to a minimum. This is done in order to retain mobility in joints particularly prone to stiffness with disuse, e.g., the shoulder, elbow and fingers. Unless they are directly involved in the trauma these joints are often excluded from the immobilisation.

UPPER LIMB FRACTURES

Fracture	Treatment and Method of Immobilisation	Special Points in Nursing Management
Clavicle (Deformity: drooping of shoulder)	Shoulders braced to stabilise the fracture either by 3 sling method or figure of 8 bandage. Inside collar/cuff sling for 2–3 weeks.	Important to keep slings tight enough to correct the deformity. Watch for signs of **pressure** on blood vessels and nerves, and in axilla, where slings may be too tight.
Neck of Humerus	*Stable:* Inside collar/cuff sling for 2–3 weeks. Outside collar/cuff sling until painfree.	Early shoulder and finger exercises.
	Unstable: 1 Manipulation. Axillary pad and inside collar/cuff sling for 3 weeks in the elderly.	Care of elderly. **Beware of stiff shoulder.** Early shoulder and finger exercises.

UPPER LIMB FRACTURES—continued

Fracture	Treatment and Method of Immobilisation	Special Points in Nursing Management
Neck of Humerus —cont.	2 Manipulation. Shoulder spica for 4 weeks in adolescent.	Plaster care. Watch for **pressure in axilla.** Bi-valve arm piece of plaster at 3 weeks. Shoulder and finger exercises.
	3 Internal fixation if fracture is irreducible. Axillary pad and inside collar/cuff sling.	Wound sutures removed at 10 days.
Shaft of Humerus	After reduction, arm is splinted to chest wall, with intervening pad. Outer plaster shell bandaged to arm. Collar/cuff sling and body bandage. Immobilisation for 6–8 weeks.	Observe circulation and peripheral nerve function. (**Radial nerve palsy.**) Finger exercises.
Supracondylar Fracture of Humerus ('Swan-neck' deformity of elbow)	*Stable:* *Undisplaced:* Inside collar/cuff sling for 3 weeks (outpatient). *Displaced:* Reduction. Inside collar/cuff sling for 3 weeks.	Common in children. Watch circulation (**Volkmann's ischaemia**). Check tension of sling. Tendency to displacement 1–4 days.
	Unstable: Manipulation. Collar/cuff sling and posterior plaster shell for 2 weeks.	Bed rest and elevation of elbow in plaster splintage. Check for circulation and displacement as above.
Medial Epicondyle of Humerus	*Undisplaced:* Inside collar/cuff sling until painfree.	Finger exercises.
	Displaced: Often associated with torn medial ligament and dislocation of elbow. Open reduction. Internal (screw) fixation. Ligament repaired. Long arm plaster for 3–4 weeks.	Plaster care. Removal of sutures 7–10 days. Finger exercises. Encourage gentle, active use of elbow after removal of plaster to restore function.
Head of Radius	*Marginal:* Inside collar/cuff sling for 2 weeks.	Shoulder and finger exercises. **Restrict early elbow exercise to avoid stiffness later.**

UPPER LIMB FRACTURES—continued

Fracture	Treatment and Method of Immobilisation	Special Points in Nursing Management
Head of Radius —*cont.*	*Depressed or Comminuted:* Excision. Inside collar/cuff sling. May also be associated with fracture of ulna, dislocation of elbow, or dislocation of inferior radio-ulnar joint.	Sutures out by 10th day. Shoulder and finger exercises. Restrict early elbow exercise.
Olecranon	*Stable:* Long arm plaster for 6 weeks.	Finger and shoulder exercises. Restrict early elbow exercise. Care of limb in plaster.
	Unstable: Internal screw fixation. Plaster for 4–6 weeks. May be associated with fracture or dislocation of head of radius.	Care of limb in plaster. Finger and shoulder exercises. Restrict early elbow exercise. Removal of sutures at 10th day.
Radius and Ulna (both bones of forearm)	*Stable:* Long arm plaster for 8–10 weeks.	Finger and shoulder exercises. Observe circulation. (**Volkmann's ischaemia.**)
	Unstable: Internal fixation of both bones (bone plate and screws). Long arm plaster for 8–10 weeks.	Care of limb in plaster. Elevation of limb for first 24–48 hours. Removal of sutures, 7–10 days.
Colles' Fracture (Lower end of radius and ulna. 'Dinner-fork' deformity)	*Stable:* Colles' forearm plaster for 4 weeks. *Unstable:* Manipulation. Dorso-radial plaster slab for 12–48 hours. Complete plaster and retain for 4–6 weeks.	**Check circulation and plaster initially for pressure on thumb and ante-cubital fossa.** 'Grip' should not compress hand. Finger and shoulder exercises.
Scaphoid	Scaphoid forearm plaster for at least 6–8 weeks.	Care of limb in plaster. Watch for pressure in the antecubital fossa. Change to close-fitting plaster after swelling subsides. Observe **circulation** carefully, particularly in the **thumb.**

Fractures of the Lower Limb

The lower limbs **support body weight.** It is most important in these fractures or in fracture dislocation to **restore** the **correct anatomical position of the bones and joints** to conserve their weight-bearing function. **Reduction with good alignment and full leg length is most important if deformity, shortening and loss of function are to be avoided** Deformity can result in faulty union, and on full weight-bearing refracture may occur. Mal-alignment of joints causes mechanical stress and predisposes to osteoarthritis. The initial management during the first 2–3 weeks, involving frequent clinical assessments, careful observation of splintage and plaster casts together with radiological examination, is vital to the success of the fracture union. The principles of complete fracture immobilisation are more closely observed than in the case of the upper limb with the exception of femoral fractures. Although a hip spica seems the obvious method of immobilising the joint above and below a femoral fracture it does not successfully control the position of the bone fragments. The Thomas's splint and traction method allows for more precise control of this fracture although the hip joint is mobile. In all fractures of the lower limb, whenever instability is a significant problem, there is an indication for internal fixation in order to prevent malunion.

It is important in fracture treatment to **nurse the patient on a firm bed with fracture boards under the mattress** as there is a tendency for joints (particularly the hip joint) to sag under the weight of splintage.

FRACTURES OF THE LOWER LIMB

Fracture	Treatment and Method of Immobilisation	Special Points in Nursing Management
Neck of Femur (Deformity: swollen hip and thigh. Shortening of limb. Foot externally rotated)	Internal fixation by nail and plate, or sometimes by low angled Smith Petersen nail in transcervical fractures.	Care of elderly patient. Suction drain for 48 hours. **Up to sit early** (1st or 2nd day). Removal of sutures 10–14 days. Early weight-bearing with walking aid at 2 weeks if painfree. Watch for signs of **deep venous thrombosis.**
	Unstable sub-capital fractures: Replacement arthroplasty with sliding traction until painfree.	**Anterior wound; avoid external rotation. Posterior wound; avoid internal rotation.** Suction drain for 48 hours. Care of elderly. Up to sit once pain and wound reaction settled. Removal of sutures at 14 days. Walking aid and weight-bearing 2–3 weeks.

FRACTURES OF THE LOWER LIMB—continued

Fracture	Treatment and Method of Immobilisation	Special Points in Nursing Management
Upper Third Shaft of Femur	*Stable:* Sliding traction (Russell) for 10–16 weeks.	Patient is propped up a little to relax pull on proximal fragment. Care of limb in traction.
	Unstable: Transverse. Internal fixation. Intramedullary nail. Bed rest. No traction. Limb rests on splint or is cradled between sandbags. After 6 weeks, progressive mobilisation until weight-bearing.	Suction drain for 48 hours. Removal of sutures, 12–14 days. Care of skin. Active exercises of toes, foot and ankle. Passive movement of patella.
	Unstable: Comminuted. Böhler Braun splint and sliding traction until stable at 3–6 weeks. Thereafter Thomas's splint and fixed traction until 12–16 weeks.	**Watch for pressure from splint on perineum.** Patient propped up a little to relax pull on proximal fragment. Care of limb in traction.
Middle Third Shaft of Femur	*Stable:* Fixed traction. *Unstable but reducible:* Sliding traction for 3–4 weeks until stable, then fixed traction for 8–12 weeks until united.	Management of patient in traction. Passive movements of patella. Knee flexion piece at 6 weeks.
	Unstable and irreducible: Internal fixation. Intramedullary nail or bone plate and screws.	Suction drain for 48 hours. Wound sutures removed, 12–14 days. Active toe, foot and ankle exercises. Passive movements of patella. Progressive knee flexion exercises once sutures removed.
Lower Third Shaft of Femur (supracondylar)	*Stable:* Fixed traction. Thomas's splint with knee flexion piece or Böhler-Braun splint.	Care of limb in traction. **Special check for signs of developing drop-foot.** Passive movements of patella. Progressive knee extension exercises.

FRACTURES OF THE LOWER LIMB—continued

Fracture	Treatment and Method of Immobilisation	Special Points in Nursing Management
Lower Third Shaft of Femur (supracondylar) —cont.	*Unstable:* Sliding traction for 3–6 weeks. Fixed traction up to 12–16 weeks. or	Care of limb in traction. **Special check for signs of developing drop-foot.** Passive movements of patella. Progressive knee exercises. **Cautious ankle movements** (plantar-flexion), to avoid calf muscle pull on distal fragment.
	Internal fixation. Supracondylar nail plate.	Suction drain for 48 hours. Wound sutures removed, 12–14 days. Active toe, foot and ankle exercises. Passive movements of patella. Graduated knee exercises.
Lower Femoral Condyles	Adequate reduction. *Immobilisation:* 1 Long leg plaster or Thomas's splint and fixed traction for 6–8 weeks.	Care of limb in plaster or traction. Weight-bearing plaster at 6 weeks. Knee mobilising exercises on removal of plaster or splint.
	2 Internal fixation and either plaster or splint immobilisation.	Wound sutures removed, 7–10 days. Graduated knee exercises after 2–3 weeks.
Patella: 1 Indirect injury 2 Direct injury: Stellate or comminuted fracture	*Young:* Internal (screw) fixation. Long leg plaster cylinder for 2–4 weeks. *Elderly:* Patellectomy. Long leg plaster cylinder for 2 weeks. *Operation:* Patellectomy and repair of quadriceps tendon. Long leg plaster cylinder for 2 weeks.	Care of limb in plaster. Trim plaster where necessary, e.g. to allow freedom of foot and to relieve friction in groin. Suction drain for 48 hours. Bivalve plaster at 2 weeks and retain posterior shell support initially. Graduated knee exercises.
Tibial Table (condyles)	*Stable:* Long leg plaster for 6 weeks. Initially haemarthrosis may require aspiration.	Pain, tension under plaster, swelling of toes, suggest haemarthrosis. Knee exposed by window in plaster to

FRACTURES OF THE LOWER LIMB—continued

Fracture	Treatment and Method of Immobilisation	Special Points in Nursing Management
Tibial Table (condyles) —cont.		relieve tension. Trim plaster if necessary to ensure freedom of toes and relieve friction in groin. Knee flexion exercises after 6 weeks.
	Unstable: 1 Closed manipulation and sliding skeletal traction through tibia. Splint with knee flexion piece for 6–8 weeks. Initially haemarthrosis may require aspiration.	Pain and swelling of knee indicates **haemarthrosis.** Knee exercises as pain settles. Commence progressive weight-bearing after 6–8 weeks as knee function is restored.
	or 2 Open elevation of depressed fragment. Supporting bone graft. Long leg plaster for 8–12 weeks.	Iliac crest wound (bone graft donor site). Analgesia to control pain, otherwise breathing restricted and chest infection may result.
	or 3 Internal screw fixation where large condylar fragment. Long leg plaster for 2 weeks.	Trim plaster if necessary to allow freedom of toes and relieve friction in groin. Sutures removed 14 days. Early knee mobilising exercises. Progressive weight-bearing after 6–8 weeks.
Tibial Shaft and fibula)	*Stable:* Long leg plaster up to 16 weeks. Weight-bearing plaster at 6–10 weeks.	Plaster care. Trim plaster if necessary round groin and toes to allow free movement. On removal of plaster, toe, foot, ankle and knee exercises as outpatient.
	Unstable: Internal fixation and long leg plaster. *or* Manipulation and Steinmann pin through each fragment. Long leg plaster incorporates pins and provides stability.	**Elevation of bed and limb until swelling settles.** Care of limb in plaster. Plaster care. Trim plaster if necessary round groin and toes to allow free movement. Watch circulation.

FRACTURES OF THE LOWER LIMB—continued

Fracture	Treatment and Method of Immobilisation	Special Points in Nursing Management
Ankle 1 Pott's fracture (lateral malleolus of fibula) 2 Bimalleolar 3 Trimalleolar	*Stable:* Below-knee plaster for 6–8 weeks. Weight-bearing plaster after 3 weeks.	Outpatient treatment. Measure for crutches. Discharged non-weight-bearing. Instruction in care of limb and plaster.
	Unstable: Internal screw fixation of medial malleolus. Where necessary, screw fixation of the posterior malleolus and screw or bone plate fixation of the lateral. Plaster immobilisation up to 12 weeks.	**Elevation of bed and limb until swelling settles.** Plaster care. Trim plaster where necessary to allow free knee flexion and free movement of toes. Plaster changed, sutures removed 14th day. Non-weight-bearing until fractures stable at 6–10 weeks.
Metatarsals and	Well moulded below-knee plaster necessary to maintain reduction of metatarsal fracture.	Care of limb in plaster. Watch circulation and peripheral nerve function.
Phalanges	'Hood' extension to below-knee plaster in phalangeal fractures.	**Particular observation of circulation to toes.** Ischaemia or gangrene of the affected toe can occur.

FRACTURES OF THE SPINE

Wedge or Compression fracture of Vertebral Body (usually dorsal) (Deformity: angular kyphosis)	*Stable fracture:* Bed rest on a firm bed until pain settles (3 weeks). Graduated back extension exercises until posture normal. Plaster jacket support if pain severe for 6–12 weeks. Period of hospitalisation about 4–6 weeks.	In order to minimise pain, change patient's position carefully, i.e. maintain relationship of spine to pelvis by rolling the patient from side to side. Avoid flexion of spine.
Fracture of Vertebral Body with damage to Neural Arch and Articular facets	*Unstable fracture:* 1 *Fracture without displacement: Conservative management:* Bed rest on a firm bed. After pain settles (3–4 weeks) plaster jacket for 3–6 months.	As above. Potentially unstable therefore avoidance of flexion of spine more important.
	Operative management: Internal fixation (spinal plate) where there is greater risk of displacement.	Removal of sutures at 10 days. Gradual mobilisation. Redevelopment of spinal

FRACTURES OF THE SPINE—continued

Fracture	Treatment and Method of Immobilisation	Special Points in Nursing Management
Fracture of Vertebral Body, etc.—*cont.*	Sometimes augmented by plaster jacket support once patient can stand erect. Plaster retained for 3–6 months.	muscles and rehabilitation of patient important (physiotherapy and occupational therapy).
(Spinal cord and nerve roots exposed to damage if vertebral displacement occurs. Usually dorso-lumbar spine)	2 *Fracture with displacement and partial paraplegia:* *Method (a):* Where there are signs of recovery, conservative management as above. Active and passive movements of limbs encouraged. Regular assessment of progress. Plaster jacket support before patient fully mobile.	**Avoid flexion of spine.** Several nurses required to change patient's position. Stryker frame or revolving bed may be used to allow for adequate care of skin. Care of paraplegia (see p. 150).
	Method (b): Internal fixation to avoid risk of further displacement and to facilitate nursing management. Plaster jacket support when patient can stand erect. Retained for 3–6 months.	Patient nursed on firm bed. Turned carefully until pain settles and recovery of movement and sensation. Sutures removed at 14 days. Passive movements in paralysed areas. Active movements increased with signs of recovery.
	3 *Fracture with displacement and total paraplegia:* *Method (a):* **Conservative management** but **no plaster.** Passive physiotherapy in paralysed areas. Active exercises with emphasis on full development of muscle power in the arms to increase mobility and independence.	Intensive nursing care of the paralysed patient (see p. 150). Rehabilitation very important both mentally and physically (see Chaps. 27 and 28).
	Method (b): **Operative management.** Internal fixation of the fracture by a spinal plate to facilitate movement of the patient. Passive physiotherapy in the paralysed areas. Active exercises with emphasis on full development of muscle power in the arms to increase mobility and independence.	Sutures removed at 14 days. Intensive nursing care of paralysed patient and rehabilitation as above.

FRACTURES OF THE PELVIS

Fracture	Treatment and Method of Immobilisation	Special Points in Nursing Management
Undisplaced fracture of pelvic ring, e.g. fracture of an ischio-pubic ramus or fracture of the anterior superior iliac spine.	*Stable Fracture:* Bed rest on a firm bed until pain settles. Gradual mobilisation until patient regains muscle tone.	General nursing care.
Displaced fracture of pelvic ring, i.e. ring broken anteriorly and posteriorly producing an unstable section of the pelvis which usually includes the hip joint. Shortening of the affected leg may occur.	*Unstable Fracture:* 1 Initial manipulation under general anaesthesia to reduce displacement. 2 Sliding traction either to reduce fracture or to maintain reduction (10–12 weeks). Graduated physiotherapy.	Care of traction. Watch for complications such as dropfoot, haematuria in urethral damage, paralytic ileus (see p. 151). Gradual weight-bearing after 8–12 weeks.
Fracture of the Acetabulum with **Dislocation** of the **Hip Joint** (Central dislocation of the hip joint. The head of the femur is driven through the acetabulum).	1 Open reduction and sliding skeletal traction. *or* 2 Sliding skeletal traction for 4–6 weeks. Graduated physiotherapy.	Sutures removed at 14 days. Care of traction. Nursing care as for fracture of the pelvis.

14 LIGAMENTOUS INJURIES, DISLOCATIONS AND FRACTURE DISLOCATIONS

LIGAMENTOUS INJURIES

The stability of a joint is largely dependent on the muscles controlling it in the first instance and ultimately on the integrity of its ligaments. Where an **unexpected force** is applied to a joint and the muscles are taken 'off guard' the ligaments may be injured. This may vary from a minor sprain to a complete rupture. In a sprain the ligament is stretched but is intact; a rupture may be partial or complete. The distinction is important for the prognosis and it is essential that a major ligamentous injury is not mistaken for a minor one, e.g. a total rupture for a partial rupture or strain. The differentiation is made on clinical and radiological grounds. The history of the **mechanism of injury** indicates the type of ligamentous lesion to be expected. **Clinical examination** may, however, still leave doubt. More detailed examination of the integrity of the ligament or ligaments by the application of stress to them is possible under either local or general anaesthesia. **X-ray** pictures of the **joint** are taken while the **stress** is being applied. If the ligament is intact the bones will retain their normal relationship; if ruptured an obvious change will be observed.

Minor ligamentous injuries are extremely common, particularly in sport. In most instances these are successfully treated in the casualty outpatient department and are therefore included in Chapter 17. Severe force applied to the taut ligaments of a joint in the young results in **partial** or **total rupture** of one or more ligaments. A similar force sustained by the same joint in the elderly is much more liable to produce bony damage within the joint. On the one hand the bone is hard and resistant while, on the other, it is softened because of osteoporosis. **Rupture of ligaments is associated with instability.** This is more apparent in the weight-bearing joints, particularly in the knee and ankle.

Injury to the Ligaments of the Knee Joint

The knee joint is stabilised by four ligaments. Medial or lateral movement of the femur on the tibia is controlled by the strength of the **medial and lateral collateral ligaments** which are structures external to the joint. Forwards or backwards movement is prevented by the integrity of the **cruciate ligaments** which are attached to the condyles of the femur and tibia within the joint.

The knee is more exposed to direct trauma on the lateral rather than on the medial side, which is relatively protected by the other leg. When the lateral side of the joint is subjected to injury the strain or stretching occurs at the medial side

This explains why partial or complete rupture of the medial ligament is one of the common injuries of the joint.

Total Rupture of the Medial Ligament. This is a serious injury as there is complete instability of the knee on weight-bearing. Early repair of the ligament is essential to restore stability. The limb is immobilised in a plaster cylinder with the knee in extension. Quadriceps exercises are commenced on the 1st post-operative day. Sutures are removed in 10 days either through a 'window' or at the change of plaster. After 3 weeks the plaster is bivalved and the posterior shell retained for support during rest or ambulation. The patient then starts knee flexion exercises. In the 4th week he may be measured for crutches and allowed to walk non-weight-bearing on the affected limb. Weight-bearing is delayed until 90° of knee flexion is obtained.

If repair of the ligament is not undertaken early, recurrent instability of the knee results. This means that the patient's mobility is restricted and arthrodesis of the joint may be necessary to restore stability.

Anterior Cruciate Ligament Injury. A rotational injury to the weight-bearing limb which damages the meniscus may also produce rupture of the anterior cruciate ligament. In other instances, the ligament may be torn along with the medial and sometimes the lateral ligaments. An isolated injury to the cruciate ligament can occur where the femur is forced backwards on the tibia, or the knee joint hyperextended.

Treatment depends on whether the injury is isolated or associated with rupture of other supporting structures. Provided the quadriceps function is good an isolated injury is generally left untreated. The instability is not significant enough to demand repair of the ligament, which in any case does not restore total knee function. If other structures are damaged, however, their treatment is the initial consideration. Where the degree of ligamentous damage is considerable the cruciate ligament may be repaired along with other ligaments in an effort to provide as stable a joint as possible. The lower limb is immobilised in a plaster cylinder with the knee in slight flexion for about 4–6 weeks. Knee function is thereafter improved by graduated exercises.

Lateral Collateral Ligament. Although the lateral ligament is the stabilising joint support on the outer side of the knee joint its function is not as important as that of the medial ligament. Most of the stresses and strains to which the joint is subjected are absorbed by the medial ligament. The significance of rupture of the lateral ligament is in its association with **traction lesions of the lateral popliteal nerve.**

Existence of the torn ligament does not produce undue instability in the joint. An attempt is made, nevertheless, to repair the ligament in order to restore full knee function. If there is also rupture of the cruciate ligament, repair of the lateral collateral ligament is desirable to improve the stability of the joint. The limb is immobilised in a plaster cylinder for 3 weeks and thereafter in a posterior shell until knee function is satisfactory. Where popliteal nerve damage exists early exploration of the nerve is undertaken to diagnose the type of lesion and to assess the degree of damage. In a few cases primary nerve suture is possible. Generally, where a traction lesion has occurred, it may be more effectively treated as a secondary elective operation.

Posterior Cruciate Ligament Rupture. This rarely occurs as an isolated injury. It is usually one of the four ligaments torn where there is complete dislocation of the knee joint.

Ligamentous Injury of the Ankle Joint
Rupture of the Lateral Collateral Ligament. The most important injury producing instability of the ankle joint is complete rupture of the lateral collateral ligament. This results in marked swelling and bruising of the whole ankle, particularly on the lateral side. Pain is acute and limp is severe, due to a marked tendency to unprotected inversion at each step. X-ray examination is essential to confirm the diagnosis. Where pain is severe, special stress films may be required under a local anaesthetic. Treatment must be adequate initially, otherwise the injury recurs. Complete immobilisation in a padded below-knee plaster cast is necessary for 2-4 weeks. Once the swelling has settled, a close-fitting plaster is applied for a further 6 weeks. Thereafter mobilising ankle and foot exercises are performed, eversion in particular.

Rupture of the Medial Collateral Ligament. The medial ligament of the ankle joint is usually torn in association with one of the fractures of the joint. Treatment is therefore linked with the management of the fracture.

DISLOCATIONS
Dislocation is the **displacement of a bone from its natural position in a joint.** Although the majority of cases are traumatic, congenital and pathological dislocation can also occur. Congenital dislocation (*see* Chapter 2) is not uncommon. Pathological dislocation may follow inflammation, e.g. septic arthritis, or spastic paralysis where there is weakness in a group of muscles with overaction of the opposing group, e.g. cerebral palsy.

In **trauma** the injury causes tearing of the ligaments holding the joint in position. The muscles are stripped off their attachments allowing the bones forming the joint to slip out of position. The whole area fills up with blood which gradually becomes organised into scar tissue. This binds the bones and soft tissues (ligaments and muscles) in the position of dislocation. They are then most difficult to replace in their proper anatomical position. The process is well advanced by 10 days and completed by about 20 days. The dislocation is therefore reduced while the blood is still in the fluid or haematoma state.

Other factors such as shock, obstruction to circulation and pressure on nerves make it vital that the dislocation be reduced as soon as possible, otherwise additional complications arise, e.g. severe shock, ischaemia or paralysis.

Sometimes in traumatic dislocation the ligaments remain intact and are either pulled from their attachment thus avulsing a flake of bone, or there is a definite fracture of one or both bones forming the joint, i.e. **fracture dislocation.**

COMMON DISLOCATIONS OF THE UPPER LIMB

Dislocation	Treatment and Method of Immobilisation	Special Points in Nursing Management
Shoulder (Deformity: Forward displacement of head of humerus. Angulation of shoulder due to lateral projection of acromion process)	Reduction, axillary pad, inside collar/cuff sling—3 weeks in young adults; 10 days in elderly. X-ray check on reduction. (May be associated with deltoid palsy, fracture of tuberosity or rupture of rotator cuff tendon.)	**Collar/cuff sling should be comfortable** and not obstruct circulation or constrict the neck. It **should, however, be difficult for the patient to remove.** Graduated physiotherapy after removal of sling.
Acromio-clavicular Joint (Deformity: Downward displacement of acromion process leaves angular projection of the clavicle)	Stabilisation of the joint: 1 Unreduced. Conservative management. Simple inside collar/cuff sling till pain settles. Scar tissue forms round the displaced joint so stabilising it. 2 Operative Treatment. Open reduction and internal (screw) fixation. Inside collar/cuff sling for 3–4 weeks. X-ray check of reduction at intervals.	Collar/cuff sling should be comfortable, and must not obstruct circulation. Physiotherapy. Wound sutures removed, 10–12 days. Graduated physiotherapy once collar/cuff sling is removed.
Elbow (Deformity: Backward projection of olecranon and radial head producing a large posterior swelling)	*Stable:* Reduction, inside collar/cuff sling. Elbow in a little flexion. *Unstable:* Reduction, padded long arm plaster for 3 weeks. X-ray check at intervals.	Observe swelling, **check circulation** and **peripheral nerve function.** Care of plaster. Ensure free movement of fingers. Check upper end of plaster for pressure or friction. Extend or trim plaster as necessary. On removal of plaster **vigorous physiotherapy is avoided,** otherwise stiffness results. Free use of elbow is encouraged with gradual recovery of movement.

COMMON DISLOCATIONS OF THE UPPER LIMB—continued

Dislocation	Treatment and Method of Immobilisation	Special Points in Nursing Management
Fingers Interphalangeal joints (Deformity: Finger shortened. Dislocated joint appears swollen)	Reduction, dorsal strapping over a pad in flexion. 2–3 weeks.	Check strapping is not too tight. Observe circulation. Graduated physiotherapy on removal of strapping.

COMMON DISLOCATIONS OF THE LOWER LIMB

Dislocation	Treatment and Method of Immobilisation	Special Points in Nursing Management
Hip (Deformity (posterior dislocation more common): Swelling of the hip. The limb is flexed, adducted and internally rotated)	*Stable:* Reduction. Sliding traction. Regular X-ray for signs of redislocation or avascular necrosis of the femoral head.	Care of traction. May need drop-foot splint appliance if there is sciatic palsy. Watch for signs of deep venous thrombosis.
	Unstable: Open reduction. Internal fixation of acetabular marginal fragment. Sliding traction. Periodic X-ray check to exclude avascular necrosis of femoral head.	Suction drain for 48 hours. Wound sutures removed, 12–14 days. Watch for signs of deep venous thrombosis.

DISLOCATION OF THE CERVICAL SPINE

Dislocation	Treatment and Method of Immobilisation	Special Points in Nursing Management
Cervical spine Instability at the inter-articular facets with or without a fracture of the vertebral body. May produce	*Immediate Treatment:* *Conservative:* Skull skeletal traction (p. 104). Gradual reduction. *Operative:* 1 Manipulation under general anaesthetic. Immediate reduction. Position maintained by skull traction.	Care in handling traction. Help with feeding patient. Respiratory paralysis with quadriplegia—**observe breathing.** Remove excess secretions by suction. Patient may require tracheostomy and assisted

DISLOCATION OF THE CERVICAL SPINE—continued

Dislocation	Treatment and Method of Immobilisation	Special Points in Nursing Management
partial or total quadriplegia.	*or* 2 Open reduction of locked facets. Immobilisation for 6 weeks in skull traction. *Secondary Treatment:* *Operative Stabilisation:* Usually done after period of 6 weeks immobilisation. 1 **Posterior fusion:** Internal fixation of the two vertebrae concerned by wiring of the spinous processes and bone grafting of the laminae. 2 **Anterior fusion:** Bone grafting of the vertebral bodies concerned. In both methods further immobilisation by skull traction for 3 weeks. Cervical collar, or 'Halo' traction (see p. 104) thereafter until 12 weeks. Regular X-ray checks of position.	ventilation. General **care of paralysed** patient (see p. 150). **Physiotherapy—** passive in paralysed areas, active in areas showing signs of recovery. **Rehabilitation.** Sutures removed at 14 days.

FRACTURE DISLOCATIONS

These can involve any joint. They are more difficult to treat successfully than either fractures or dislocations because the basic principles of fracture treatment differ from those of dislocation although initially both require rest. Later, after about 3 weeks, a joint requires increasing freedom of movement to regain full function. The fracture, however, still requires rest, often for many more weeks. It is difficult to satisfy both. The nearer a fracture is to a joint the more difficult it is to treat successfully even by open operative methods. Very often the fragments are friable, small and difficult to reduce. This is a serious disadvantage to the restoration of joint function. Perfect reduction is necessary if full function is to be regained and osteoarthritis later avoided.

Fracture with an Associated Dislocation

Sometimes in fractures of either the radius or the ulna, an excessive force produces dislocation of a related joint. Radial fractures may have an associated dislocation of the inferior radio-ulnar joint; in fractures of the ulna there is often a dislocation of the head of the radius. Similarly, although a fracture of the shaft of the fibula does not usually require treatment it may be part of a more major injury involving the inferior tibio-fibular joint. Each of these combined injuries is referred to generally by the name of the person who first recognised its significance.

Monteggia Fracture. This is a fracture of the ulna with dislocation of the head of the radius.

Galeazzi Fracture. This is a fracture of the shaft of the radius with dislocation of the inferior radio-ulnar joint.

To ensure stability in the Monteggia and Galeazzi fractures treatment involves reduction of the dislocation, internal fixation of the fracture and the application of a long arm plaster. If the circulation appears satisfactory during the early post-operative period the patient is discharged. Further treatment is continued in the outpatient department.

Inferior Tibio-fibular Diastasis. Where fracture of the fibula is associated with rupture of the inferior tibio-fibular ligament subluxation of the ankle joint results; this instability is referred to as a diastasis. Treatment is by reduction of the sub-luxation and internal screw fixation of the lower fibular fragment to the tibia. Immobilisation in a below-knee plaster is necessary for 8–12 weeks. A walking heel is applied to the plaster after 8 weeks.

15 PERIPHERAL NERVE INJURIES

The Peripheral Nerves
These nerves form the **communication system between the central nervous system and the periphery.** The spinal cord, although a continuous structure, is described in segments corresponding to the cervical, thoracic, lumbar and sacral segments of the vertebral column. At either side of each cord segment a sensory nerve root enters posteriorly, and a motor nerve root leaves anteriorly. These combine to form a mixed peripheral nerve which divides and subdivides until its terminal branches end in the skin, muscle, joints or organs which are controlled by that particular segment of the cord. As these nerves form smaller branches some of them become more motor or more sensory depending on their function in that particular area of the body. The radial nerve for example is almost completely motor supplying the extensors of the wrist and fingers and has only small sensory branches innervating the skin of the dorsum of the hand.

In the skin, muscles and around the joints are special receptor nerve endings which respond to different stimuli. Superficial sensations such as pain, heat and light touch, and deeper perceptions as of pressure, position and vibration are transmitted to the central nervous system by the sensory branches of the peripheral nerves. As the sensory fibres approach the spinal cord they are dissociated from the motor fibres to form the posterior nerve root which is composed completely of sensory fibres. These nerves have their cell station in a ganglion on this posterior root. From this ganglion another fibre enters the postero-lateral aspect of the spinal cord. Here the fibres are organised further. They all travel to the sensory area in the brain. Some ascend in the posterior column while others cross immediately in the cord and reach the brain via the anterior tract.

The motor impulses are initiated in the cells of the motor cortex and are carried via the upper motor neurones to end in the anterior horn cells of the spinal cord. New neurones then carry the motor impulses from the cord and travel along with the sensory fibres in the peripheral nerves to activate the muscles supplied by that particular segment. These are the **lower motor neurones,** the motor part of the peripheral nervous system.

It is important to know that **trophic nerves** which are part of the autonomic nervous system also have their smaller branches running in the peripheral nerves and these control the blood vessels and sweat glands of the skin in the areas of nerve distribution.

As the peripheral nerves are the link between the central nervous system and the periphery they also form part of the reflex arc, and this is significant where there is nerve damage.

Terms used in the Description of Nerve Damage

Neurotmesis Complete anatomical division of a nerve producing total loss of its function distal to the injury.

Axonotmesis This is a lesion in continuity, i.e. although some of the supporting structure is preserved or intact there is always damage to the fibres or axons in the nerve so that true degeneration occurs peripherally (distally).

Neuropraxia There is a transient block due to a minimal lesion. Although an incomplete paralysis exists it is temporary as there is no peripheral nerve degeneration. It is a physiological interruption of nerve conduction with predominantly a loss of motor function and with little wasting. Any sensory changes of paracsthesia and the loss of motor function usually recover in 6–8 weeks.

PERIPHERAL NERVE DAMAGE

This can affect a peripheral nerve almost anywhere in the body. Some nerves are, however, more vulnerable than others because at certain points in their course they are very superficial. Injury results from **pressure, stretching, cutting, crushing, ischaemia** i.e. lack of blood flow, or **injection.** The result may vary from contusion with transient symptoms and signs to complete rupture with permanent paralysis of a particular group of muscles and loss of sensation of a specific area of skin. In a mixed peripheral nerve, the symptoms and signs of damage involve both the sensory and motor components. Sensory disturbance may vary from paraesthesia to anaesthesia. Loss of motor function may be confined to muscle weakness or extend to total paralysis in a particular group of muscles. Atrophy or wasting of the soft tissues in the area of the sensory and motor changes may also be apparent.

Pressure on nerves can be an unfortunate complication in the nursing management of a patient in hospital. The common causes are **splintage,** i.e. Thomas's splint or plaster casts, the **misuse of crutches,** particularly in a thin patient, or **pressure from a fragment of bone in a displaced or comminuted fracture.** The more serious nerve injuries are associated with **violent trauma** causing stretching, cutting or crushing of a nerve. The injury may result in either a **partial or complete nerve lesion.** There are three possible results: the lesion may recover completely after a long period of conservative management; it may not recover without surgical repair; even with surgical intervention damage may be irreparable.

Conservative Management of Peripheral Nerve Injuries

It is important to appreciate that, although the pain, paraesthesia and motor weakness are experienced initially in the distal digits of either the hand or foot, the **source of pressure responsible for the lesion is situated more proximally in the limb,** e.g. at the elbow or knee. These areas therefore should be inspected carefully and pressure **relieved immediately** in order to avoid serious damage to the nerve, e.g. by alterations in external splintage or by remanipulation of fractures. The application of corrective splints is necessary if permanent changes in muscles and joints with persistent deformity are to be prevented, e.g. a 'cock-up' splint in radial nerve palsy and a drop-foot splint in lateral popliteal nerve palsy. **The splintage must be removed several times daily and passive movements given** if joint function is to be maintained. Electrical muscle stimulation helps to retain muscle tone until eventually full muscle tone and joint movement are regained. Where the nerve injured has a large sensory component and there is resultant extensive sensory loss, in the hands and feet in particular, the wearing of protective clothing is essential especially once the patient is discharged, e.g. gloves or padded boots.

Operative Management

Primary Nerve Suture. Where a wound is complicated by division of a peripheral nerve, an attempt to resuture the nerve may be made during the course of wound repair. The cut ends of the nerve require to be held together by suturing the two ends of the torn sheath. This is a delicate procedure and the sheath often tears resulting in poor approximation. It is therefore sometimes considered necessary to delay the surgical treatment. The retraction of the torn ends of the nerve is prevented by loosely suturing the nerve sheath to the adjacent muscle.

Secondary Nerve Suture. Surgical repair of the nerve may be attempted: in a complete lesion once the wound has healed; in an incomplete lesion where there is failure to improve within three months; in subjects who develop excessive pain, i.e. **causalgia;** in patients who present with a nerve lesion after an interval from the time of original injury.

Some nerves are more easily sutured than others. The terminal digital ones are particularly difficult, often impossible to suture as they are thread-like in structure. Where deformity has led to lengthening of the course of a nerve producing a traction lesion, e.g. valgus deformity of the elbow causing stretching of the ulnar nerve, **transposition of the nerve** may relieve the tension and restore function.

If the lesion is irrecoverable, particularly in the upper limb, the deformity may be corrected by transplantation of the tendon of a less important functioning muscle into that of a paralysed one thus compensating for its loss of power. For example, the insertion of the ulnar wrist flexor is divided and reattached to the extensor tendons of the fingers in the drop hand deformity of radial nerve palsy. In the lower limb, tendon operations are less satisfactory. Where possible a bony operation is performed. For example, in order to compensate for drop-foot deformity in lateral popliteal nerve palsy a **Lambrinudi triple arthrodesis** fuses the three main joints of the foot in a permanent but more functional position.

Significant Features of Common Nerve Injuries

Radial Nerve. This nerve is particularly exposed to damage in the axilla and upper arm. In the axilla pressure from crutches may produce crutch palsy in which the origins of either the radial or ulnar nerve may be contused. In the upper arm displaced fragments in fracture of the humerus can cause damage to the radial nerve. The lesion is usually partial and recoverable. It is recognised by the patient finding difficulty in extension of the elbow and dorsiflexion of the wrist and fingers. There may be a tingling sensation over the dorsum of the hand towards the base of the thumb. In crutch palsy elbow crutches are substituted to relieve the pressure and a 'cock-up' splint is always applied to support the wrist (*see* Appendix *Fig. 49b*).

Lateral Popliteal Nerve Palsy. This nerve is especially vulnerable as it passes postero-anteriorly round the neck of the fibula. Damage is usually produced either by pressure or traction. **Patients nursed in Thomas's splints** are particularly exposed to this lesion if the leg is insufficiently controlled and is allowed to rotate externally. The head of the fibula then rests against a tight sling, a firm pad or even the outer bar of the splint. **Pressure from an inadequately padded or badly moulded plaster cast** can also give rise to nerve damage. A thin patient may develop the lesion with the limb simply resting on a firm mattress. Where recognition is early the lesion is partial and recovers completely. Delay in appreciating a developing lesion may result in complete and permanent nerve palsy. The lateral popliteal nerve is more motor than sensory.

The symptoms and signs to be observed in the foot are weakness in dorsiflexion and tingling or burning sensation in the dorsum, particularly at the base of the first and second toes. The nerve at this stage is still viable. Once it is completely damaged there is anaesthesia of the skin and a **true drop-foot deformity.** This picture of complete nerve palsy is seen in traction lesions of the lateral popliteal nerve where there is rupture of the lateral collateral ligament of the knee and in fractures of the lower end of femur and upper end of tibia.

Where the lesion is caused by pressure this must be relieved immediately. The position of a limb in a splint can be altered, a firm pad may be removed and tight slings readjusted. **Pressure under a plaster is relieved by the removal of a window,** at least 6 in. x 4 in. (15 cm x 10 cm) over the head and neck of fibula. Signs of pressure, i.e. redness of the skin, will be seen and the patient may feel instant relief. If this method of treatment fails the plaster should be removed and the limb inspected. A fresh plaster is then applied with adequate padding to protect the head and neck of fibula. When there is **weakness or loss of dorsiflexion of the foot,** it must be **supported by a corrective appliance.** The support may either be a sling or footpiece incorporated in a Thomas's splint to keep the foot in dorsiflexion or an extension of the plaster to form a toe platform in plaster casts. Physiotherapy is important, progressing gradually from passive movements of the toes and dorsiflexion of the foot to active exercises as recovery continues. Where drop-foot deformity is permanent various devices can be incorporated in below-knee calipers to resist the tendency for the foot to drop. If these prove unsuccessful surgery is the only alternative.

Median Nerve. This nerve is susceptible to damage by pressure from the bone fragments of a displaced fracture. The nerve is compressed, e.g. in front of the elbow in supracondylar fracture, in front of the lower end of the radius in Colles' fracture or in front of the wrist in carpal tunnel syndrome. It can also be divided by incisional wounds in the region of the wrist. Pressure lesions tend to be partial while incisional ones are more likely to be complete. A complete lesion of the median nerve severely affects the function of the hand. There is loss of sensation in the radial 3½ fingers and a **claw-like deformity** of these fingers and the thumb. This may be corrected by a hand splint. Where there is anaesthesia of the fingers a **protective glove** should be worn to avoid burns or other damage to the skin and soft tissues. Physiotherapy is necessary to maintain joint function and muscle tone.

Ulnar Nerve. In the ulnar nerve, although it is a mixed nerve, motor function is more important than sensory function. The nerve supplies most of the small muscles of the hand, providing only sensory branches to the little finger and the adjacent half of the ring finger.

The damage is usually by lacerations of the anterior inner aspect of the wrist. Pressure on the nerve producing a partial lesion may be a complication of: fractures of the humerus or of both bones of forearm; crutch palsy; pressure on the inner side of the elbow in a long arm plaster cast. It is recognised by **tingling or numbness particularly in the little finger and a weakness of grip.** Treatment is by a **hand splint** (*see* Appendix, *Fig. 49a*) to prevent claw deformity of the little and ring fingers and by physiotherapy to maintain joint function and muscle tone.

Digital Nerves. These nerves are the sensory terminal branches of the median and ulnar nerves, and they are the receptor organs for the sense of touch. Damage to them is common after cuts of the fingers by glass, scalpel blades or tin cans. The result is either partial or total division of the nerve. Partial lesions of digital nerves are actually the more difficult for the patient to accept because of hyperaesthesia in the area of the tip of the finger due to the development of a **neuroma** which is extremely troublesome. Treatment presents many problems. Total division of a digital nerve leaves an area of numbness which in the thumb and index fingers can be a disabling feature destroying the pincer action. For this reason surgical suture of these particular nerves is sometimes attempted but is often unsuccessful. A partially successful operation may only produce the effect of a partial lesion which is most undesirable for the patient.

Sciatic Nerve Palsy. This nerve is formed in the sciatic plexus in the pelvis from which it emerges behind the hip joint in the inner, lower quadrant of the buttock. It then runs down the back of the thigh, in the lower part of which it divides into the medial and lateral popliteal nerves. Damage to it occurs in posterior dislocation of the hip. The nerve is either contused or crushed by a bony fragment broken off from the acetabulum or the head of the femur. Sciatic nerve palsy is also **one of the dangers of intra-muscular injections into the buttock.** To avoid this, these injections should be given into the upper outer quadrant.

The effects of this lesion are those of a combined medial and lateral popliteal nerve palsy. The important features are **total anaesthesia of the skin of the sole of the foot and a flail foot** due to paralysis of all the muscles controlling it. Because of the length of this nerve recovery cannot be expected for some 18–24 months. If paralysis is complete only those parts of the lower limb supplied by the femoral nerve will have any function. As the function of the knee is not impaired a **below-knee caliper** is sufficient to control the flail paralysed foot. **A soft, wool-lined felt boot** is necessary to avoid pressure on anaesthetic skin. The hygiene of the foot, care that socks are unwrinkled and inspection of shoes for small stones are all important. Pressure sores may develop otherwise. If the nerve fails to recover the apparatus will be required permanently (*see* Appendix, *Fig. 50c*).

16 HAND INJURIES

These include fractures of the metacarpals and phalanges, joint dislocations, tendon injuries and damage to the soft tissues.

The hand is a very useful instrument. The fingers are named rather than numbered to avoid confusion (thumb, index, middle, ring and little finger). The thumb opposes the other four fingers and allows the hand to grasp objects with a 'claw-like' action. Loss of the thumb results in 50 per cent loss of the functional efficiency of the hand. The thumb, index and middle fingers (radial side) are used in the **pincer action** involved in gripping a pen or in precision movements. The middle, ring and little fingers (ulnar side) are used in the **grasping action** associated with the coarser activities of manual labour. Obviously the length and breadth of the hand are important. The longer the fingers and the broader the hand, the better is the grip. Utilisation of all the fingers is necessary in some activities, e.g. playing musical instruments. There is a close functional co-ordination between the brain and the hand.

Hand injuries are of three main types: crush injuries; incisional wounds; fractures or dislocations. Sometimes the trauma produces a combination of these.

Crush Injuries
Crushing (or bursting) injuries produce open fractures in which the soft tissue damage is severe, often with damage to blood vessels and nerves. The injury may have included amputation of a segment of one or more fingers.

The hand receives its blood supply via several blood vessels and unless the injury is extensive there is sufficient reserve to provide a collateral circulation. The main problem in these injuries is, therefore, the control of bleeding. Where the vascular damage is severe, amputation of segments of one or more fingers may be necessary because the part is non-viable. **As much of the finger as possible is conserved in order to maintain the function of the whole hand.** Although the patient's occupation influences the extent of surgery performed the cosmetic effect is, nevertheless, considered.

Nerve damage in the hand involves the median and ulnar nerves, and their branches. Repair of a divided nerve by nerve suture is often undertaken in an attempt to restore function.

Incisional Wounds
Incisional wounds of the hand caused by glass, knives, etc. often involve division of tendons as well as nerve and blood vessel damage. **Tendon injuries** may be partial or complete. In a partial lesion, unless the tendon is liable to rupture,

surgical repair is unnecessary. The wound is cleaned and sutured. In a divided tendon there is complete loss of function. This necessitates tendon repair by primary suture. Where this is contra-indicated because of the situation and nature of the lesion, the wound is primarily cleaned, sutured and allowed to heal. At a second operation the divided tendon is then replaced by one taken from a less important site, i.e. free tendon graft.

Fractures

Fractures of the **metacarpals and phalanges** may result from direct or indirect injuries. These are either stable or unstable.

Stable fractures are **lightly splinted** until painfree. Fracture of a finger may be splinted by the adjacent finger by bandaging them together (**Garter strapping,** *Fig. 31a*). Fractures of the metacarpal bones are splinted either by a **pad and bandage** or a **light anterior plaster slab support** (*Fig. 31b*).

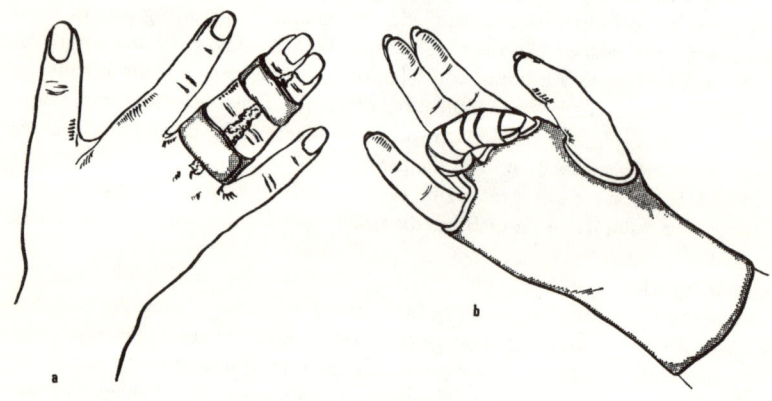

FIG. 31   (*a*) Garter strapping
(*b*) Anterior slab support

Unstable fractures require **reduction** and **manipulation** prior to immobilisation. The method of immobilisation is similar to that of stable fractures but usually more adequate in order to prevent redisplacement of the bone ends. In all fractures of the hand it is important to **prevent joint stiffness by short term immobilisation** (2–3 weeks) with immediate exercises of the unsplinted fingers and the fractured ones whenever painfree.

Dislocations

Dislocation of the finger joints may be simple or in the form of a fracture dislocation. Simple dislocations are reduced by gentle steady traction with or without an anaesthetic. The fingers are then **bandaged in flexion** over a pad to maintain the reduction for 2–3 weeks. **Fracture dislocations** may be treated similarly but where they are unstable **internal fixation** is the method of treatment which offers least restriction and permits early functional activity.

Occasionally, **isolated ligamentous injuries** occur leaving instability or weakness in a finger. Although natural repair can occur with plaster splint immobilisation for 2–3 weeks **surgical repair** is more certain.

Reconstruction of the thumb may be attempted where the functional efficiency of the hand has been gravely diminished by the severe destruction or loss of the thumb. Where a stump remains it can be built up by grafting a pedicle of abdominal skin to it and later incorporating a bone graft from the iliac crest. If the thumb is completely absent, it may be replaced by the index finger which is rotated through 90 degrees so that it opposes the middle, ring and little fingers. The main problems of these operations are: deficient sensation of the abdominal skin of the new thumb; pressure from plaster splintage; failure of circulation due to tension on the blood vessels; non-union of the bone graft in the reconstructed thumb or of the metacarpal osteotomy graft in the index finger transposition.

Nursing Problems in Hand Injuries

The main problems are: **obstruction to circulation** by swelling; numbness due to nerve damage; **pressure sores** from plaster splints; infection in compound injuries; **post-traumatic stiffness.** It is important therefore to remove rings immediately on admission or before elective operation. Post-operatively, the limb is elevated to minimise swelling (*see Fig. 47b*).

The circulation to the fingers should be checked frequently and any obstruction dealt with immediately. Swelling, blue discolouration or pallor, tingling sensation, lack of feeling or inability to move the fingers are important warning signs. As early as a few hours after operation, gentle active finger movements of unsplinted fingers are commenced. This limits swelling and avoids stiffness. Pyrexia indicates infection. Residual haematomata after hand injury and hand surgery easily become infected. It is therefore quite common practice in compound injuries for the patient to be given prophylactic antibiotics. Once the wound has healed and dressings or plaster removed, the physiotherapist continues with treatment to restore complete function wherever possible. If the wound fails to heal, regular daily dressings, sometimes over a prolonged period, may be required. Various desloughing agents are available to effect slough separation so that the denuded area can be covered by healthy granulation tissue over which the new epithelium grows. Stiffness is more difficult to avoid in delayed wound healing because, mechanically, bandaging limits movement and the patient is also reluctant to use the painful finger.

17 THE MANAGEMENT OF MINOR INJURY PROCEDURES IN THE CASUALTY DEPARTMENT

The Casualty Department is a central reception area for those patients in urgent need of treatment. In less urgent situations they would normally be seen by appointment in the appropriate clinic of the outpatient department, i.e. medical, surgical or specialty. The patients with whom we are concerned are those who have sustained an injury of bone, muscle, joint or soft tissue. The **injuries** may be **minor, major** or **multiple.** Multiple injuries need not always be major, e.g. multiple lacerations. A single injury need not be minor, e.g. a complicated fracture of femur. Trauma, however minor, produces some degree of **shock,** i.e. the systemic reaction to the injury, and one should remember this in the treatment of outpatients. The injuries are usually the result of an **accident in the home, at work** or **on the road.**

Outpatients and their Injuries

Children are usually the victims of fractures. Greenstick fractures, fractures of both bones of forearm, supra-condylar fractures of elbow, spiral fractures of tibia and fracture of the clavicle are among the more common injuries. The elderly are more susceptible to fractures of the surgical neck of humerus and Colles' fracture. The working age group sustain injuries such as fractures of the scaphoid, crushing and bursting injuries of the hand by machinery and of the feet by heavy objects falling on them. Manual workers involved in heavy lifting or pushing are liable to suffer acute strains of the back. The active sports enthusiast may be subjected to direct blows producing fractures or dislocations, e.g. tibia in football, or acromio-clavicular joint in rugby. Twisting injuries of joints are very common. Damage to the ligaments of the knee in football, the ankle in ski-ing, the spine in golf or cricket are but a few examples. The housewife is also prone to falls in the home, particularly when 'spring-cleaning' and decorating. Her injuries vary from simple strains to fractures and dislocations.

Types of Injury

Soft tissue injuries fall into five main categories.

1 Simple contusions and bruises
2 Incisional wounds and lacerations
3 Ligamentous lesions

4 Crushing and bursting injuries of hands and feet
5 Simple fractures

Simple Contusions and Bruises. These are localised areas of swelling with temporary impairment of function. Pain is relieved by **rest,** perhaps with the aid of a **supporting bandage or sling** and mild **analgesia.** The patient can be instructed to apply cold compresses to the contused area in an attempt to reduce swelling. Skin discolouration develops as the blood diffuses into the tissue planes and may be quite extensive. Contusion injuries recover rapidly and completely with minimal treatment. The marked tissue reaction associated with more serious underlying structural damage, e.g. fracture, may give a similar appearance. It is always important to exclude such possibilities before the injury is treated as a simple contusion.

Incisional Wounds and Lacerations. These are treated either under local or general anaesthesia depending on their severity. Simple wounds will only require **thorough cleaning and suturing.** Complicated wounds may necessitate the additional repair of other structures, e.g. **repair of extensor tendons,** which is more comfortable for the patient if done under general anaesthesia.

Ligamentous Lesions. These include 'sprains', partial (i.e. 'strains') or complete rupture of ligaments. The pain may simulate that of a simple fracture and X-ray examination is usually a routine method of excluding the presence of such. There is obvious loss of function, and protective muscle spasm. The treatment depends on the degree of the ligamentous damage. **Strain of the ligaments** may be treated by the **temporary support** of an **elasticated** type of **firm bandage** in order **to control swelling and relieve pain. Analgesia** will also be necessary initially. Where the **spinal ligaments** are strained the patient will require to **rest in bed** at home until the pain settles. Thereafter, **spinal exercises** should assist a rapid recovery in 4–6 weeks.

More serious damage, e.g. **partial rupture of ligaments,** may necessitate the application of a firm supporting strapping. For example, in the ankle, stirrup strapping or a plaster cast may be applied to provide immobilisation until the pain is relieved and the muscle function restored. Injection of a **local anaesthetic, hydrocortisone** and **hyalase** into the tender spot may be used to relieve pain. Where a ligament is completely ruptured the patient is usually admitted to the orthopaedic or accident unit for elective repair. (*See* Chapter 14.)

Crushing or Bursting Injuries. Such injuries may be confined to the skin and underlying muscle. The damage may, however, be extensive, necessitating the removal of sections of dead tissue. Repair of the remaining tissues may then be difficult and **plastic surgery** may indeed be necessary. As these wounds are prone to slough formation and infection because of the devitalised tissue, the patient will require **regular frequent supervision at a soft tissue clinic.** Healing may be slow. Initially **analgesia** is necessary to relieve the pain produced by the tension of the tissues as a result of the reaction to injury. Even an apparently minor injury of this nature cannot be treated too lightly as amputation may be the result if complications do arise. More serious crushing injuries of hands and feet involving the important underlying structures, tendons, nerves, blood vessels and bones, will be treated in the accident unit. Sometimes there is a special unit which deals with hand injuries.

Simple Fractures. Undisplaced simple fractures are managed by the application of a plaster cast without anaesthesia being necessary. Simple displaced fractures which after reduction under anaesthesia appear potentially stable are often treated in the outpatient department. Where such a fracture is found to be unstable the patient must be transferred to the accident unit for observation of the fracture and if necessary for further treatment to avoid shortening of the limb.

Nursing Management of Outpatients

All patients require reassurance and a simple explanation of the treatment they are to receive. Even although a general anaesthetic is unnecessary, the patient may be asked to approve of his treatment by signing a special permission form. This safeguards not only the medical and nursing staff, but also the patient, especially in large busy outpatient departments. Children, wherever possible, should have the comfort of the presence of at least one parent. The nurse often has the responsibility for the preliminary cleansing of the skin prior to the administration of local anaesthesia and suturing of wounds. Sometimes it is necessary to shave the area of skin in the region of the wound, e.g. scalp wounds. She can give the patient added comfort during a period of treatment by supporting the limb or by talking quietly and reassuringly to him. In the treatment of injuries in children, although ideally a mother is the obvious person to comfort her child, she may find this too distressing in which case the nurse herself must substitute.

Anti-tetanus toxoid for passive immunity is given routinely to outpatients with open wounds. It is administered by intramuscular injection, the initial dose being given at the time of treatment and a subsequent dose six weeks later. The patient either may be given an appointment to attend a special clinic in order to receive this injection or be directed to his own general practitioner.

Sometimes **antibiotic therapy** is required. An intramuscular injection of a long-acting broad spectrum antibiotic is administered after the wound is sutured and arrangement for completion of the course made with the patient's own doctor.

Observation of the patient's general condition during treatment is important. Irrespective of how brave patients wish to appear many cannot tolerate the general hospital casualty environment and fainting is a common reaction.

Some modern outpatient departments have a special hostess 'instruction to patient service', but where this is not available the nurse must substitute. The patient, or his parent in the case of a child, must know when and where further treatment is to be given. Some injuries require hospital outpatient supervision, e.g. fractures at a fracture clinic. Others require medical supervision which can be given by the patient's doctor at home. Although in general stitches are removed at 10 days, facial sutures are taken out earlier e.g. in 5-7 days; others, e.g. in the foot, may be left for 12-14 days. Wound infection is the obvious complication. The patient should be informed of the significance of throbbing pain, moisture, heat under a dressing or staining through it. Any of these features demands a medical check either by the patient's doctor or at a soft tissue clinic.

Outpatient Treatment Under General Anaesthesia

The manipulation of simple fractures and the treatment of more complicated lacerations require the administration of a short general anaesthetic. The patient will be admitted to a special pre-operative ward or area in the casualty department. Explanation of the reasons for admission and anaesthetic must be given both to inform and to reassure the patient. The written permission by the patient, or the parent in the case of a minor (under 18), is necessary for operation and anaesthetic. It must be ascertained that the next of kin is notified. A parent may wish to wait with his child over the period of operation. Arrangement for discharge is often made at this stage so that relatives wishing to leave the patient know when to return. **A patient should never be allowed out of hospital unaccompanied after a general anaesthetic.** An adequate **period of starvation** is arranged prior to the proposed time of operation. **Skin preparation** may be necessary before the administration of **premedication.** The casualty doctor obtains from the patient a short relevant **medical history.** The nurse will **test the urine** for the presence of abnormal constituents and record the **temperature, pulse** and **blood pressure. Care of personal belongings** is extremely important. These patients are unprepared for their hospitalisation and many may have large sums of money or other valuables in their possession. In some outpatient departments the modern railway 'luggage lock-up' system is used which affords an efficient method of safekeeping. The locker should be carefully marked with the name of the patient and his hospital number. Dentures can be placed in containers and stored with the individual's belongings. After operation the patient is received in a recovery area or ward and supervised until he has completely recovered from the effects of the anaesthetic. It is always advisable to have the discharge of the patient approved by a member of the operation team.

Instructions should be given to the patient and his guardian regarding the immediate post-operative care. Where **plaster** has been applied he must be told to protect it until dry and keep that limb elevated for 24-48 hours. Instruction in **maintenance of joint function** and the discarding of supporting slings etc. should be given to the patient on discharge. He should also be cautioned about the **development of circulatory problems,** e.g. blue discolouration of the extremities, coldness, numbness, or pain under the plaster. The patient should cover the extremity with a glove or sock and raise his limb higher for a short period. Unless there is a marked improvement in half-an-hour he should be seen by his own doctor or return to the outpatient department immediately for the necessary plaster adjustment. **All patients with newly applied plaster casts should be given an appointment routinely to attend the fracture clinic on the**

following day and have the plaster checked. Subsequent appointments are then arranged to assess progress until treatment is complete. Where the nature of the operation has been soft tissue repair these patients are required to attend a soft tissue clinic for further care and treatment. Each patient is issued with a clearly completed appointment card on which it is also helpful to have written detailed post-operative instructions.

RECEPTION, RESUSCITATION AND DIAGNOSIS

Patients with major multiple injuries are the immediate responsibility of the accident team on duty. They are received on to a special trolley which can be tilted in any direction. It can, if necessary, be used as an operating table. The patient is often in a **serious state of shock.** The preliminary precaution of receiving him on to a special trolley avoids the necessity of his later transfer to a bed or operating table, which may produce aggravation of an existing critical condition. The trolley is also designed to accommodate equipment for resuscitation. It contains a casement fitting to take **X-ray** cassettes and a **drip stand to support bottles of intravenous fluid.** A space is provided to contain **apparatus for oxygen administration,** i.e. a Polymask or Edinburgh mask. A charged **oxygen cylinder** with mask and tubing, a spare cylinder and valve keys should be near at hand. **Breathing apparatus,** i.e. an AMBU resuscitator and mouthpiece or mask is available on the trolley should assisted ventilation be required. A portable AMBU **suction pump** and disposable catheters are also an essential part of the resuscitative apparatus. Additional **equipment for intubation** should be available, i.e. **laryngoscope,** a selection of **endotracheal tubes, a syringe for inflating the cuff, pressure forceps** to clamp the inflated cuff and a **standard adaptor** to allow the endotracheal tubes to be attached to other equipment, e.g. a ventilation machine. A **mouth gag,** a selection of **airways** including mouth-to-mouth airways, **swabs** and a **lubricant** are also required. A variety of **syringes** and **needles** should be available.

In modern hospitals patients with major injuries are admitted directly to the intensive therapy area of the accident unit. Otherwise they must be monitored closely in a specially equipped resuscitation area which in some hospitals is attached to the casualty department. The reception area should be at **theatre temperature** level so that the patient can be completely exposed for detailed examination.

First aid is given either at the site of the accident or in the ambulance. Once the patient arrives in hospital intensive resuscitative measures are commenced immediately by trained staff using modern hospital equipment and technique. **Treatment at this stage is no longer first aid but definitive.**

The efficient management of the 3 B's (Breathing, Bleeding and Breaks) is vital to the survival of the patient.

Breathing

This must be unobstructed or the patient will die. The **airway is cleared** of any blood or secretions using readily available suction apparatus. The **tongue must be pulled forward,** the patient nursed with his **head to one side** and, if necessary, an airway inserted. Any cyanosis or irregular noisy breathing indicates respiratory impairment which may necessitate intubation and oxygen administration.

Cardiac and Respiratory Collapse. When a patient is admitted in this state it is often impossible to ascertain the length of time he has been pulseless and apnoeic. **Immediate life-giving measures** are necessary. The **airway** must first of all be sucked **clear of secretions,** the patient quickly **intubated** and **artificial respiration** commenced using the AMBU **manual respirator.** At the same time **external cardiac massage** is necessary to stimulate heart action. The ratio of cardiac massage to respiration rate is 3 : 1. Once the patient shows signs of survival he is then quickly **attached to a pre-set ventilating machine** to assist his breathing and to allow for further investigations to be carried out. There is often an urgent need for **drug stimulants** e.g. adrenaline and calcium chloride. Sometimes **electro–cardiac stimulation** is required to restart the heart action or, if the heart is acting abnormally, to correct the rhythm by electric shock, i.e. **defibrillation.** Initially the **cardiac function** must be **monitored** closely by a special machine as there is always the immediate possibility of further cardiac arrest. Other injuries, no matter how serious, are of secondary importance at this stage. **Arterial puncture** is done to find out the state of the oxygenation of the blood. **Sodium bicarbonate** is administered where there is **acidosis** associated with hypoventilation of the patient during the period of cardiac and respiratory failure. Once cardiac and respiratory function is restored these patients require skilled continuous special medical supervision and nursing care in an **intensive therapy unit** for a preliminary period prior to their general management in an intensive care area of the accident unit.

Bleeding

While the patient is in a state of severe shock bleeding will not necessarily be a major problem. Blood must be obtained for **emergency cross-matching.** Temporary **supportive fluid** is given by venepuncture or, where necessary, by **intravenous** 'cut-down' in order to raise the blood pressure. The fluid used is one with a high molecular weight which minimises the escape of fluid into the tissues, e.g. Macrodex. As soon as whole blood is available it is substituted. Frequent **recordings of the pulse** and **blood pressure** are made and charted to assess the state of shock. A **fluid balance chart** is essential to record accurately oral and intravenous fluid replacement and fluid loss by urine, vomit and suction. Bleeding from open wounds is controlled by a **simple pad and bandage** or **by an inflatable splint. Obvious bleeding points** can be **occluded by artery forceps** until the patient is fit for more definitive treatment.

Breaks

Fractures may be simple or compound, single or multiple, minor or major. They may be associated with dislocation of joints. **Temporary immobilisation** of fractures by **sand-bags** or **by inflatable splints** is often the simplest means of relieving discomfort until the patient is fit for fracture treatment under general anaesthesia. It is unwise, purely as a first aid measure prior to resuscitation, to subject a patient to any procedure which is painful so aggravating the degree of shock present, e.g. application of a Thomas's splint in fracture of the femur. All fractures are treated as soon as the patient is sufficiently resuscitated to allow for an anaesthetic to be given. **The principles of fracture treatment may require modification because of other injuries.**

Dislocated joints greatly aggravate shock. If the patient is not fully conscious simple dislocations are often easily and quickly reduced, and this may alleviate shock. Reduction of a dislocated hip, however, cannot be attempted until the patient is fully relaxed under general anaesthesia. Early reduction is necessary or the patient's state of shock will not improve significantly.

Examination for Other Injuries

The **skull** is examined for bruises or wounds indicating head injury. The presence of a fracture is generally confirmed by X-ray examination. The **neck** should also be examined radiologically. Assessment of the level of consciousness is made and charted. The **ears and nose** are inspected for bleeding or for leakage of cerebrospinal fluid. **Pupils** are examined and reflexes tested together with the **patient's response to sensory stimuli.** Regular **blood pressure** and **pulse** records indicate also the severity of the head injury.

Chest. Abnormal irregular breathing after the airway has been cleared may indicate chest injury. Respiration may be painful in the conscious patient. On inspiration **lung expansion** may be absent on one or both sides of the chest. X-ray will show **fractured ribs.** Lung collapse can be due to **haemothorax** or **pneumothorax.**

Oral and Maxillo-facial Injuries. As well as other injuries there may be fractures of the facial bones. These can occur in one or other of the following sites or sometimes in a combination of two or three of them; the **mandible,** the **zygomata** (cheek bones), the **maxillae** or the **nasal bones.** The last three sites constitute what is termed the middle third of face. An oral or maxillo-facial surgeon conducts the treatment and management of these injuries.

Spinal Injuries. The conscious patient may be obviously **paraplegic** or **quadriplegic.** The level and degree of cord or nerve root damage is ascertained by the testing of reflexes and sensation. X-ray examination will reveal **fractures** or **fracture dislocation.**

Obviously the longer a paralysed patient is left immobile the sooner skin sores develop. The nursing techniques used in changing such a patient's position adequately and safely must be adopted early.

Abdominal injuries. Bruising of the abdominal wall, particularly in association with **shock in excess** of that expected from the obvious injuries, may indicate damage to abdominal viscera, e.g. **spleen, liver, kidney** or **bowel.**

Pelvic Injuries. Fractures of the pelvis **increase shock** because of the severity of pain and the extent of blood loss. This is always considered when calculating fluid replacement. Assessment of **urethral and bladder neck damage** is important. **Bruising of the perineum, oedema of the tissues** by extravasated urine, **bleeding from the external urethral meatus, haematuria** or the **inability of the patient to void urine** are all important observations. The risk of further complication by infection associated with catheterisation is not usually taken at this early stage. It is often delayed and done later if necessary under aseptic conditions. **Displaced fracture** of the posterior wall of the pelvis may **damage the origins of the sciatic nerve** resulting in **a drop-foot lesion** or total sciatic palsy.

Fractures of Limbs. These require treatment as early as possible to relieve pain and to avoid later complications. Initially they are probably among the least significant of injuries in a patient with other severe and multiple injuries.

Degloving Injuries. Extensive skin loss from a limb can occur following an accident in which a pneumatic tyre runs over the limb. This is termed a degloving injury. The skin is stripped off the limb in much the same way as one strips off a glove, turning it inside out. The injury usually includes damage to bone or joint.

TREATMENT AND NURSING MANAGEMENT

During the early stages of treatment the patient is nursed in a specially-equipped intensive care area. Intelligent basic nursing care is the main principle of treatment. A patient should not be left unobserved. The conscious patient requires a lot of comfort and reassurance as he is usually extremely anxious. Children with multiple injuries are particularly frightened of dying or losing a limb. The nurse with a calm confidence can often allay their fears and help them to accept the necessary treatment. The knowledge that one or both parents are in the vicinity often gives the child added confidence and encouragement.

The initial observations include maintenance of an unobstructed airway. Suction may be required to keep the **air passages free from secretions,** particularly if the patient is unconscious. Sterile disposable catheters are used, each once only. The patient should be positioned with his head to one side in order to encourage the drainage of secretions from the mouth. **Temperature, pulse, respiration** and **blood pressure** must be recorded frequently as this is a positive means of establishing whether or not the patient's condition is improving. **A record of fluid intake and output** must be kept accurately. Intake includes all fluids administered whether orally, via naso-gastric tube or intravenously; output consists of the total fluid loss in the form of urine, vomit, suction or blood drainage. The patient should be watched carefully for signs of reaction to **blood transfusion.** The early signs may be an elevation in temperature, rapid pulse and flushing of the skin, perhaps with accompanying rigor. The labels on each bottle of blood administered must be carefully checked with the name of the patient, if known, and his hospital number. The time of administration and dosage of all **drugs** is entered carefully on a drug therapy chart. Although the relief of pain is essential to reduce shock the selection and administration of analgesic drugs is carefully regulated by the medical staff so that important symptoms and signs of injury are not masked.

Fracture Care
The principles of fracture treatment, i.e. reduction and immobilisation, are followed as closely as the condition of the patient permits. Some modifications may be necessary. For example, a fracture which would normally be treated conservatively may be fixed internally because of other fractures either in the same limb or other limbs. In addition it makes nursing procedures less distressing for the patient and management easier for the nurses in their attempt to avoid any further complications, e.g. skin sores. The nursing management will involve care of splintage, plaster immobilisation or internal fixation (*see pp.* 159, 168, 192).

Head Injuries
When a patient has sustained a head injury serious enough to justify his admission to hospital **close observation,** particularly in children, is most important. **Dramatic changes can occur within a short space of time.** The following table (*p.* 142) gives a guide to the main patterns of change that are recognisable in the management of head injuries.

Special Observations in the Care of Head Injuries. Undue **restlessness** is often an early sign of increasing intra-cranial pressure. As well as frequent records of **temperature, pulse, respiration** and **blood-pressure** a special chart must be kept and details recorded of the **level of consciousness,** the size of the **pupils** and their reaction to light. Consciousness is classified into four levels:

1 Fully conscious
2 Response to simple commands
3 Response to painful stimuli
4 Lack of response to any stimulus, i.e. unconsciousness

These special observations are entered at 10–15 minute intervals until the patient has recovered **full consciousness with all parameters normal.** In this way the problem of the lucid interval is overcome. **Any change from the previous assessment** must be reported immediately to a doctor as well as being entered in the chart. A patient's condition may alter so significantly within minutes that death can be imminent unless there is immediate surgical intervention to relieve the compression of the brain. This is a neurosurgical emergency procedure.

Where a patient is admitted with a severe head injury and there is a steady deterioration in his condition, an intravenous infusion of **Mannitol** 20 g in 100 ml sterile water may be given as a temporary measure prior to neurosurgery. Mannitol is an invert sugar which does not participate in sugar metabolism and exerts its effect by its osmotic action. Fluid is withdrawn from the tissues, including the brain, and excreted in a considerable diuresis. It is imperative to have the patient catheterised previously with an in-dwelling catheter and closed drainage system.

RECOGNISED PATTERNS IN HEAD INJURY

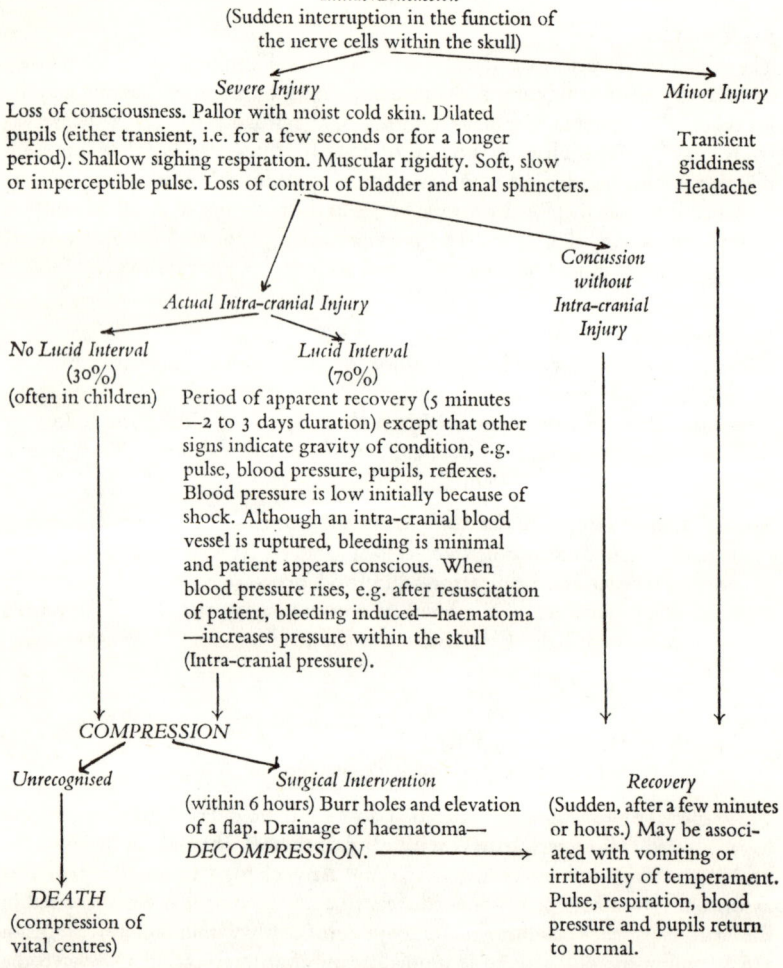

Initial Concussion
(Sudden interruption in the function of
the nerve cells within the skull)

Severe Injury   *Minor Injury*
Loss of consciousness. Pallor with moist cold skin. Dilated
pupils (either transient, i.e. for a few seconds or for a longer   Transient
period). Shallow sighing respiration. Muscular rigidity. Soft, slow   giddiness
or imperceptible pulse. Loss of control of bladder and anal sphincters.   Headache

Concussion
without
Actual Intra-cranial Injury   *Intra-cranial*
                                                       Injury

No Lucid Interval   *Lucid Interval*
(30%)   (70%)
(often in children)   Period of apparent recovery (5 minutes
                      —2 to 3 days duration) except that other
                      signs indicate gravity of condition, e.g.
                      pulse, blood pressure, pupils, reflexes.
                      Blood pressure is low initially because of
                      shock. Although an intra-cranial blood
                      vessel is ruptured, bleeding is minimal
                      and patient appears conscious. When
                      blood pressure rises, e.g. after resuscitation
                      of patient, bleeding induced—haematoma
                      —increases pressure within the skull
                      (Intra-cranial pressure).

COMPRESSION

Unrecognised   *Surgical Intervention*   *Recovery*
                      (within 6 hours) Burr holes and elevation   (Sudden, after a few minutes
                      of a flap. Drainage of haematoma—   or hours.) May be associ-
                      DECOMPRESSION. ——————→   ated with vomiting or
                                                                  irritability of temperament.
DEATH   Pulse, respiration, blood
(compression of   pressure and pupils return
vital centres)   to normal.

The limiting factor in the use of this agent is the dehydration it produces. The
infusion therefore is rarely repeated, but if it is considered necessary to do so, six
hours must elapse between each infusion and the total period should not extend
beyond 36–48 hours.

Chest Injuries

Where a lung is partially or completely collapsed by air or blood **chest drainage**
is required immediately. In **pneumothorax** air rises to the upper chest; con-

sequently a fine catheter is inserted into the third intercostal space. In **haemo-thorax,** blood gravitates to the lower chest and is more viscous so a wider gauge drain is inserted into the eighth or ninth intercostal space. In each case the **chest drain** is connected to a **closed simple water seal drainage system** (*Fig. 32a*). This is a modified syphon system which maintains a constant negative pressure in

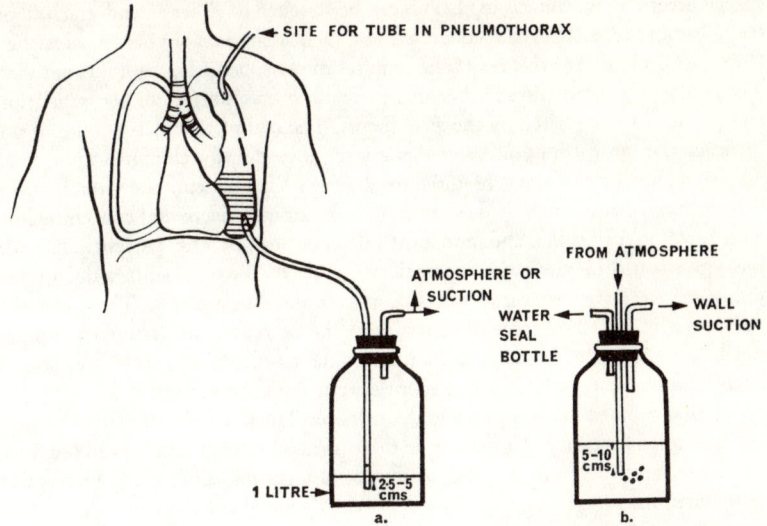

← SITE FOR TUBE IN PNEUMOTHORAX

ATMOSPHERE OR
↑ SUCTION

FROM ATMOSPHERE

WATER ←
SEAL
BOTTLE

→ WALL
SUCTION

1 LITRE →   2·5–5
cms

5–10
cms

a.   b.

FIG. 32 (*a*) Closed simple water seal drainage system
(*b*) Wangensteen system for suction drainage

the pleural cavity allowing the contents to drain off and the lung to expand. The chest tube must be 'milked' frequently to keep the blood draining freely and avoid blockage. A close watch must be kept on the level of fluid in the under-water tube in the bottle; the level fluctuates with each respiration. Electric con-tinuous suction at very low pressure may be attached using the **Wangensteen valve drainage** system (*Fig. 32b*) which avoids direct suction being applied to the pleural cavity.

Adequate **analgesia** is essential to control pain. This allows intensive chest **physiotherapy** to be carried out and makes expectoration easier. Good colour, regular unassisted breathing, the ability of the patient to cough effectively and a generalised relaxation of his behaviour indicate satisfactory progress. If the chest X-ray film is also satisfactory the drainage tube is clamped for a trial period prior to removal. The entry wound into the chest cavity must be completely sealed with an occlusive waterproof dressing.

Disturbances in the blood gases produced by the lung contusion require the patient to have continuous controlled **oxygen therapy** via a face mask until the results become normal.

Close constant observation of the patient is essential. Cyanosis, pallor, confusion, excessive perspiration, noisy breathing, restlessness and the inability to cough sputum all indicate respiratory difficulty which demands immediate attention. Should ventilation via an oral tracheal airway be unsuccessful, **tracheostomy** may be necessary with perhaps assisted artificial ventilation.

Assisted Breathing in Chest Injuries. Where artificial ventilation is required a special breathing machine is used. This can be attached to either an endotracheal or tracheostomy tube. The main concern is that the patient does not become detached from his machine. For this reason he requires direct supervision 24 hours per day. The machine is automatic and the rate of respiration, volume of air per inspiration and pressure are regulated by the anaesthetist. The complete understanding of the intricacies of this form of intensive therapy requires special training. A nurse need not panic, however, if she is required to observe such a patient. She should ignore the machine about which she has no knowledge or experience and concentrate on basic nursing principles and **constant observation of the patient.** The **air passage should be cleared of secretions** regularly. Two nurses or a doctor and nurse are necessary to carry out this procedure satisfactorily. The patient is momentarily detached from the machine; the secretions are removed using a sterile catheter attached to a suction machine regulated at gentle pressure. A sterile disposable polythene glove worn during the procedure is an added aseptic precaution as infection must be avoided. **Prophylactic antibiotic therapy** may be considered necessary. The patient in this distressed state should be well **sedated;** the nurse must therefore watch carefully for any complicating signs. **Ineffective ventilation** is soon recognised by the patient's general cyanotic or pallid appearance, his rapid pulse and obvious perspiration.

Clearing of the air passages by suction may cause a tracheostomy tube to slip. The air inspired is then directed into one bronchus and only one lung is ventilated. It is a useful practice for a nurse to be able to listen over the lungs with a stethoscope and hear air entering both lungs each time after the airway has been cleared. Thus **absence of air entry into one lung** can be detected. The worst, but most unlikely, catastrophe that can happen is for a machine to fail. Time cannot be lost tracing a fault. If a nurse acts immediately and intelligently the patient need not be in any real danger. **There must always be an alternative method of ventilation readily accessible.** There is insufficient time available to plug in and set another machine. Manual artificial respiration can be quickly established using an **AMBU resuscitation bag** which has a standard fitment for attachment to all tracheostomy and endotracheal tubes. The respiratory rhythm must correspond to normal respiration. As long as the emergency has been dealt with expeditiously the patient will survive. Once the breathing rhythm is controlled the nurse, if acting alone, can summon help by whatever alarm system has been organised for this purpose.

Oral and Facio-maxillary Injuries

Different techniques are used in the treatment of each type of fracture. There are also various nursing procedures carried out in each case.

Fracture of the Mandible. If the mandible is stable and undisplaced, fixation may be unnecessary. A jaw bandage may be applied for temporary support only. Soft diet and analgesics are prescribed. In **displaced fractures** where there is mobility, tenderness, swelling and bruising, some means of fixation is necessary and is maintained for four to six weeks depending on the age of the patient, the site of the fracture and the amount of displacement. Fixation methods are based on securing the teeth together in the position in which they normally occlude (**inter-maxillary fixation**). Most of these procedures are done in theatre with the patient under general anaesthesia. The methods include: (a) **interdental eyelet wiring,** (b) special bars wired to the teeth and to each other, i.e. **arch bar wiring,** (c) **cast cap splints** made from impressions taken of the patient's dentition and later cemented to the teeth. Wires or elastic bands are passed round hooks on the opposing splints thus connecting the jaws together.

When teeth are absent intermaxillary fixation is obtained by using **Gunning splints** which resemble dentures without teeth. These splints are wired to the mandible and maxilla before being wired together.

Intermaxillary fixation may be supplemented by direct wiring of the bone fragments either through an incision made inside the mouth or through the skin of the neck. The fracture is exposed and the bone ends have holes drilled in adjacent sites. After reduction of the fracture, wire is passed through these holes and is tied firmly thus maintaining the reduction. Sometimes a special **bone plate** is **screwed** to the reduced bone ends in which case intermaxillary fixation may be unnecessary. A pressure bandage applied to the external incision sites may help reduce post-operative swelling of the area.

Where the patient's jaws are wired or fixed together he cannot open his mouth and thus presents special nursing problems. He should therefore be nursed **prone with his head to one side.** This allows for **secretions to drain from the mouth.** Gentle suction can be applied to the mouth to remove blood or mucus which may have collected. It is preferable that as soon as his condition permits, the patient should be nursed sitting up. **Suction apparatus** and **wire cutters** must be available at the bedside. The patient may vomit and with his jaws fixed together could easily inhale the vomitus. In this event it may not be possible to clear the mouth with suction, so the rubber bands or wires fixing the jaws must be cut to allow the free passage of vomitus from the mouth. Routine oral hygiene is essential. As the patient is unable to masticate his food because the jaws are immobilised the normal salivary cleansing of the mouth will not take place. He is also unable to clean his teeth in the usual way. The nurse must therefore **irrigate the patient's mouth** briskly every four hours using a dental syringe or Higginson's syringe and a 1 per cent solution of sodium bicarbonate and glycothymoline. (1½ teaspoonfuls to 500 ml of water = 1% solution.) The solution should be as hot as the patient can tolerate comfortably. The **syringe nozzle should be put at the back of the mouth** so that the water jet is directed forwards over the teeth or splints thus washing debris out of the mouth into the receiving bowl. **Vaseline should be applied to the lips** to prevent them from becoming dry and cracked. The

splints should be **cleaned gently** each day with a **soft toothbrush.** As soon as the post-anaesthetic period is over the patient is given a **high protein fluid diet.** This is fed to him initially in a feeding cup but with a little practice the patient can suck through a straw. It is advisable to chart the fluid intake in order to make sure his diet is supplying adequate nourishment.

The oral surgeon will examine the patient daily to check the position of the jaws and to ensure that he is not having any discomfort from the splints. Once there is evidence that the fracture is uniting he can be discharged and attend the hospital as an outpatient. The wires or splints are normally left in position for four to six weeks. They are removed under local anaesthesia in the outpatient department.

Fracture of the Zygoma (Cheek bone). Surgery is indicated when a patient complains of infra-orbital anaesthesia, trismus or diplopia, or when on examination there is obvious flattening of the cheek prominence. Under general anaesthesia the **displaced zygomatic fragment is elevated back into position** using a special elevator. The fracture is approached through a skin incision in the temporal region. Once reduced this fracture should be stable. If unstable, **1 in. (2.5 cm) ribbon gauze** soaked in Whithead's varnish may be packed **into the antrum** to retain stability. Sufficient packing is inserted to maintain the orbital floor at the correct level and to push out the flattened cheek prominence. The packing is removed in 10–14 days. The end of the ribbon gauze is left protruding into the mouth to facilitate its removal. **Intermaxillary wiring** may also be used to immobilise a fractured zygoma. The method used is similar to that described in the treatment of fracture of the mandible. The wires are left buried permanently.

Patients who have sustained a fracture of the zygoma usually have a 'black eye' and localised swelling of the soft tissues. **Bathing the eyes with saline** every four hours helps to reduce the oedema. The patient is given a **soft diet** and **mouthwashes four-hourly** if an antral pack has been inserted. For the first 48 hours following elevation of a fractured zygoma a firm pressure bandage is applied round the head to prevent a haematoma developing under the suture line. Great care should be taken to **avoid direct pressure over the cheek prominence after operation as this may lead to redisplacement.** Skin sutures are taken out in 5–7 days.

Fracture of the Maxilla. The maxilla and associated parts of the facial skeleton may be fractured at several levels separating the 'middle third' of the face from the rest of the skull. The maxilla may be pushed backwards into the nasopharynx, causing airway obstruction, forcing the mandible open and preventing the teeth from meeting in the front of the mouth. The cheek bones, orbital walls and nasal bones are often involved at the same time. The **displaced bony complex** must be **reduced using special maxillary disimpaction forceps** and restored to its proper relationship to the skull above. The reduced complex must then be fixed to the cranium, i.e. **craniomaxillary fixation.** Finally, in order to be sure that the teeth are properly related to each other in both jaws, **intermaxillary fixation** is also applied. Splints are usually used, and the upper splint carries a projecting bar which protrudes from the mouth and is attached to the cranium by a plaster headcap, by a halo frame or by supra-orbital bone pins. Metal rods with special connecting joints are used to attach the projecting bar to the halo, headcap or pins.

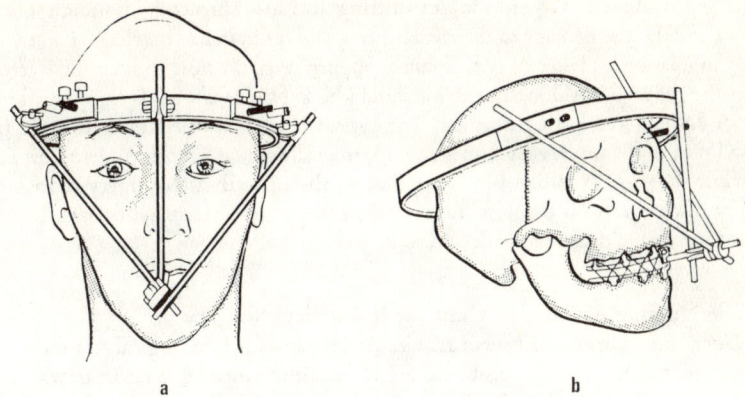

FIG. 33   (a) Craniomaxillary fixation ('Halo' frame)
(b) Oblique view of skull showing (a) combined with intermaxillary fixation

(*Fig. 33a and b.*) All pin entry sites must be kept clean and sprayed with an anti-biotic mixture three times a day. When a halo is used a small rolled towel provides a comfortable support for the nape of the neck when the patient wants to rest his head. Other methods of craniomaxillary fixation employ wires passed through the tissues in the cheek; these connect the splinted teeth below to the cranium above.

The surgeon **checks the joints of the splintage** daily to see that they are kept tight. If the nurse notices that one or both joints have worked loose, she must notify the oral surgeon. This is important because the resultant mobility of the joint leads to displacement of the fracture. The nursing care is similar to that of fracture of the mandible. If the rod projecting from the mouth rests on the upper lip thus liable to cause pressure, it requires readjustment and the surgeon should be informed. **Oral hygiene** is again very important. A **high protein fluid diet** is given.

Where there are fractures of the 'middle third', the nurse must also check specifically for leakage of **cerebro-spinal fluid from the nostrils** and report at once should this occur. It signifies a dural tear. The fluid is water clear and the volume is sometimes increased by dropping the head forward. As there is always a risk of meningitis it is imperative that **prophylactic chemotherapeutic drugs** are given.

Fracture of the Nasal Bones. In a fracture of the nasal bones, there is often deviation of the septum or collapse of the nasal bones with associated soft tissue injury to the nasal mucosa. The fracture will require to be reduced by manipulation of the nasal bones under general anaesthesia. Following this, **tulle gras packing** is inserted into both nostrils to help maintain the correct position and prevent the occurrence or recurrence of a haematoma. This is left in position for 48 hours. The nurse should remove the packing carefully to prevent **epistaxis** occurring. The patient is advised to **avoid violent sniffing and sneezing** with his mouth shut as this could cause damage to the nasal mucosa and result in haemorrhage. Following manipulation a plaster of Paris splint is applied over the nose to hold the fracture in the reduced position. The splint should be kept on for one week, thereafter it can be removed during daytime. The patient is advised to continue wearing the splint at night to prevent damage to the nose should he happen to lie on his face while sleeping. **A gauze bib is applied to the nostrils** after surgery to soak up any discharge from the nose. Initially the bib should be changed frequently and, as soon as the discharge ceases it can be removed altogether.

The Nursing of Patients Unfit for Immediate Surgery

When, on admission, a patient requires resuscitation before surgical treatment can be undertaken the main problems are the **maintenance of a clear airway** and the **control of haemorrhage.** Respiratory distress can be due to oedema of the tongue or due to its falling backwards as in a fracture of the mandible. In this case a suture may be passed through the tongue. Pressure forceps are applied to the ends of the suture to **pull the tongue forwards.** Haemorrhage can occur in fractures of the maxilla with bleeding into the pharynx. Wherever possible the patient is nursed in the **prone position with his head to one side.** This facilitates the drainage of blood from the mouth and allows the tongue to fall forwards. Routine **oral hygiene** is carried out and the mouth kept as clean as possible. If the patient has severe respiratory impairment **tracheostomy** will be performed. Where soft tissue injuries have been sutured, the **suture lines should be cleaned with 'cotton buds' and Cetavlon 1 per cent or Normal Saline every 4 hours.**

Degloving Injuries

Sometimes it is possible to suture the degloved skin back into position. The skin must be viable. If it has been completely sheared off the limb it will have lost its blood supply and will be non-viable. Before replacing and suturing skin which is viable it has to be suitably cleaned and any fat removed. If additional skin is required to cover the limb, **split skin grafts** can be taken from other limbs or from the abdomen. These grafts are either sutured into position or laid on the area of skin loss and covered by a pressure dressing.

Skin grafts normally require about five days to 'take'. The dressing is then removed and the area cleaned up. The **donor area dressing** should be left undisturbed for 10-14 days by which time it should separate easily. On no account should the nurse pull off the dressing forcibly as this will damage the granulating surface and cause haemorrhage in the area. If after 14 days the dressing has not separated spontaneously it should be soaked off. The best method to do this, provided the patient is fit, is in a warm bath.

Where the area of skin loss is extensive it may be necessary to apply skin grafts in several stages.

While the graft is 'taking', the patient is kept on complete **bed-rest** especially if the degloved area is on a lower limb. When he is fit enough to be allowed up a **firm supporting bandage,** i.e. Bisgaard, should be applied to the lower limb. This is applied before the patient actually gets out of bed and is removed once he is back in bed.

Care of the Unconscious Patient
Such a patient is completely dependent on the nurse to keep him alive as he is totally incapable of any voluntary movement. She is therefore responsible for maintaining a **clear airway, feeding** him, **changing his position, caring for his skin,** attending to **bladder** and **bowel function** and assisting with passive **physiotherapy.**

If there is any tendency to vomit a **naso-gastric tube** is passed and the stomach contents aspirated. A deeply unconscious patient without a cough reflex must have a naso-gastric tube in position.

The patient should be nursed on alternate sides to allow drainage of secretions from the air passages and also allow equal lung expansion. His skin must be kept clean, dry and powdered, his bed free from wrinkles and crumbs and his position changed at least every two hours.

Water-proof backed disposable hip sheets are useful to collect any faeces, although during the first day or two bowel movement is not usually a problem. However, if consciousness is not restored within 2–3 days, an enema will be necessary to evacuate the bowel.

A **urethral catheter** is inserted with a closed system of drainage to drain the bladder. This gives an accurate measurement of the urine passed and also keeps the patient's skin dry and less liable to the development of sores. The skin round the external urinary meatus must be cleaned daily with an antiseptic solution and the catheter changed about every successive third day until consciousness and bladder control is regained.

At first the patient is given **intravenous fluids** or blood transfusion to replace quickly the fluid lost as a result of his injuries. If his state of unconsciousness continues he requires to be fed with more **calorific foodstuffs** which can be given through the naso-gastric tube. The tube should be cleared after each feed by passing some water through it. It is changed completely every second day and inserted through the other nostril to try and prevent excoriation of the skin and mucus membranes. **Vaseline or lanolin** will help **protect the nostril. Care of the mouth** is essential as salivation is diminished because of lack of mastication. Accurate records of the patient's dietary **intake and fluid output** must be kept to ensure that the necessary daily requirements are being fulfilled. Supplementary **vitamins,** are important additives to the daily diet.

Prophylactic antibiotics are sometimes given. Regular specimens of urine, and sputum if any, should be sent for bacteriological examination so that **infection** can be recognised and treated early.

Passive exercises of all the limbs are easily remembered if done routinely with each **change of the patient's position.**

Care of the Paralysed Patient

This patient is also largely dependent on the aid of the nursing staff to meet not only his physical needs but also to help him psychologically. Hemiplegia, paraplegia or quadriplegia are the main clinical pictures of paralysis.

Paralysed patients are more successfully nursed on a **turning bed** which alters their position from the supine to the prone alternately. Thorough **care of the skin** in the paralysed areas is essential as sensory perception is absent and the patient cannot feel discomfort such as crumbs in the bed. The paralysed limbs may be positioned on soft foam pillows rather than allowed to rest on a firm bed. Plaster of Paris is not used where there is absence of sensation. **Maintenance of joint function** is necessary and passive movements of the joints through their total range must be done frequently to avoid contractures.

Retention of urine is often a hazard which, if untreated, may lead to cystitis. **Catheterisation** using a strict aseptic technique is usually required with closed bladder drainage until the patient can be taught how to control the rhythm of emptying the bladder. **Constipation** is another problem requiring enemata to empty the bowel. Later a similar pattern of controlled bowel evacuation can be developed. **Haematuria,** often indicating renal stones, is not uncommon and patients should be encouraged to drink as much as possible, a minimum of $1\frac{1}{2}$ **litres of fluid per day.** A 'pint' of lager or stout, given occasionally, is often a pleasant effective means of producing a diuresis as well as being a mild appetite stimulant. **Bacteriological examination of the urine** should be done frequently and **antibiotic therapy** given when necessary.

There are many facilities available nowadays which help the disabled to regain a degree of independence. The nursing staff and medical social worker can co-operate in helping them to benefit from these. The medical social worker is often the patient's main support in this situation as she can help tremendously in the organisation of rehabilitation, and resettlement where possible.

Internal Abdominal and Pelvic Injuries

These are often associated with severe multiple injuries. Extreme **restlessness** is sometimes an early sign. The **blood pressure fails to rise** even with intravenous replacement therapy. The **pulse is rapid and feeble.** The **abdomen may be distended and rigid** due to guarding muscle spasm with the presence of blood or urine in the abdominal or pelvic cavity. The organs commonly damaged are the **spleen, bladder, bowel and liver.** A severe back injury may involve damage to one or both kidneys with resultant renal failure. This must, therefore, always be considered a possible cause for **failing urinary output,** particularly if there is haematuria.

Injury to the lower spine or pelvis may cause interference with the function of the autonomic nervous system. Paralysis of the sympathetic nerves results in smooth muscle paralysis, loss of peristalsis and dilatation of the small bowel, i.e. **paralytic ileus.** It is recognised by recurrent or persistent vomiting, often in small amounts, the inability to pass flatus, distension of the abdomen, absence of bowel sounds on auscultation and the general effects of dehydration. This must be regarded as an acute emergency. A **naso-gastric tube** must be inserted immediately and the contents of the small bowel aspirated by continuous gentle **suction.** At the same time the **intravenous administration of fluid** is important to correct dehydration. There is usually a deficiency in the electrolytic balance. The type of fluid given is controlled by daily estimation of the blood electrolytes. An accurate record of all oral and intravenous fluid, together with fluid loss by urine and suction, is of great value in determining progress. After the emergency has been relieved and there are obvious signs of recovery, i.e. lack of aspirate and the return of bowel sounds, the patient is gradually weaned on to small amounts of oral fluids. The naso-gastric tube can then be removed and when the oral fluid intake is adequate the intravenous administration of fluids can be discontinued. The patient thereafter progresses from light to normal diet.

CASUALTY ARRANGEMENTS FOLLOWING A MAJOR DISASTER

In the event of a major disaster all central accident units within the area will be involved in the first aid management, casualty treatment and definitive accident surgery of the injured. All accident units, therefore, have a prepared programme of action in anticipation of such an emergency. The following paragraphs outline briefly the way in which a hospital might adapt to meet such a situation.

The matron's office is notified by the accident registrar that the police or ambulance service have informed him of a major disaster. Two or more nurses with casualty experience are seconded to stand by.

All accident medical staff are contacted in their homes by the receiving accident consultant. He decides whether or not to send an initial team to the disaster site. The team includes at least one accident surgical registrar, one anaesthetic registrar and two or more casualty nurses. Travel to the site is by ambulance.

The nurses and doctors must be familiar with the accident equipment. This consists of plasma (and substitutes), emergency pack, which contains all materials necessary for the administration of intravenous fluids and the dressing of wounds, and emergency anaesthetic equipment. The emergency accident equipment is checked monthly.

The duties of the initial team are the assessment of injuries (severity and numbers), resuscitation and primary treatment (3 B's, *see p.* 137) and the relaying of information to the receiving accident consultant surgeon at the base hospital.

The matron's office will be in liaison with the medical superintendent and accident consultant surgeon. Through them the matron will be in contact with the accident site, all medical and non-medical staff on duty and those 'standing by'. X-ray, blood transfusion, biochemistry and kitchen staff will be alerted by the telephonist. Additional clerical staff will be allocated by the records officer. Communications are maintained between the hospital and accident site by the police.

Reception of the injured is into the casualty department which is used as a clearing station and assessment area. Major cases are transferred to the accident unit and intensive therapy area, and minor ones into the casualty wards. The number of nursing and medical staff will be varied as required by the duty nursing superintendent and accident consultant.

Documentation must be closely supervised by the nursing staff, especially if there are several unconscious patients. Numbered and named wrist bands will be attached to all patients. If the name is unknown the admission number will be used for identity and emergency blood sample labels will bear the same number. This admission number will also be used to identify blood which has been cross-matched.

Resuscitation will be carried out in this area under the supervision of the accident surgeon and anaesthetist, in close liaison with the nursing staff. The accident theatre and other emergency theatres as required are opened and manned by nursing staff and orderlies 24 hours a day until the emergency is under control.

The medical superintendent or hospital secretary is responsible for co-ordinating the service. In liaison with the matron he ensures the availability of beds. If necessary relatively mobile and other suitable patients are transferred to temporary accommodation elsewhere within the hospital. He arranges also for extra porters to move patients and beds; he advises the catering officer of the total number of extra patients and hospital personnel requiring food. Co-operation with the press is essential but to avoid confusion all enquiries should be directed to the medical superintendent's office where official information is available.

PART II

Basic Orthopaedic Nursing Techniques and Rehabilitation

19 TRACTION METHODS AND PLASTER OF PARIS TECHNIQUES

TRACTION METHODS

Skin traction is a method of applying an indirect pull to a particular part of the skeleton. In **skeletal traction** the force is acting directly on an appropriate part of the skeleton. The mechanism may be a **fixed** or **sliding** (balanced/continuous) force. Irrespective of which part of the body is being treated in traction or which mechanism is used, the same basic principles of nursing care can be applied.

Requirements for the Application of Traction in Fractures of the Femur

1 For **skin preparation:**
   Warm water in a basin, soap in a dish, a razor, cotton wool swabs, a towel and disposal bag.
2 Tincture of Benzoin compound aerosol spray.
3 Scissors, a needle and thread and safety pins.
4 A tape measure.
5 A Thomas's splint (a metal splint with a padded ring covered by pigskin).
6 Cotton slings made from cotton strips 6–8 in. (15–20 cm) wide and 12–14 in. (30–35 cm) long.

7 **Skin traction requirements:**
   (a) Extension adhesive plaster (one-way transverse stretch to accommodate the circumference of the leg but which does not yield longitudinally) made up as roller bandages. For convenience these may be prepared with a length of strong twill or lampwick stitched into the free end ready for use when required.
   (b) A spreader bar and extension cord.
   (c) Non-adhesive orthopaedic felt and 4–6 in. (10–15 cm) roller bandages (crêpe or domette).

or

A complete pre-packed skin traction kit. This contains two lengths of adhesive extension strapping already joined by a wooden spreader bar. The lower ends of the strapping and the spreader are lined with foam rubber to give protection to the malleoli. From the spreader there is a cord extension for attachment to the splint or weights. A weak elastic bandage is included to encircle the area of strapping thus holding it in position.

8 **Skeletal traction requirements:**
A sterile pack containing gauze swabs, drapes, a selection of Steinmann pins, an introducer, scalpel and forceps. Antiseptic lotions to cleanse the skin.
9 A Balkan bed-frame, cross bars, pulleys and extension cord.
10 Bed elevator, weights and weight carriers.
11 Böhler's stirrup and outer pin guards.
12 Knee flexion piece.
13 $\frac{1}{2}$ in. (1.25 cm) zinc oxide tape.

The Application of a Thomas's Splint

The application of a splint in the treatment of fractures of the femur is done by the surgeon and his assistant. The assistant controls any tendency for the limb to rotate by grasping the heel and foot and exerting manual traction. **The ring of the splint must correspond accurately to the measurement of the circumference of the patient's thigh.** This measurement is taken at the level of the line joining the ischial tuberosity and the greater trochanter. The splint must also be **long enough** to allow **free movement of the foot.**

The correct size of splint is then slipped on to the leg and the ring is pushed into position where it rests at the level of the ischial tuberosity and against the soft tissues of the groin. The skin under the ring is eased backwards and forwards to confirm that it is not too tight. A sling is made by doubling a cotton strip over the inner bar of the splint; holding the two free ends together the doubled layer is then brought under the limb and over the outer bar where it is folded back on itself and pinned in position. **Three or four slings may be necessary** for each splint to support a limb. The slings are always **pinned on the outer side** where they are easily accessible for adjustment. In order to form one continuous platform **the adjacent slings are pinned together** with one curved pin. When pinned separately they tend to slide apart allowing that area of the limb to sag. It is important to prevent the proximal sling from slipping as this will cause alteration in the position of all the others. This can be simply done by attaching a tag of $\frac{1}{2}$ in. (1.25 cm) zinc oxide adhesive tape to the outer bar of the splint immediately below the ring. The **position of the proximal sling** is maintained by fastening the first pin through both it and the tag (*see Fig. 25*). Canvas or perhaps plaster of Paris supports may be used in preference to cotton slings. A **knee flexion piece** may be added to the splint to support the limb in such a position that the knee is slightly flexed.

The Application of Skeletal Traction

This is a **sterile procedure** requiring a theatre or sterile dressings room technique. Where a fracture is stable or if displacement is minimal it may be permissible for the Thomas's splint and traction to be applied under light premedication combined with local anaesthesia for the insertion of the Steinmann pin. In the majority of patients who are generally fit it is kinder to do this procedure under light general anaesthesia.

Method. The area is draped with sterile towels. The surgeon's assistant maintains traction on the limb keeping it clear of the sterile area. At the level of the tibial tuberosity the leg is cleansed with antiseptic lotion and a small cruciate incision is made in the skin to allow entry of the pin. It is usually inserted from the medial side and as it appears under the skin on the lateral side of the leg a second cruciate incision is made through which it emerges. The points of entry and exit are sprayed with plastic skin dressing. An outer pin guard is slipped over the pin on either side to avoid injury to the patient's other leg or to anyone handling the splint.

In **fixed skeletal traction** (*Fig. 34b*) a length of extension cord is attached to either side of the pin, the free ends being fixed to the U-piece of the Thomas's splint. To prevent excoriation of the skin at the points of entry and exit of the pin, inner pin guards (of metal or sorbo-rubber) may be interposed between the skin and the extension cord. Alternatively a Böhler's stirrup of the correct size to thread over the protruding ends of the pin is fitted. Fixed traction is effected by extending a length of cord from the loop of the stirrup to the U-piece of the splint. A knee flexion piece is attached to the Thomas's splint which allows the

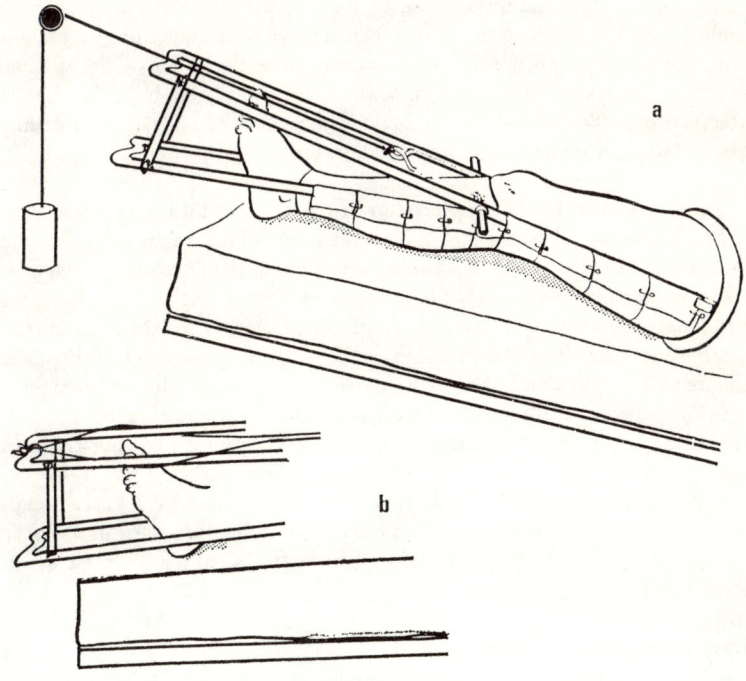

FIG. 34   (*a*) Sliding skeletal traction
(*b*) Fixed skeletal traction

knee to be flexed sufficiently to lower the foot below the line of the extension cord.

In **sliding skeletal traction** (*Fig. 34a*) a Böhler's stirrup and knee flexion piece are essential. The extension cord from the loop of the stirrup passes over a pulley system towards the end of the bed where a weight carrier supporting the necessary weights is attached. The weight is estimated provisionally by the surgeon according to the degree of traction he considers necessary. The **foot of the bed** is then **elevated** so that the patient's tendency to slide in the direction of incline acts as the counter traction.

The Application of Skin Traction

This is a procedure which is often done in the ward except when it is applied after reduction of a fracture under general anaesthesia in theatre. While an assistant controls the limb the skin is washed, shaved and dried. The spraying of Tincture of Benzoin compound on to the skin overcomes its natural oiliness and allows for close adhesion of the strapping. The ankle is encircled by a strip of $\frac{1}{2}$ in. (1.25 cm) thickness non-adhesive orthopaedic felt 2–3 in. (5–7 cm) wide, to protect the skin over the malleoli from pressure and friction.

The lengths of skin extension strapping are applied one on each side of the limb from a point above the malleoli to the level of the fracture; the inner strip is applied slightly anterior to the medial malleolus while the outer one lies posterior to the lateral malleolus. Small oblique slits made at the edges of the strapping at various levels allow it to conform to the contour of the limb. Wrinkles in the strapping must be avoided. To maintain its position and adhesion to the skin a crêpe bandage is applied from the ankle upwards.

Important Points in the Application of Fixed and Sliding Traction

In **fixed traction** a Thomas's splint is essential. In **sliding traction,** the bed must be elevated so that the patient's tendency to slide in the direction of incline acts as the counter-force to the pull of the weights. A Thomas's splint is usually applied but is only an accessory to provide comfortable support for the limb. In fixed traction the wicks from the strapping or the cords from each end of the skeletal pin are pulled tightly and fixed to the U-piece of the splint. The tendency for the limb to rotate externally in the splint is controlled by the method of application of the strapping already described and the **special system of tying the cords** (*see Fig. 25*).

In sliding skin traction the wick from each adhesive strap is buckled through a spreader bar. An extension cord from the centre of the bar is then passed over a pulley at the foot of the bed and a carrier bearing the calculated weight is attached (*see Fig. 26*).

Suspension of the Thomas's Splint

The aim is to give the patient more freedom of movement and to facilitate certain nursing procedures, e.g. straightening or changing a drawsheet. The splinted limb, whether in fixed or sliding skin or skeletal traction, is treated as one unit.

The additional cords and pulleys used in its suspension neither interfere with this unit nor influence the type and function of the traction mechanism.

There are various methods of suspending a splint although only two methods are described here. The splint may be suspended using either a complete or partial balance system.

Complete suspension of the splint requires four individual cords, pulleys and weights (*Fig. 35a*). These are fixed two on each side of the splint, one proximally and the other distally. The free ends of the four cords are led over a pulley system to the foot of the bed where the necessary weights are attached in order to suspend the splint. This fully balanced system is only suitable for suspension of a limb in fixed traction.

As rotational movement of the splint is restricted by a **partially balanced system** it is a more convenient method of suspension where the limb is in sliding traction (*Fig. 35b*). The distal end of the splint is elevated 3–4 in. (7–10 cm) off the bed so that the patient's heel is free from pressure. This is done by tying each end of a length of cord about 20 in. (50 cm) to either side of the distal end of the splint thus forming a loop. From the centre of this loop a cord is extended over a pulley system beyond the foot of the bed and sufficient weight is attached to suspend the end of the splint at the required height. A similar suspension system using longer cords is assembled at the proximal end of the splint. Its function is to counterbalance the weight of the limb in the splint as the patient lifts his buttocks off the bed.

Nursing Management of a Patient in Traction

Daily observation is necessary to make sure that the **traction** is **functional.** The **splint must be in position** against the area of the ischial tuberosity and the surrounding soft tissues, particularly in fixed traction. All **knots on the extension cords must be secure** and these are better taped with ½ in. (1.25 cm) zinc oxide plaster. **Weights** must not be resting on any part of the bed but should remain **freely suspended.** The Balkan frame and beam should be checked to make sure that **all nuts and bolts are tight** so preventing collapse of any part of the framework. Extension cords must be examined for areas of friction, e.g. where they pass over pulleys; **frayed cords** are replaced where necessary. Where a nurse is in doubt or where the frayed extension cord is an integral part of the traction mechanism, she should then inform the doctor who will carry out the replacement. If skin traction is used the overlying crêpe bandage should be removed occasionally and the **skin strapping examined to make sure it has not slipped.** The skin is also inspected carefully for any signs of **skin reaction.** Where a **Steinmann pin** has been inserted its points of entry and exit should be examined daily for signs of **inflammatory reaction.** If any discharge is present it must be reported to the doctor immediately and a swab of the discharge sent to the bacteriology department for culture. Where a Böhler's stirrup is attached to the pin the screws holding it in position should be checked and tightened when necessary.

If the patient is uncomfortable and slides upwards or downwards in bed the

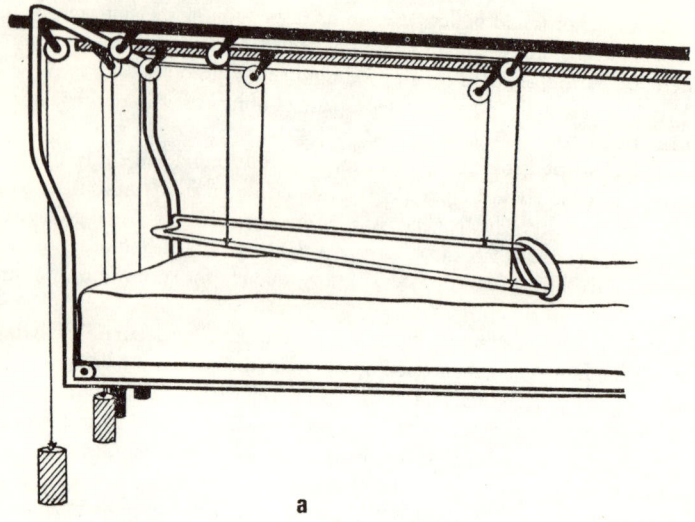

a

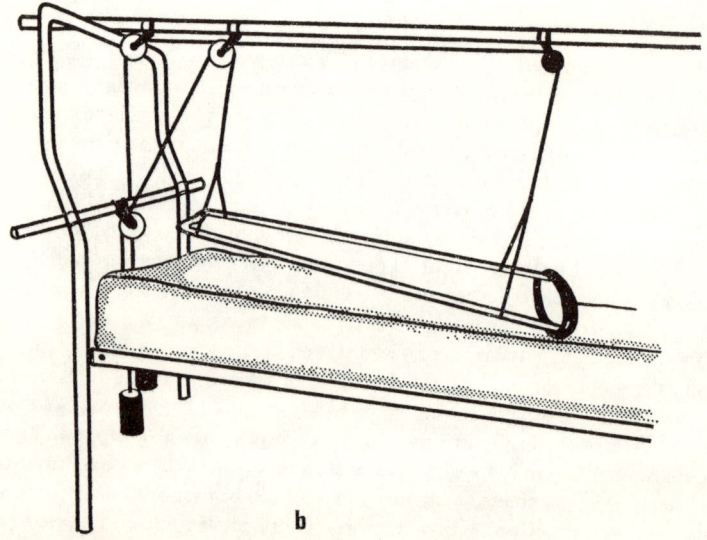

b

FIG. 35   Suspension of a Thomas's splint
(a) Complete suspension
(b) Partial suspension

weights are not **correctly balanced** and will require some adjustment. Re-adjustment of the traction weight may also be required where X-ray shows inadequate reduction of the fracture. Movement of the patient's bed must be done with care so that the weights do not swing about freely and possibly interfere with the function of the traction.

Where **movement of the pin** occurs, or at the first suggestion of any inflammatory reaction, it is **removed** and is **reinserted more distally,** e.g. through the lower end of tibia. It is not inserted proximally as the infection may subsequently travel up to infect this track as well. If the fracture is uniting the pin may be removed completely and skin traction applied for the remainder of the period of immobilisation.

Particular care of the limb in traction is important. Initially when there is considerable swelling of the limb **observations** should be made at least **four-hourly.** The **skin under the ring of the splint** must be inspected carefully so that pressure sores are prevented. It should be manipulated in the direction of the abdomen on one inspection and towards the toes on the next. A sprinkling of talcum powder helps to keep the skin dry and less likely to stick to the splint, especially while the limb is swollen.

During the regular nursing care of the limb it is important to **encourage the patient to do the exercises** taught to him by the physiotherapist, particularly toe, foot and ankle movements and later quadriceps and knee flexion exercises. Any **inability to dorsiflex the foot** should be mentioned immediately to the doctor.

The **slings** should be examined and if they are too tight the tension must be altered in order to avoid damage to the skin and underlying structures. Those which are most likely to cause trouble are the proximal sling under the thigh, the sling immediately behind the knee and the sling under the ankle.

If the ring of the Thomas's splint is causing **pressure on the skin in the groin** prompt attention is necessary or a sore will rapidly develop. In sliding traction pressure in the groin is easily relieved by moving the splint about 5 cm out of the region. The splint is only a means of supportive immobilisation in this instance. In fixed traction where the splint is part of the traction mechanism any attempt to remove it from the groin renders the traction ineffective. The solution therefore is to convert the mechanism to sliding traction temporarily and to angle the suspension cords away from the patient so that the ring will be directed away from the groin. Once the skin has healed fixed traction may be restored.

When a patient is lying in traction dry or **hard skin** tends to develop on the foot of the exposed limb. Obviously the patient cannot attend to this himself so routinely, once or twice weekly, it is the nurse's responsibility to inspect the feet and remove any hard skin using oil if necessary. Toenails should also be trimmed and sometimes **chiropody** is required.

Care of the patient in general is essential. At the four-hourly inspection of the limb the patient's draw-sheet should be pulled through and any crumbs or other debris removed. At first three nurses will be required to assist the patient;

two to help lift him and one to pull through the draw-sheet. Once the patient recovers he is often able to lift himself by grasping a patient helper device attached to the bed. He will also need similar assistance to manoeuvre himself on and off a bed-pan. After the patient has used a bed-pan the **skin** must be left clean, dry and well-powdered. The patient should be bed-bathed daily. **Hair washing** is done when necessary. Women in general are usually grateful for this service. Morale may be further improved where there is a hairstylist service available.

Splints are left on for varying lengths of time depending on: the age of the patient; the type of fracture; its normal healing period. **Removal of splintage** will depend on the clinical and radiological assessment of the fracture by the surgeon. Because of the danger of osteomyelitis a Steinmann pin if used is usually removed at 6 weeks. If skeletal traction is still required the pin is resited more distally. However, by this time the fracture is often stable and skeletal traction unnecessary; further immobilisation is continued in fixed skin traction.

During the period of immobilisation it is essential to maintain the general well-being of the patient. **Diet** should contain ample protein, vitamins and calcium to allow for tissue repair and new bone formation. Fats and carbohydrates are controlled to avoid obesity, which is undesirable particularly when the patient becomes ambulant. Sufficient roughage should be included in the diet to stimulate bowel function which becomes sluggish because of the immobilisation of the patient. An **adequate fluid intake** of 3–6 pints ($1\frac{1}{2}$–3 litres) daily is extremely important to maintain urinary tract function. General **maintenance physiotherapy** is essential to avoid stiffness of joints and weakness of muscles outwith the immobilisation.

The **length of treatment varies.** Where it is prolonged it is only natural that some patients will become depressed and perhaps difficult. This should be anticipated where possible and some means sought to occupy their time; perhaps an **occupational therapist** can help in the solution of such problems. Many patients, because of the long period of time away from home and work, have social and financial difficulties. This is often a matter which can be rectified easily after discussion with the **medical social worker.** The nurse gets to know the nature and individual interests of her patients, and by tactful grouping can often create a very pleasant atmosphere in the ward.

Complications of Traction Immobilisation

(a) **In relation to the fracture treatment: Non-union** of the fracture can be the result of excessive traction for a prolonged period of time. **Mal-union** can be caused either by ineffective traction and inadequate check X-rays, or by a badly fitting splint, e.g. one becoming too loose after the swelling subsides.

(b) **In relation to traction apparatus: Pressure** from splints and slings is not uncommon in the initial treatment, and if unrelieved can lead to **skin sores** which may involve underlying structures, e.g. the tendo Achillis. Pressure on the lateral popliteal nerve predisposes to **drop-foot deformity. Skin reactions** to adhesive plaster may necessitate substitution by a sorbo-rubber, non-adhesive extension strapping. In skeletal traction, **infection in the pin track** resulting in osteomyelitis is a serious complication. **Chronic oedema** can occur due to badly placed pads and tight bandages.

(c) **In relation to the general care of the patient: Bed sores** will result if there is inadequate care of the skin. Immobilisation of the patient in bed can predispose to constipation, **urinary stasis** and **infection,** and if immobilisation is prolonged, **renal calculi** can also develop. **Stiffness** of previously supple joints can occur due to inadequate physiotherapy. In the elderly in particular, **chest infection,** e.g. hypostatic pneumonia, and **deep venous thrombosis** are often complications. Deep venous thrombosis may develop quickly if, for example, supporting pads are badly placed, particularly those which rest immediately behind the knee in fractures of the lower end of the femur.

PLASTER OF PARIS TECHNIQUES

Plaster Room Requirements
1 A mobile metal trolley with a metal or glass surface.
2 In the drawers of the trolley:
   (i) A selection of bandages, i.e. plaster, orthopaedic wool and conforming gauze bandages.
   (ii) Orthopaedic felt and stockinette or tube gauze.
   (iii) A tape measure for measuring slabs.
   (iv) Böhler's plaster scissors, plaster knives, shears, spreaders and evertors.
   (v) Black wax pencil for marking plaster casts.
   (vi) Assorted wedges, cork or wood, for the correction of angulation of fractures.
3 Waterproof aprons, rubber gloves and boots.
4 Mackintoshes and newspapers to protect both the patient and his surroundings.
5 A pail filled with tepid water, which is held in a special fitment at the side of the trolley.
6 A fulcrum or wedge support for the limb.
7 Flat waterproof pillows.
8 Rubber walking heels, and Böhler's walking irons.
9 An oscillating electric plaster saw.

Explanation to the Patient
In a conscious patient it is important to give a preliminary explanation of the routine involved in plaster application and other relevant information:
1 The reason for its application.
2 The way in which the patient will be positioned and how the plaster will be applied.
3 The approximate period of immobilisation and the activities permitted.
4 The extent of the plaster and the restriction of movement produced.

Positioning of the Patient

The position of the patient is of special importance in the correct application of a plaster cast. The first essential is that the patient must be **relaxed.** Where the muscles are relaxed the outline of the limb is regular and smooth and a close-fitting plaster is easily applied. If the patient is tense the plaster cast is applied over contracted muscles; when he relaxes his muscles the plaster will no longer conform to the contour of the limb and is therefore less efficient. The patient may either lie comfortably in the supine position which is convenient for the application of most plasters, or sit at ease in a chair, e.g. in the application of some upper limb plasters. **An assistant is required to support the weight of the limb** and maintain it in the correct position by holding either the fingers or toes. The patient should not be asked to hold his own limb in the elevated position because in so doing his muscles will be contracted. On completion of the plaster it is helpful to mark with a wax pencil the position of wounds, the condition or procedure carried out and the date of application. This provides useful information for those carrying out the ward management.

Points to Note about Individual Plaster Casts

Upper Limb. A long arm plaster extends from below the axilla to the mid-palmar crease. It is applied with the forearm at right angles to the upper arm. The hand is mid-way between pronation and supination, and abduction and adduction. It is slightly dorsiflexed to allow for the normal function of the fingers. A forearm, or a short arm, plaster extends from below the elbow to the mid-palmar crease. In this plaster it should be possible to flex the elbow to 90 degrees.

Special fractures of the upper limb necessitate certain plaster modifications. A **Colles' plaster** (*Fig. 36a*) is a modification of a short arm plaster. The hand instead of being in the neutral position is in pronation, is palmar flexed and slightly deviated to the ulnar side. A **scaphoid plaster** (*Fig. 36b*) is another modification of the short arm plaster. The hand is slightly dorsiflexed and radially deviated. The space between the index finger and the thumb should be sufficient to accommodate a small tumbler. In addition the thumb is incorporated as far as the interphalangeal joint.

Lower Limb. A below-knee plaster (*Fig. 37a*) and long leg plaster (*Fig. 37b*) both extend to the metatarsal arch. The leg should be held midway between external and internal rotation. The knee, in a long leg plaster, is supported in about 5–10 degrees of flexion in order to prevent tension on the posterior capsule of the knee joint. The foot is in the neutral position, i.e. at right angles to the leg, and midway between inversion and eversion. The great toe lies in the same vertical plane as the patella.

Plaster Jackets. A full length plaster jacket (*Fig. 37c*) extends from the sternal notch to the symphysis pubis. Shorter plaster jackets extending to just below the nipple line are commonly used in the treatment of low back pain. These provide sufficient immobilisation of the lumbosacral spine and relieve the patient of the

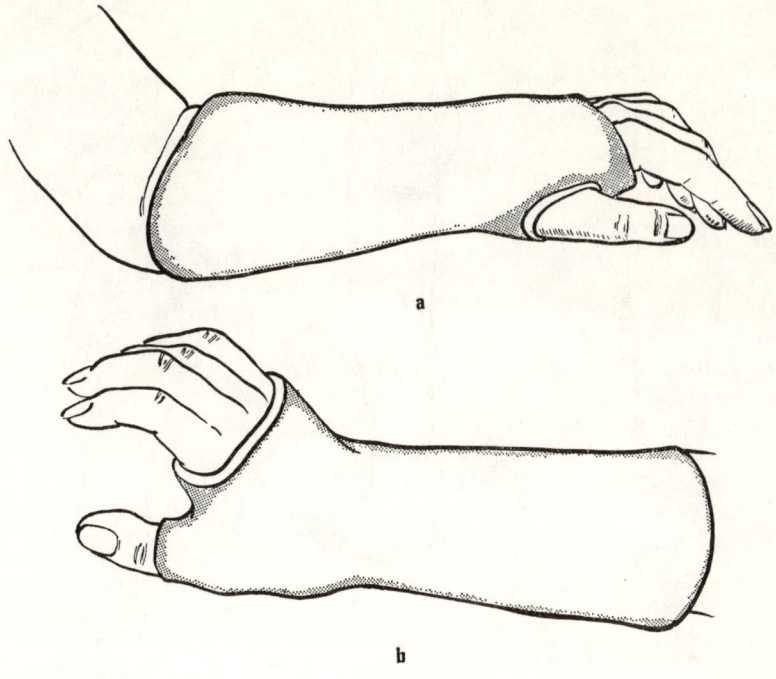

FIG. 36 (*a*) Colles' plaster
(*b*) Scaphoid plaster

weight of excess plaster. The patient stands erect with the shoulders held back and down; the spine is kept straight; the abdomen is held in; the body weight is evenly distributed on both legs which should be slightly apart.

Hip Spica. There are several varieties. A **single hip spica** (*Fig. 37d*) can incorporate either the full length of the limb (long leg spica) or the leg to just above the knee (short leg spica). A **double hip spica** may include the full length of both legs, the combination of a long and a short extension or two short leg extensions.

It is most important that the patient should be given an **enema** a few hours before the application of a hip spica for two reasons:

   1 that the patient's bowels do not act until the plaster is completely dry;
   2 to prevent a 'pseudo-ileus' where the bowel is full of faeces and gas ('meteorism').

The patient is supported on an **orthopaedic table** in the supine position. Tilting of the pelvis is avoided by making certain that the iliac crests are in the same horizontal plane. Support for the shoulders is necessary but at the same time the lower trunk must be kept free to just above the nipple line which is the upper

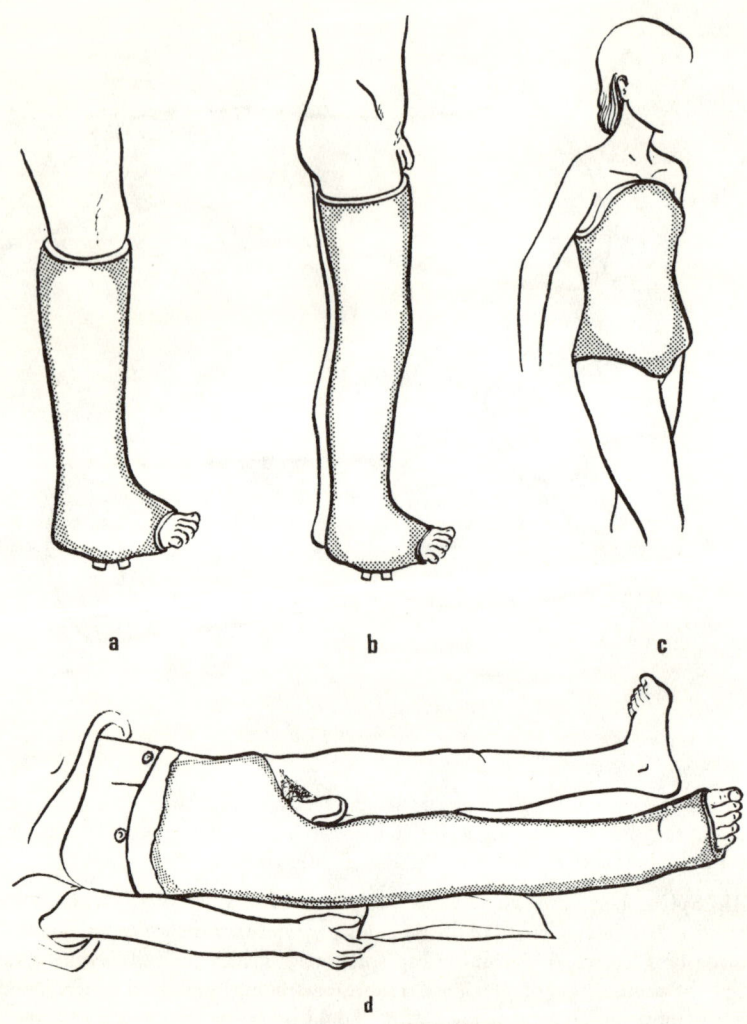

a   b   c

d

FIG. 37   (a) Below-knee plaster
          (b) Long leg plaster
          (c) Plaster jacket
          (d) Hip spica

border of the spica. The patient's arms must also be supported away from the trunk, e.g. resting behind his head. If one leg is to be incorporated it is abducted about 5–10 degrees and held in the same position used in the application of a long leg plaster. Where both legs are to be immobilised the unaffected leg should be abducted sufficiently to allow the patient to use a bed-pan easily.

Shoulder Spica. This is virtually a plaster jacket with a long arm extension. The hand is held at the level of the mouth and in a similar position to that used in the application of a scaphoid plaster. The elbow is supported at a right angle a little below shoulder level and in front of the chest.

Minerva Plaster. This is a plaster jacket with a head extension. The head is held erect and central over the midline of the body. The plaster extension supports the head at the chin and occiput.

The Application of a Plaster Cast

The limb is positioned and supported by an assistant. It is washed and dried, and shaved if necessary. **Orthopaedic felt** may be applied to encompass bony prominences and so prevent pressure on them from the plaster, particularly in a thin patient. The correct size of **orthopaedic wool bandage** is selected and applied smoothly to the limb. Any wrinkles will be reproduced subsequently in the plaster in the form of hard ridges and must be avoided. As an alternative to the application of felt in the protection of bony protruberances extra turns of cotton wool bandage may be substituted. Where the bones are particularly conspicuous a combination of both felt and wool is more practical. If the plaster is required to be close-fitting, and swelling is not a problem, the wool bandage may be replaced by **stockinette or tube gauze.** Nevertheless the bony prominences are always protected with felt or orthopaedic wool before application of the plaster.

Plaster slabs are made and applied either as a means of holding the position of fragments of a fracture during the application of the plaster bandages or as a means of strengthening a plaster cast. Using a tape measure the patient's limb is measured to obtain the correct length of slab. A plaster bandage is folded back on itself to the required length about 4–5 times and cut. This slab is immersed in the tepid water until the bubbling ceases. It is then laid soaking wet on the top of the trolley and excess moisture is removed after which the slab is quickly moulded to the limb. In order to complete the plaster the correct size of bandage is selected and applied. Each bandage is unrolled for 3–4 in. (7–10 cm) so that there is a free end to grasp once it has been immersed in the **tepid water.** When the bubbling ceases the bandage is removed from the water and compressed at each end to remove some excess moisture. It is applied to the limb with **even pressure,** like any roller bandage **from below upwards covering one third of the previous width** at each circumference. As the plaster dries fairly quickly it is necessary that each bandage is **moulded to the limb** as it is being applied. **All wrinkles should be removed** and all air expelled to avoid the presence of ridges and indentations in the dry plaster cast. Before the cast becomes too hard it is convenient to **trim away any excess plaster** which would restrict movement, e.g. round the fingers and toes.

If this is a first plaster application following an injury or operation **it should be split but not sprung.** This is a safety measure. In the event of further swelling and possible vascular obstruction it is easily and quickly sprung in the ward without distressing the patient further.

If a limb is badly swollen a supporting plaster splint or slab may be applied in preference to a complete plaster. A slab is made as described earlier and moulded usually to the posterior contour of the limb. The surface of the limb not included in the plaster is padded and the splint is bandaged in position using a conforming bandage.

The Application of Special Plasters

Plaster Jackets. Two persons are required to apply a plaster jacket. The iliac crests, sacrum, costal margins and sternum must be carefully protected with orthopaedic wool or felt, or a combination of both. The plaster technician, using 6 in. (15 cm) bandages, encircles the trunk with plaster so holding the wool and felt in position. The plaster must be moulded carefully to the contours of the patient's body. Several 6–8 in. (15–20 cm) slabs are made and applied anteriorly and posteriorly to the trunk. These must also be made to conform to the shape of the trunk. The slabs are utilised to strengthen the plaster jacket and are held in position by circular plaster bandages which complete the plaster.

Hip Spicas. The body piece is constructed in the same manner as a plaster jacket and the leg piece in the same way as a long leg plaster. The weak part of a hip spica is at the hip because of the excess leverage at this point due to the weight of the plaster. As this can be anticipated the plaster should be strengthened by the application of longitudinal and oblique slabs extending from the body piece to the leg piece, anteriorly and posteriorly. Where a double hip spica is used it is essential to join the two legs together with a plaster bar so preventing individual movement of the limbs and weakness of the plaster at the hips.

Shoulder Spica. This is applied as a plaster jacket with a long arm extension· Sometimes the armpiece is supported by an oblique strut between it and the body piece. The areas which must be well padded are the iliac crests, the chest wall, particularly on the side of the arm extension, and the medial epicondyle of the humerus. The weight of the extra plaster on this side tends to cause the trunk part of the plaster to be pushed further against the skin of the chest wall. Inadequate protection of the skin predisposes to the rapid development of a plaster sore. The medial epicondyle of the humerus requires particular protection as the ulnar nerve is superficial at this point. If this point is neglected and pressure on the nerve occurs, ulnar nerve palsy may result.

Observation of a Patient in a Plaster Cast

After plaster application the **limb should be elevated** for the first few hours especially following operative treatment or trauma. Elevation is achieved using waterproof, flat, firm pillows.

All plasters should be exposed to the atmosphere while drying, and care taken that pressure on any one part of the wet plaster is avoided. The limb in plaster should be **positioned carefully** in bed by the nurse who also assists the patient by lifting this limb when necessary until he is accustomed to the weight of the plaster.

During the first 48 hour period of a newly-applied plaster the limb must be checked regularly. An easy way to remember the important observations is by the '5 P's'.

1 **Pain,** often 'throbbing' in nature and increasing in severity.
2 **Paraesthesia,** either 'burning', 'tingling' or extreme cold sensation.
3 **Pallor** of the skin in the extremities and gross swelling of fingers or toes.
4 **Pulse,** diminished or absent in the extremity of the affected limb.
5 **Power loss.** The patient is unable to move the associated fingers or toes.

The extent of injury or nature of operation will indicate the degree of tissue reaction to be anticipated. Where it is likely to be considerable, observation of the limb ½-hourly is necessary during this initial period. When any one, or a combination of one or more of these symptoms and signs is present, the following steps should be taken immediately.

1. The limb should be **elevated** on waterproof pillows. If already raised, further elevation is necessary, e.g. by raising the foot of the bed. It is important to make sure that the patient is not 'propped up' as this will defeat the effects of elevation of the limb.

2. The limb should then be **examined every fifteen minutes** for half to one hour and reassessment made of the degree of the patient's discomfort and condition of the fingers or toes. During this period the extremities should be covered with a glove or sock as their coldness may be associated with a damp exposed plaster.

3. **If there is no improvement immediate action is then necessary.** A mackintosh cover is placed under the limb. The patient is told that his plaster requires to be split in order to relieve his discomfort; he is reassured that the procedure is not painful. Using a saw or shears **the plaster is split throughout its length and thickness.** Any existing injury to the skin or the presence of an operation wound should be considered and the plaster split away from this area if possible. Once split, the plaster is 'sprung' or spread apart using spreaders. Any orthopaedic wool bandage or underlying dressings are then divided using Böhler's scissors until the **patient's skin is visible throughout the length of the plaster cast.**

Once the obstruction has been relieved the gap between the cut plaster edges is filled or packed lightly using orthopaedic wool to prevent blistering of the skin. A non-elastic bandage is applied to complete the splint until all swelling has subsided after which the bandage is removed and the plaster completed. The limb is elevated until the patient's symptoms are relieved. This procedure may aggravate the discomfort temporarily, particularly after a recent operation so that the patient will require an analgesic.

If a patient is unconscious and unable to relate his symptoms the nurse must observe the limb in plaster closely for signs of pressure or ischaemia. Splitting of a plaster in an unconscious patient must be done with the utmost care and only by one with experience in this procedure.

Indications of the Development of Plaster Sores. The following are examples of 'distress signals' which should be immediately investigated.

1 **Itching, tingling** or a **'burning'** sensation under the plaster.
2 Sometimes the patient describes the discomfort as similar to that of a **'stone in the shoe'.**
3 **Undue heat** in one specific area experienced by the patient and also elicited on palpation of the plaster.
4 A **rise in temperature** for no other apparent reason.

The actual development of a sore can be avoided if prompt action is taken. Where there is pain or an unpleasant sensation the nerve endings in the skin are still active. If these symptoms are ignored the nerve terminals are damaged due to the continued pressure after which **pain is absent.** The skin, nevertheless, can be grossly damaged. Later there is an associated offensive odour from the plaster and only after its removal is the extent of skin damage discovered. Immediately any symptoms and signs are present an **observation window** should be cut in the plaster over the area in which the discomfort is felt. The part of the plaster removed should be examined in an effort to diagnose the cause of the pressure. If the skin is undamaged a pad of orthopaedic wool corresponding to the size of the window is applied over it. The plaster 'lid' is replaced on top and is temporarily held in place by the application of a non-elastic bandage. If the discomfort is relieved by this method the bandage should be subsequently removed and the plaster completed.

Where a sore has developed there is a wound present which requires treatment using an **aseptic technique.** A preliminary swab of the exudate should be taken and sent to bacteriology for **culture and sensitivity.** If the patient's own resistance fails to deal with the infection the appropriate **antibiotic** can be given. The type of dressing used will depend on the condition of the wound. Daily wound attention may be required until it is sufficiently healed for a dry dressing to give sufficient protection. Thereafter a sterile pad of cotton wool is placed over the dressing and the plaster completed.

Discomfort under a plaster can cause irritability with loss of appetite in an adult and fretfulness or restlessness in a child, particularly at night. Rulers, pencils and knitting needles are examples of items often used by patients to relieve itching under a plaster. This practice should be discouraged as damage to the skin and the interior of the plaster can result in skin abrasions or sores. A plaster should be inspected routinely for **cracks or deficiencies.** These should be repaired, reinforced or if necessary a new plaster applied to retain function.

Patients in Plaster Jackets or Spicas. As an orthopaedic bed is firm and a hip spica is a hard cast it is necessary to **lay the patient on waterproof pillows** so that the plaster will be adequately supported. Thus the patient's heel is not subject to friction as it does not rest on the bed. Once the **anterior part** of the plaster has **dried sufficiently** the patient should be **turned into the prone position** to allow the **posterior part to be exposed** to the atmosphere. When the plaster is dry the **margins round the groin and buttocks** should be protected by several strips of a **waterproof adhesive plaster** or sprayed with a protective plastic coating in order to prevent soiling. It is important when assisting in the lifting of a patient in a hip spica to **support the whole length of the plaster cast.** The nurse sometimes tends to concentrate on supporting only the limb extension, which produces excessive strain on the cast at the hip so that it cracks or weakens at this point.

If a plaster jacket, hip or shoulder spica is too tight, it may be split down the side which does not include a limb extension. It is then sprung and the gap filled with orthopaedic wool. A non-elastic bandage is applied to complete the plaster temporarily. Sometimes such patients suffer **abdominal discomfort or distension** and may even show signs of **paralytic ileus.** In the event of such signs, a window is cut over the abdomen often giving rapid relief or a plaster jacket may be bivalved, i.e. split down both sides.

Observation should be made for skin allergy to plaster. If this occurs the plaster has to be removed and immobilisation effected by some other means, e.g. a Thomas's splint or a non-reactive plastic splint.

Removal of a Plaster Cast

The patient is made comfortable, either lying supine on a couch or bed or seated comfortably in a chair. The whole length of **the cast to be removed is supported on firm waterproof pillows.** The patient's clothing and his immediate environment should be protected by using mackintoshes and newspapers. When using plaster instruments it is important to assure the patient that proper care will be taken in their use to avoid injury, i.e. abrasions or cuts. If an **elecric saw** is used it is important to explain to the patient that it is a vibrating and not a cutting instrument and that its noise does not mean that it will cause injury. **Plaster shears** are so designed that one cutting blade has a flat under surface. When these shears are in use this flat surface rests against the underlying wool, tube gauze or skin, acting as a protection against injury. The handle attached to this blade should be kept still and the action done with the other, so preventing the points of the shears from digging into the tissues. Where further division of underlying wool padding is necessary in order to expose the limb, special **curved scissors** (**Böhler's**) are essential for the same reason.

Most plasters are removed by **bivalving.** The anterior or posterior shell may be used for further splintage should this be necessary. These should be retained after removal until clear instruction has been given that they are no longer required. Arm plasters are bivalved usually medially and laterally, care being taken to avoid the main bony prominences. Leg plasters are bivalved on either side, with the cutting curve at the ankle directed beneath the internal and above the external malleolus. Trunk plasters are bivalved, so forming two shells, one anterior and one posterior.

After removing the plaster it is important to **support the limb.** The muscles which have become inactive will require to be strengthened and stiff joints to be mobilised gradually by physiotherapy. **Sudden or excessive active or passive**

movement is extremely painful. If a plaster is no longer required the patient, if possible, should be helped into a **bath to cleanse the skin.** In order to control oedema a **supporting elastic bandage** may be applied to the lower limb from the **toes to below the knee before the patient gets up to stand.** In the upper limb a supporting bandage, if required after removal of plaster, must only be retained for a short time as a free range of movement of these joints is extremely important.

Orthopaedic theatre technique is in many ways similar to that of a general theatre. There is, for example, the same necessity for thorough cleansing of walls, floors and furniture. The basic instruments, their care and sterilisation are the same. The nurse accustomed to general surgery will, however, find herself confronted with an apparently bewildering array of additional instruments and appliances peculiar to orthopaedic surgery. Osteotomes, gouges, tenotomes, meniscectomy knives and other **sharp instruments should be inspected regularly and sharpened when necessary.** This includes scissors which are subjected to much wear and tear in bone surgery. Many instruments have handles, screws or hinges which can become stiff and rusty if not checked regularly. Instrument Lube has proved useful in preventing this, but **oiling** may be necessary.

Although the modern orthopaedic operating table (*Fig. 38*) can be used for any surgical procedure it is especially designed to support the patient in a suitable position for operations on the hip and the application of a hip spica. It has many adaptions and fitments in frequent use which require regular oiling.

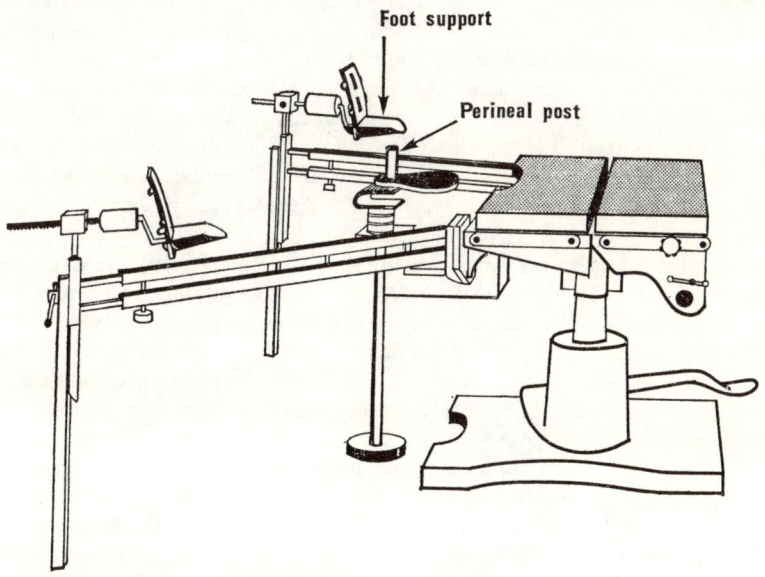

FIG. 38 An orthopaedic operating table

It is necessary to **maintain stocks of screws, nails, plates, prostheses, special sutures, etc.** according to the type of surgery performed. These are usually ordered specially and may take some weeks to obtain. A careful record of the level of stocks is therefore necessary. Methods of preparing and sterilising instruments again depend upon the facilities available. The **tray setting system** is ideal from the point of view of sterility and convenience. By having trays and additional instruments packed and sterilised beforehand it is possible to deal with emergencies at very short notice. It is sometimes thought that sharp instruments should not be autoclaved but rather immersed in a sterilising fluid. Such fluids evaporate, necessitating frequent 'topping up'. In practice therefore it has been found that the advantages of **autoclaving** outweigh the disadvantages provided that there are facilities for regular sharpening of instruments. Where equipment is prepacked any difficulty in teaching new staff is overcome by having a definite policy whereby nurses in training are present with more experienced staff when packing is being done. The accurate packing and labelling of instruments is vital to the smooth running of theatre.

Patients about to undergo elective surgery are usually prepared in a manner similar to that prior to general surgery. The specific skin preparation is now tending to be replaced by a more general skin hygiene, e.g. antiseptic baths, commenced as soon as the patient is admitted. This is followed in theatre by a more thorough local skin preparation.

In an accident unit the theatre and staff should be constantly prepared to deal with any emergency. It may be considered necessary to wear theatre dress throughout the working day in order to save time. The type of dress worn varies with each hospital. The rules are made according to the plan of the individual theatre. Some older hospitals are built in such a way that makes it difficult to have a dividing line between 'clean' and 'dirty' areas where theatre dress may be changed. Nevertheless, some sort of regulation can usually be made and should be strictly observed. It is inadvisable for staff on theatre duty to be involved in work elsewhere, e.g. the wards. Firstly, the risk of introducing infection into theatre is eliminated, and secondly, theatre is always staffed ready to deal with unexpected emergencies.

Multiple injuries may involve many specialties all requiring emergency treatment. The accident theatre must therefore be equipped to deal with such emergencies. Pre-packed autoclaved instrument kits should be available for craniotomy, chest aspiration and drainage and repair or removal of abdominal and pelvic viscera, e.g. splenectomy. A resuscitation trolley to provide an immediate means for treating cardiac arrest is, as in other theatres, an integral part of accident theatre equipment.

The reception of accident patients may present different problems. Sometimes a patient is brought directly into the theatre annexe without having been admitted to a ward. In other instances a patient may have received only the minimal preparation because of the difficulty in moving one who is already shocked and in severe pain. In these cases the patient may be fully or partly clothed and in possession of dentures, rings, watches or other valuables. He may have been given first-aid using blankets, pillows and appliances which do not belong to the hospital. The disposal of these articles then becomes the concern of the theatre staff. The patient's personal possessions should be checked and listed with the same care as when he is admitted to a ward because of the legal implications involved. Their ultimate disposal can usually be arranged with the ward sister who will be caring for the patient. Arrangement for the return of first-aid equipment will vary according to each hospital.

In some cases the patient will be dirty depending on the situation of the accident, e.g. a mining injury. Some preliminary skin cleansing by the theatre staff is then necessary before the skin preparation by the surgeon. It is useful to have basins of warm water ready containing antiseptic solutions (e.g. iodine preparations), plain swabs (not to be confused with those used during surgery which are X-ray detectable), a nail brush, a razor and towels. Cleaning is usually confined to the affected limb and is done after administration of the anaesthetic. Great care must be taken in handling the limb to ensure that the injury is not further complicated. Where there is an open wound, as in a compound fracture, shaving and scrubbing of the skin should be done in such a manner that dirt and hair do not enter the wound. The clean part is then dried and covered with a clean towel until the surgeon is ready.

Tourniquets

A tourniquet is a surgical means of stopping, by compression, the flow of blood through a blood vessel. The two tourniquets generally used in theatre are:

1 A 3 in. (7.5 cm) elasticated rubber bandage (Esmarch's)
2 A pneumatic cuff tourniquet

These are used to create a bloodless area for operations on the limbs in both orthopaedic and accident theatres. After the limb has been elevated for 1-2 minutes to allow blood to gravitate from the veins the Esmarch's rubber bandage is applied from the tips of the toes or fingers to the upper thigh or arm. The tension must be sufficient to occlude the arterial blood supply. The cuff tourniquet is applied immediately above the upper border of this bandage and inflated to just above the arterial pressure. This tourniquet has a gauge which indicates the pressure applied. In a leg, depending on the volume of soft tissue present, a pressure of up to 10 lbs (500 mm Hg) per square inch may be used although 7 lbs (350 mm Hg) per square inch is usually adequate. In an arm 5 lbs (250 mm Hg) per square inch is sufficient. Once the cuff is inflated, the Esmarch's bandage is removed and the limb lowered into position for operation.

The **time of application** must be written and displayed where it can be clearly seen in theatre. One member of the theatre staff should be delegated the duty of noting the tourniquet time and informing the surgeon when necessary after each half hour. If one hour has elapsed and surgery is incomplete, the length of time necessary to complete the operation should be estimated. It may be desirable to elevate the limb and have the tourniquet released for one minute. Some arterial bleeding will occur but in this way the dangers of ischaemia are avoided.

Sometimes it is desirable before the wound is closed to release the tourniquet in order to ligate or coagulate bleeding vessels by diathermy. This is especially important in amputation surgery. The circulation of the limb is checked immediately after completion of the operation by the surgeon, and the total time of tourniquet control noted in the patient's operation report for reference in the event of complications. If all tourniquets are kept in an obvious position in theatre it is easy to check the number present before and after the patient leaves theatre. In this way the danger of a patient returning to the ward with one still in position is avoided. Should a nurse see a patient being taken from theatre with a tourniquet still in place she should certainly make relevant enquiries immediately. It is most unlikely that it is being done intentionally.

Although a **swab count** may be considered unnecessary it is often a useful precaution for two reasons.

1 Many procedures are carried out without the use of a tourniquet. It is therefore necessary to ensure that all swabs from a previous operation have been removed from theatre. The most certain way to do this is to count them.
2 There are usually some inexperienced staff, under instruction, in theatre, especially in a teaching hospital. They should be taught the routine practice of counting swabs even in minor surgery so that this becomes automatic when major operations are in progress.

Contra-indications and Risks in the Use of Tourniquets. Where there is vascular disease, particularly with associated ischaemic changes in a limb, the use of a tourniquet is contra-indicated. Incorrect application of a tourniquet can produce complications such as deep venous thrombosis or nerve palsy (lateral popliteal and ulnar).

Tourniquet palsy is a condition which occurs where a tourniquet has been left unreleased in position for an excessive period. The patient complains of sensory upset, e.g. areas of paraesthesia (tingling or numbness) and motor weakness (loss of finger, toe, hand or foot movements). The peripheral circulation and pulse are usually satisfactory. The symptoms are due to deprivation of the tissues of blood during the period of tourniquet control. If this period were prolonged gangrene would result.

The Pre-operative Period

Pre-operative preparation for all patients is basically similar. On admission the patient should be asked specifically if he has suffered from any ailment, however minor, which would contra-indicate surgery meantime, e.g. common cold, sore throat, dyspepsia, diarrhoea, etc. An inspection for recent cuts, abrasions, septic spots or skin rash is important. The presence of any nasal, aural, urethral or vaginal discharge will delay surgery until the cause has been treated.

After admission the **patient's fitness for operation is assessed** and discussed by both the surgeon and the anaesthetist. The nurse should note any treatment which has to be continued during the period of hospitalisation and perhaps altered over the operative period, e.g. digitalis, cortisone, insulin, antibiotic therapy, etc. Sometimes in the pre-operative period an observant nurse will detect other significant features, e.g. breathlessness, cough, oedema or incontinence. These will necessitate further investigation prior to surgery.

The patient will need to have a sample of **blood removed for cell count, haemoglobin** estimation, **grouping and cross-matching. Chest X-ray** and **electrocardiogram** are often necessary in determining the fitness of the patient for surgery.

Dietary adjustment, urine examination and **bowel evacuation** are all included in the pre-operative nursing management. **Skin cleansing** is important. Antiseptic baths twice daily, with particular attention to the areas between the toes, other flexor folds and the perineum, are essential to ensure that the skin is clean. Nails should be cut short. Any other specific preparation, e.g. **skin shaving,** may be considered necessary at this stage. On the other hand this may be accepted as part of theatre room preparation. The important fact to remember is that every possible effort must be made to avoid wound infection in orthopaedic operations as the resultant chronic osteomyelitis can be disastrous for the patient.

MENISCECTOMY

Meniscectomy is the removal of one of the semilunar cartilages in the knee joint. The patient is **usually a young man,** often a footballer, between 20–40 years of age. The operation is usually short and simple although this is dependent on the nature of the lesion in the cartilage. A **tourniquet** is applied to the limb to provide a bloodless operation area. A good adjustable light is necessary to illuminate the joint clearly. As the direction of the light has to be altered frequently during the operation an attendant should stand by it to make the necessary adjustment when required by the surgeon. This operation involves **removal of the whole cartilage,** i.e. **medial or lateral meniscectomy.** During the operation the condition of the articular surfaces of the joint and the integrity of the cruciate ligaments are assessed. This will influence the post-operative management and also determine the prognosis.

Immobilisation. Three methods of immobilisation of the limb are commonly used:

1 The wound dressing may be covered by a pad of cotton wool and a supporting crêpe bandage applied.
2 A posterior splint of metal or plaster may be used to augment the support given by a simple bandage.
3 A Robert Jones bandage gives additional support and compression where this is required. It is composed of several layers of cotton wool, each alternating with a layer of domette bandage. The bandage extends from the ankle to the groin.

Physiotherapy. Quadriceps exercises are started pre-operatively and are resumed on the first post-operative day. The exercises are repeated daily, for five minutes in each hour, until muscle tone and function have fully recovered. **The importance of quadriceps drill' cannot be over-stressed to the patient** as his progress is dependent on re-education of the quadriceps muscle. The nurse must therefore encourage the patient to practise the exercises taught to him by the physiotherapist.

Ambulation and Discharge. When the patient has regained sufficient tone in the quadriceps muscle to stabilise the knee he progresses from partial to full weight-bearing and if wound healing is complete he is discharged on the tenth post-operative day. Sometimes the patient still requires the support of crutches or a walking stick. Outpatient physiotherapy must always be arranged for him in order that he may regain full knee function.

Prognosis. In the absence of any complications the patient should have virtually a perfect knee and be able return to work in 6–8 weeks. On the other hand, if the operative exploration reveals chondromalacia patellae or torn cruciate ligaments the knee function will not be satisfactory. The patient may as a result require rehabilitation and resettlement. While still in hospital he is interviewed by the medical social worker who can be of valuable assistance in arranging for his retraining after discharge.

Complications. Synovial effusion. A reactionary effusion occurs due to the operation itself and the retraction of the synovial membrane by instruments. This reaction is often mild and symptomless. The effusion, however, may distend the knee joint, causing **pain** and **interference with quadriceps exercises.** Although there is marked local discomfort there is no general systemic reaction and the **patient is not ill.** Aspiration of the joint may be necessary. The procedure requires a strictly aseptic technique.

Haemarthrosis. After operation bleeding occurs from the small vessels cut during the procedure. Coagulation usually occurs naturally. Where a larger vessel is cut bleeding may be excessive and distend the joint, causing **extreme pain** and **general systemic reaction. The patient is ill.** The knee is very swollen and tense. Pressure on nerves and blood vessels can occur if the knee is grossly distended under a firm bandage. Paraesthesia of the lower limb and foot results. The bandage should be cut longitudinally throughout its layers and on the opposite side to the wound. A fresh bandage is applied on top with less tension. **Recurrent haemarthrosis** is usually investigated by **surgical exploration of the knee** under general anaesthesia and the bleeding vessel ligated. If the source of bleeding cannot be located a suction drain may be inserted and left in place until the haemorrhage stops.

REMOVAL OF A LOOSE BODY (OR LOOSE BODIES) FROM A JOINT

This procedure is necessary where there is pain, instability and locking of a joint. The predisposing factors can present at any stage in life. The operation is usually short and simple but loose bodies tend to be displaced even by the slightest movement of the joint. After the patient's limb has been draped in theatre the exact **location of the loose body is revealed by X-ray examination before the incision is made.**

Immobilisation. An occlusive wound dressing, often with the addition of a supporting bandage, is sufficient. After operation on the elbow joint a collar and cuff sling may be worn for a few days post-operatively until pain settles.

Physiotherapy. After **operation on the elbow** the patient may initially wear a sling which should be removed after pain settles and free use of the joint allowed at regular intervals during the day. **In the knee joint,** post-operatively there is little interference with quadriceps muscle function. With gentle exercise rapid recovery is usual within the first 3–4 days.

Ambulation and Discharge. The removal of an obvious loose body from the **elbow joint** may be arranged as an outpatient procedure. The patient is allowed home after a sufficient post-anaesthetic recovery period has elapsed, and provided he is fit for discharge.

Where the **knee joint** is involved the patient remains in hospital after operation. As the function of the quadriceps muscle improves he progresses from non-weight-bearing using crutches to full weight-bearing at 7–10 days. Often where removal of the loose body has been simple the patient is discharged early. He is supplied with crutches on discharge, given instructions in quadriceps function exercises and asked to attend as an outpatient for the removal of sutures.

Re-attachment of a Loose Body. In osteochondritis dissecans, particularly in the knee joint, a loose body undamaged by repetitive trapping in the joint may be re-attached to its original position. This is achieved by using a Smillie's pin as a means of internal fixation. The knee is thereafter immobilised in a long leg plaster cylinder. This is changed after 10–14 days when the sutures are removed. When the plaster is discarded completely after 3 months the joint is explored under general anaesthesia; if union of the fragment has occurred the pin is removed.

Prognosis. This depends entirely on the condition of the knee joint and the cause of the loose body formation, e.g. chondromalacia patellae or osteochondritis dissecans. The operation will cure the symptoms associated with that particular loose body; it does not necessarily guarantee, however, that the joint will remain free from further loose body development, particularly where there is present a condition such as chondromalacia patellae. Other operations such as patellectomy or synovectomy may be required later to treat the primary condition.

Complications. Although complications seldom occur any to be anticipated are similar to those following meniscectomy.

PATELLECTOMY

Where **disease** of the patella leaves a patient crippled by the chronic symptoms of retropatellar discomfort with either painful or painless 'clicking' of the joint unrelieved by conservative surgery, excision of the patella may be considered. In **trauma** it is not possible to treat adequately 'stellate' or comminuted fractures of the patella without the later development of osteoarthritis. For this reason these fractures are treated by patellectomy. The age of the patient varies from the adolescent or young adult with chondromalacia to the middle aged or elderly with osteoarthritis. Operation is short and is done with **tourniquet** control of the bleeding. The patella is a sesamoid bone in the extensor tendon of the quadriceps muscle which covers the knee anteriorly. It is quite simple to 'shell' out leaving the tendon intact. The subsequent blood clot formed in the gap becomes organised and the resultant fibrous tissue fills the space. In trauma the expansions of the extensor tendon on either side of the patella may also be damaged. After the patella has been removed a plastic repair of these structures will provide the additional strength required.

Immobilisation. Where there is disease of the patella the muscular expansions are undamaged after surgery and the complete support of a long leg plaster cylinder is less important. The limb may be immobilised in one of the three ways described for meniscectomy. Following patellectomy and repair of the extensor tendon damaged by trauma, the protection of a long leg plaster cylinder is necessary for 2 weeks.

Physiotherapy. This is similar in both instances. A programme of graduated exercises is planned, for example:

1st week: Knee exercises are withheld. Toe, foot and ankle exercises are encouraged and these maintenance exercises are continued throughout the entire post-operative period.

2nd week: Static quadriceps exercises are commenced.

3rd week: The patient practises straight leg raising.

4th week: Gentle knee flexion is permitted and graduated exercise of the joint is continued until full flexion is achieved. By this time the patient is often attending physiotherapy classes as an outpatient.

Ambulation and Discharge. The patient may be allowed to sit out of bed in the 2nd post-operative week with the leg supported in such a way that extension of the knee is maintained. When knee flexion reaches 90 degrees the patient is fitted with crutches and is allowed partial weight-bearing on the affected limb. Full weight-bearing is avoided at this stage because of the danger of rupture of the repaired tendon by any sudden excessive stress. The patient is discharged at about the 6th post-operative week and continues to have physiotherapy as an outpatient.

Prognosis. Although, after operation, a few patients may retain some discomfort it is more tolerable than the previous pain and 'clicking'. They find sudden starting and stopping difficult, e.g. in the act of running. A patient whose job involves climbing or running up and down stairs may require further rehabilitation and resettlement.

Complications. The nature of the operation predisposes to the development of **haemarthrosis. Infection** of the haematoma can result in a septic arthritis. **Rupture of the repaired tendon** may occur if the knee is prematurely subjected to excessive stress.

ARTHRODESIS

Where a joint is damaged by disease or injury to such an extent that pain, stiffness or instability cause severe disability, fusion of the joint may have to be considered, i.e. arthrodesis. The operation is more successful in the 20–40 age group than in older people whose general mobility is limited by stiffness of other joints. The smaller the joint, e.g. an interphalangeal joint, the easier is the operation. Arthrodesis of the hip and shoulder, the freely movable joints, is more difficult to achieve successfully and post-operatively requires greater supervision. The small joint fusions are done with tourniquet control of the bleeding. In hip and shoulder operations, however, haemostasis has to be achieved surgically at each stage, so prolonging the procedure. Persistent bleeding would otherwise further shock the patient and increase the dangers of operation. Blood must be available for replacement therapy and a careful swab and instrument count is necessary particularly in hip surgery.

Types of Arthrodesis

An **intra-articular arthrodesis,** inside the joint capsule, is done in degenerative conditions, e.g. primary osteoarthritis or secondary post-traumatic arthritis. **Extra-articular arthrodesis** is useful after inflammatory conditions where it is desirable to by-pass the infected joint, e.g. tuberculous disease of the shoulder or the hip joints. The success of antibiotic and chemotherapeutic drugs has increased the tendency to perform intra-articular arthrodesis as the method of choice.

Procedure. In **intra-articular arthrodesis** the joint is exposed and dislocated to allow the articular surfaces to be removed. The raw bone ends are then opposed in the neutral functional position for that particular joint. Some means of **fixation** is necessary to maintain complete immobility until fusion occurs, e.g. Charnley clamp, staples, interphalangeal fusion (*Fig. 39*). In the larger joints this may be augmented by a **plaster support. Bone grafts** in the form of cancellous bone

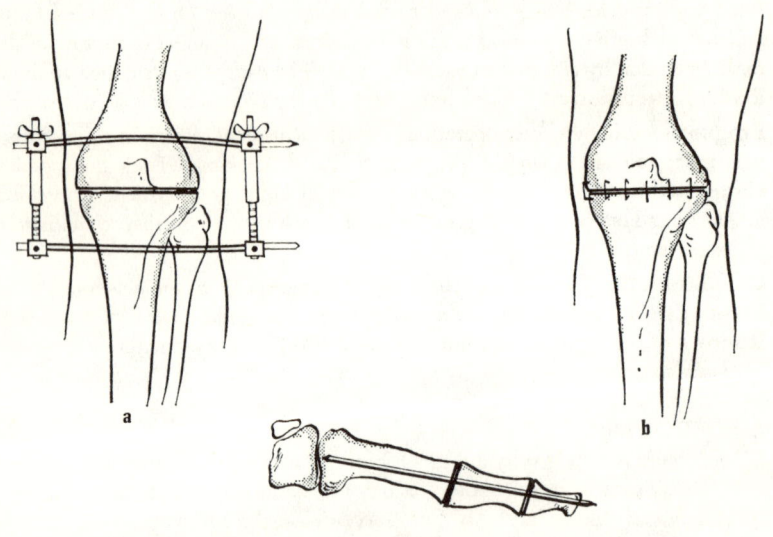

FIG. 39   Arthrodesis
(*a*) Charnley clamp
(*b*) Staples
(*c*) Interphalangeal pin

chips or strips taken from the iliac crest or upper end of the tibia are packed in and around the larger joints to assist fusion (*Fig. 40*).

Post-operative Management. In surgery of the larger joints immediate post-operative observation is initially related to the recovery of the patient from the anaesthetic. Blood replacement is linked closely with the blood pressure level and pulse rate. The nurse must record the pulse and blood pressure half-hourly until the surgeon or anaesthetist is satisfied that the blood loss has been replaced.

The nursing management of newly-applied plasters is extremely important, particularly in the larger joint fusions as tissue reaction will be more marked after an extensive operation (*see pp.* 168–71, Plaster Care). The anticipation of severe pain and its adequate relief is also extremely important.

Immobilisation. This is usually achieved by means of plaster splintage. Plaster casts are changed after about 2 weeks and removed completely where there is radiological and clinical evidence of fusion. In the Charnley clamp extra-articular fixation used in arthrodesis of knee, the limb is bandaged into a Thomas's splint. The Steinmann pins are removed at 6 weeks. If necessary, a long leg plaster cylinder is substituted until fusion is complete.

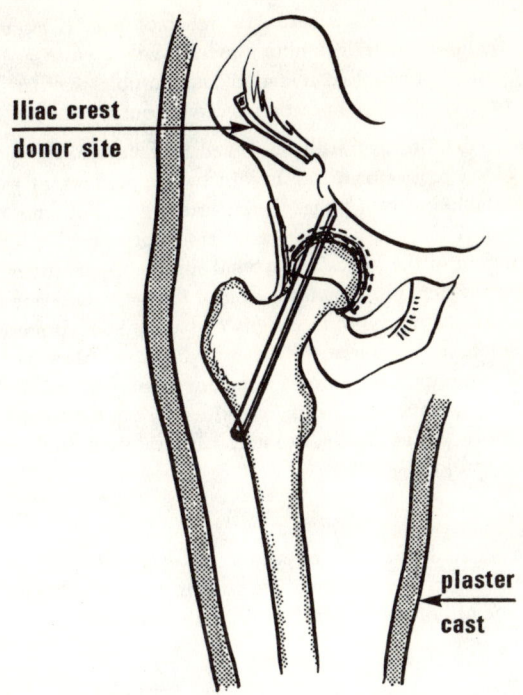

FIG. 40   Arthrodesis of hip. Trifin nail with cancellous bone chips and slivers.
Hip spica external support

Physiotherapy. Maintenance exercises of muscles and joints are important so that other joints are kept functional to compensate for the joint arthrodesed. Movement of the fused joint must be avoided. Breathing exercises will be particularly important for patients in plaster beds, hip spicas and where a bone graft has been removed from the iliac crest.

Ambulation and Discharge. After the change of plaster and removal of stitches the patient, even in a hip spica, should be able to sit out of bed; the plaster must be completely dry. The patient in a plaster bed will remain there for about three months. Weight-bearing with the aid of crutches is dependent on the joint arthrodesed, the procedure involved and the clinical assessment of progress. The stage at which a lower limb plaster is converted to a weight-bearing one is dependent on stability and on clinical and radiological appearances of union. Often the patient is discharged non-weight-bearing and returns as an outpatient for regular assessment. A patient with foot (triple arthrodesis), toe, ankle or wrist fusions should be home in 2–3 weeks; a knee arthrodesis by 6 weeks; shoulder or hip in 6–8 weeks; a spinal fusion not usually before two months.

Prognosis. Where arthrodesis is successful relief of pain is assured. Such an operation may radically alter locomotion which will require a great deal of readjustment by the patient. Rehabilitation and possible resettlement must be considered, perhaps even before operation is carried out.

Complications. Bleeding is usually suggested by failure of the blood pressure to rise despite blood replacement transfusion; by the presence of pallor, a rapid pulse, excessive staining through the plaster, bruising of the skin or marked re-actionary oedema. This presents either as a circulatory problem or as extreme tension in the region of the joint. The wound sutures appear to embed into the skin. Pressure on the nerves by the distension of the soft tissues and compression within the rigid plaster may produce signs of paraesthesia. **Infection,** delayed union or non-union can complicate any joint arthrodesis. After successful fusion some patients later complain of **pain in adjacent joints.** Added strain is exerted on adjacent joints to compensate for the one stiffened, e.g. backache from lumbo-sacral strain in arthrodesis of the hip, or interphalangeal strain in fusion of the first metacarpophalangeal joint.

OSTEOTOMY
Osteotomy is a method of correcting a bony deformity such as severe bowing of the legs or mal-union of a fracture. The bone is surgically divided and, where necessary, a wedge of bone is removed to allow the bone ends to be opposed in a stable corrected position.

Osteotomy in Osteoarthritis of the Hip
The two main clinical features of osteoarthritis of the hip joint are pain and deformity. The pain is produced by the reaction of the joint to the disease process; the deformity is the result of protective muscle spasm initially and capsular contracture later. The hip assumes a position of flexion, adduction and either internal or external rotation. Osteotomy not only allows correction of deformity but also relieves pain by improving the joint mechanics so that stress is transferred from the affected areas.

McMurray's osteotomy (*Fig. 41*) is often done in the 35–60 age group. The patient is placed on the orthopaedic table. A lateral incision is made in the soft tissues over the upper third of the femur. Under X-ray control the bone is divided transversely just above the lesser trochanter. The distal fragment is then displaced medially and the deformity slightly over-corrected by swinging the lower limb back into its normal position. If the adductor muscles have become contracted and resist correction of the deformity, these are divided by tenotomy.

Immobilisation. (i) Internal Fixation. It is desirable, whenever possible, to avoid immobilisation of the adjacent joints in a plaster. This can be achieved, particularly in the femoral osteotomies, either by the use of conventional internal fixation (*Fig. 42a*) or the more modern compression devices (*Fig. 42b*).

If the method of internal fixation used provides adequate stability external splintage will be unnecessary. After the post-operative pain and wound reaction has settled, the patient is allowed to sit up. In 4–5 days he is allowed to sit out of bed. If wound healing is satisfactory the sutures are removed at 14 days. In the absence of pain or other complications, e.g. deep venous thrombosis, the patient

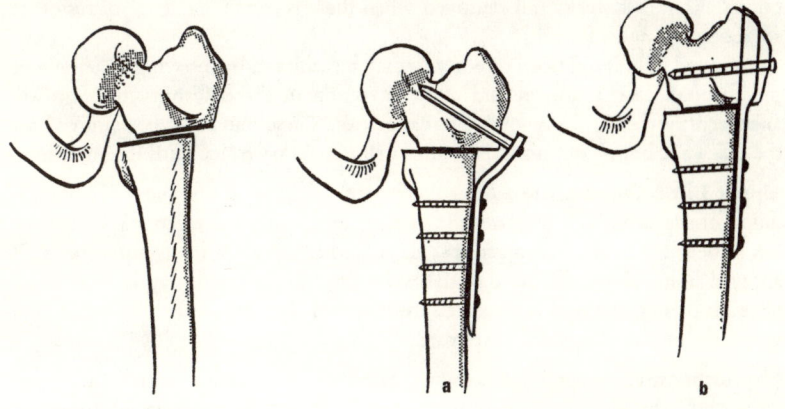

FIG. 41 McMurray's
osteotomy

FIG. 42 Fixation in McMurray's osteotomy
(*a*) Conventional nail and plate
(*b*) Compression device

may be fitted with crutches to allow limited weight-bearing on the osteotomised limb. As clinical and radiological union progress favourably the patient is allowed partial weight-bearing with crutches. Full weight-bearing is only encouraged when there are definite signs of fusion present.

(ii) **Plaster Splintage.** Plaster immobilisation is only used where an intertrochanteric osteotomy is difficult to fix internally because marked flexion, adduction and rotational deformity all require correction. In such patients a single hip spica is applied with the limb in the slightly over-corrected position. After 3 weeks when the osteotomy site is beginning to heal the plaster is changed, the limb brought into a more neutral position and a close-fitting plaster is applied. The initial position of the limb in the over-corrected position tends to prevent the recurrence of the deformity during the early post-operative period. A double hip spica provides the ideal method of immobilisation, but the dangers associated with such extensive restriction of activity in the older age group contra-indicate its application.

After the change of plaster the patient in a single hip spica may be assisted out of bed to rest on a settee or sit in a suitable high chair or on a stool. Later at about

6 weeks he is fitted with crutches and taught to walk without bearing weight on the side of the osteotomy. The plaster immobilisation is maintained for 3 months until fusion is certain. Progress to partial and eventually to full weight-bearing depend on the stability of the osteotomy site and the clinical and radiological evidence of fusion.

Where osteotomy is performed near a joint internal fixation may be difficult to apply, e.g. round the knee in lower femoral or upper tibial osteotomy. The limb will be immobilised in a well-moulded padded plaster or in a Thomas's splint. The plaster is usually changed at two weeks, converted to a weight-bearing one at about 6–8 weeks and removed when there is certain evidence of fusion at sometime around 12 weeks.

Increased stability in tibial osteotomy may be achieved by inserting a Steinmann pin through each fragment and after correction of the deformity the pins are anchored by the rigid support of a plaster cast. These pins must be removed by the 6th week but plaster immobilisation will remain necessary until fusion occurs.

Upper Limb Osteotomies. After these operations, e.g. at the elbow due to mal-union of supracondylar fracture, the patient sits up after the reactionary swelling has settled. He is allowed up in 4–5 days, and if there are no complications, is allowed home about the 7th day. Between the 10th and 14th day he returns to have his plaster renewed and sutures are removed. Union is usually sound in 6–8 weeks, when the plaster can be discarded.

Physiotherapy. General maintenance exercises of all joints and muscles are important. Hip exercises are restricted until the wound heals in McMurray's osteotomy. In all other osteotomies, exercise of muscles in proximity to the bone division are withheld until fusion is moderately advanced.

Complications. Apart from those complications associated with immobilisation the main problem which may arise in the post-operative period is **recurrence of the deformity.** It occurs usually where an attempt has been made to limit the extent of the immobilisation because of other circumstances, e.g. the age of the patient. As in the healing of a fracture, **delayed or non-union** may occur. Where osteotomy is undertaken in the treatment of osteoarthritis the joint **pain** and **stiff-ness may persist** despite the effort made to lessen the stresses on the joint. **Deep venous thrombosis** is always a possible complication. Other **vascular** or **neurovascular complications** may be produced during the correction of the deformity if one of the bone fragments presses on a blood vessel or nerve.

ARTHROPLASTY

Arthroplasty is the excision of a joint. It is usually done for arthritis, either osteo-arthritis or rheumatoid arthritis. The aim is to relieve pain and stiffness and at the same time retain joint mobility. The age group varies according to the type of arthroplasty. Surgical technique is important. There are three types of arthro-plasty: (a) excision, (b) mould or cup and (c) replacement.

In **excision arthroplasty,** the opposing surfaces of the joint are removed producing a pseudarthrosis or false joint. In **mould arthroplasty,** a cap or cup of an inert metallic alloy is inserted between the opposing bony surfaces. **Replacement arthroplasty** may be partial or total. **Partial replacement** of one side of the joint involves substituting a prosthesis for one of the bone ends forming the joint, e.g. the head of femur or radius. It may be either a metallic device (Austin Moore or Thomson's femoral head prosthesis) or one composed of plastic material (radial head prosthesis). In **total replacement** both the bone ends forming the joint are replaced by a prosthesis, i.e. a complete artificial joint. There are many prosthetic joint devices available, each designed to suit a particular joint. Examples of such prostheses are:

1 **A flexible plastic implant** used to replace finger joints.
2 **Metallic joint components,** as used in the McKee/Farrer total hip replacement; the Waldeus knee prosthesis; the Shier's knee and elbow devices.
3 **A combined metallic and plastic prosthesis,** as used in the Charnley hip replacement, where the acetabular component is made of plastic and the femoral replacement of metal.

Excision Arthroplasty

This operation is done in the metatarsophalangeal joint of the great toe (Keller's arthroplasty), the hip and in the elbow. The result of the operation allows mobility at the expense of stability.

Keller's is the most common of the excision arthroplasties performed, usually in the 40–60 age group. It is important for the patient to understand that as a result of the operation, although pain is relieved, the toe will be shorter and weaker than normal.

Post-operative Management. (Keller's arthroplasty.) **Immobilisation** may be by means of a crêpe bandage applied over firm wool padding, by a below-knee plaster or even by a simple plaster slipper.

Physiotherapy. Physiotherapy is started as soon as pain settles or plaster immobilisation is removed. Active plantar flexion exercises of the toes are encouraged. These prevent a flexion deformity of the big toe by redeveloping the muscle power and also help to maintain the transverse arch.

Ambulation and Discharge. Commencement of weight-bearing varies according to whether the operation is unilateral or bilateral. Where it is unilateral the patient may be up non-weight-bearing using crutches at the end of the first week, provided there is no discomfort and temperature is normal. In the second week partial weight-bearing on the heel may be allowed. Full weight-bearing is permitted after the sutures are removed at 14 days. The patient may, however, be discharged earlier once he is confident in crutch walking. In bilateral operations the patient must remain in hospital and avoid weight-bearing until the immobilisation and sutures are removed at the 14th day.

Prognosis. This is good in most cases as long as the patient does not subject the toe to a great deal of physical activity.

Complications. Painful flexion deformity may be due to an inadequate arthroplasty in which insufficient bone was removed. Revision surgery may be successful. If this fails arthrodesis will be required.

Mould or Smith-Petersen Cup Arthroplasty

This prosthesis is used in the hip joint. The cup is interposed between the head of the femur and the acetabulum after the articular cartilage has been removed from both surfaces, and the parts are remodelled. It retains both mobility and stability in the hip and may give considerable relief of pain. Neither mould nor excision arthroplasties need be confined to the elderly. They can be undertaken in middle-aged adults. The operation is a major one and surgical technique is important.

Post-operative Management. Immobilisation. Sliding skin traction with a gentle pull of 2–3 lbs (1–$1\frac{1}{2}$ kilos) is a useful method of controlling movement of the limb, while at the same time counteracting painful muscle spasm. The traction is removed after two weeks.

Physiotherapy. This is particularly important in cup arthroplasty. Maintenance exercises ensure retention of joint function and these are begun immediately. Careful passive hip exercises are necessary until wound healing is complete. After a fortnight a purposeful graduated programme of active hip exercises is started. The aim is to restore at least the former range of movement, more if possible, and to redevelop lost muscle power.

Ambulation and Discharge. During the third week, the patient practises active intensive mobilising exercises. In the fourth week he is allowed up; he starts partial weight-bearing using a walking aid. The patient is discharged once he is independent and continues his physiotherapy both at home and at outpatient classes. Partial weight-bearing using crutches, sticks or a walking aid is continued over a prolonged period. Full weight-bearing is encouraged only when muscle recovery is complete and when the patient can walk without a limp.

Prognosis. In some patients pain is relieved and movement retained for years. In others recurrence of pain and joint stiffness necessitate revision surgery. Sometimes the operation fails to relieve the symptoms. In the middle age group, mould or cup arthroplasty may be more beneficial than the alternative arthrodesis of the hip. Total hip replacement surgery has, however, more appeal to patients in the older age group where the prolonged period of physiotherapy is less acceptable.

Complications. Infection is a serious complication demanding early recognition and treatment by prolonged continuous antibiotic therapy. Removal of the cup may be necessary before healing can occur. **Dislocation of the hip** is suggested when post-operative pain is excessive or recurs, and is associated with deformity of the hip. X-ray will confirm dislocation. Either manipulation under a general anaesthetic or open reduction will be required. Care should be taken in changing the patient's position to avoid dislocation of the hip, by maintaining the normal relationship between the limb and the trunk, particularly with regard to rotation.

Partial Replacement Arthroplasty (e.g. Austin Moore's (*Fig. 43a*) or Thomson's)
This procedure is often undertaken in subcapital fractures of the neck of femur or where internal fixation of transcervical fractures has failed. The acetabulum must be relatively normal. The patient is usually in the 70–80 age group. The operation although relatively major can be fairly expeditiously performed, an important factor when considering surgery in the elderly. The approach is either a posterior or lateral one and the stump of the neck of femur is dislocated. This allows the head fragment to be removed by using a corkscrew. The femoral neck stump is trimmed. Bone cement may then be inserted into the medullary cavity of the femur after which the shank of the femoral head prosthesis is hammered into position. The prosthesis is then reduced into the acetabulum at which stage the joint should feel stable.

Post-operative Management. Immobilisation. This is similar to that used in the management of cup arthroplasty.

Physiotherapy. Apart from maintenance exercises, in this age group the main accent is on early walking rather than on building up muscle power.

Ambulation and Discharge. Although it is desirable to limit activities which may delay wound healing in the first two weeks the age of the patient makes compromise essential. Where possible the patient should be sitting in a chair towards the end of the first week. Walking with an aid or crutches should commence in the second week, or earlier if this is feasible. Transfer to convalescent wards can be arranged during this period. Discharge home is possible as soon as the patient is independent. This could be as early as three weeks, particularly if there is help available at home.

Prognosis. Where the operation has been technically sound and uncomplicated the outlook is good. The procedure has the advantage that, as the femoral head is removed, the associated complication of avascular necrosis requiring revision surgery will not arise. On the other hand, it is a more major operation than a simple nail and plate fixation of the fracture and the convalescence can be more troublesome.

Complications. During the insertion of the prosthesis in a difficult operation the **shaft of the femur may fracture.** The limb will then require immobilisation in sliding or fixed skin traction until union occurs in about 12 weeks. **Wound infection** may occur because of either the extensive nature of the surgery or the proximity of the wound to the perineum; this will require full doses of the appropriate antibiotic. In the incontinent patient it is the usual practice to avoid catheterisation because of the danger of introducing infection where none is present, or further introducing bacteria in an already infected urine. In those patients where hip surgery is urgent, however, i.e. fractures of the neck of femur, there is insufficient time to sterilise the urine therapeutically. An indwelling catheter attached to a closed sterile drainage system is necessary. Bladder drainage is always collected at the opposite side of the bed to the wound. Antibiotic cover is essential. This management of the incontinence is maintained until wound healing appears satisfactory whereupon the cause can be thoroughly investigated and treated.

Post-operative perineal care is an important factor in the prevention of wound contamination, particularly where the patient is obese, where there is urinary or faecal incontinence or in the presence of vaginal or urethral discharge. Regular cleansing of the perineum twice or thrice daily using an antiseptic soap followed by thorough drying of the parts is necessary. The application of an antibacterial dusting powder may give added protection.

Failure of the wound to heal properly usually indicates that the infection is deep-seated. **Removal of the metallic prosthesis** is necessary under these circumstances before healing will occur, the operation thus being converted into a pseudarthrosis. Telescoping of the hip with **shortening of the limb** results. A raised shoe and two crutches or sticks will be required for walking. Such patients are often, however, surprisingly painfree.

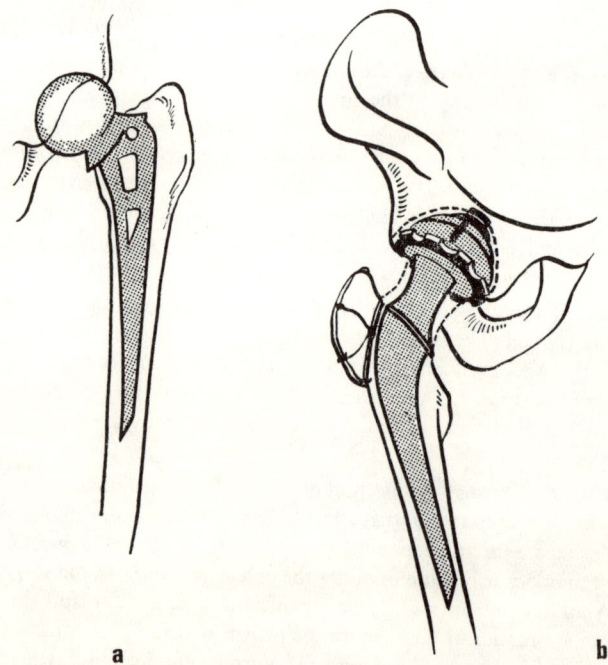

FIG. 43   (a) Partial replacement arthroplasty (Austin Moore)
(b) Total hip replacement (Charnley)

Skin sores, chest and urinary infection, stiffness of joints and **vascular complications** may occasionally arise particularly in a heavy or obese patient.

Redislocation of the hip can occur as in cup arthroplasty and the same precautions are taken in positioning the patient in order to avoid this complication.

Total Replacement Arthroplasty

In the 60+ age group, where disease or injury has so damaged a joint that function is severely impaired, total replacement arthroplasty may be considered necessary. Although an artificial joint is created the prostheses used have special low friction properties which ensure adequate joint function with the relief of pain and minimal surface wear on the opposing surfaces of the false joint. The indefinite durability of the synthetic materials used tends to limit the scope for the use of the operation in the younger age group.

The artificial replacement of a joint, where indicated, is determined by the availability of a suitable prosthesis for that joint. The principles of post-operative management are the same for all replacement arthroplasties, but obviously the larger the joint the more major the operation, e.g. total hip replacement.

Total Hip Replacement (*Fig. 43b*). Using an anterior, lateral or posterior surgical approach the hip joint is dislocated by external rotation of the limb. The femoral head and acetabulum are each replaced by a prosthesis which is bonded to the respective prepared surfaces using bone cement. The new hip joint is then assembled, stability is tested and the wound is closed.

While infection is always a serious hazard in hip surgery its consequences in this type of operation are particularly difficult to eradicate because the prostheses are cemented into position. It may be advisable, therefore, to admit the patient early so that the presence of any infection in the perineal area may be detected and treated before surgery is contemplated. Antiseptic baths twice or three times daily, where feasible, may be given from the time of admission to the day of operation as additional skin preparation.

Post-operative Management. Immobilisation. Both **legs are kept in abduction,** being separated by soft pillows. This relaxes the main hip muscles and encourages wound healing. In the lateral approach to the hip the greater trochanter is divided in order to improve access to the joint and facilitate dislocation of the head of the femur. It is reattached after insertion of the prostheses. Close apposition of the trochanteric fragment to the femur is essential if fusion is to be successful. The positioning of the legs in abduction therefore relaxes any pull on this fragment.

Physiotherapy. The elderly are particularly prone to joint stiffness because of relative inactivity. The aim in physiotherapy is to **maintain** the **function of all joints.** During the **2nd week hip abduction exercises** are commenced. These are performed either with the limb suspended in **abduction slings** or with the use of **modified skates** strapped to the patient's legs; the skates travel on a firm board placed across the bed.

Ambulation and Discharge. If wound healing is satisfactory, the patient will be allowed **up to sit** during the **second week** and he may learn to stand and become **ambulant within 14 days.** Thereafter, the emphasis is on re-education in walking with the use of a walking aid or elbow crutches. **Hydrotherapy** is of particular benefit in re-establishing total mobility. If the patient is walking confidently after 3–4 weeks he will be discharged.

Prognosis. The marked relief of pain, the increased range of joint movement and the improvement in walking make this rather major operation worth-while for many patients, irrespective of the uncertainty as to its long term results.

Complications. Perineal bruising and **oedema** may be marked in the first 2–3 post-operative days. In a male patient a scrotal support may relieve discomfort and control swelling. As in all arthroplasties, **redislocation of the joint** may occur and is avoided by careful positioning of the limb relative to the trunk on the side of operation. **Deep venous thrombosis** and **pulmonary embolism** are serious complications associated with the first three post-operative weeks. By this time the patient should be mobile and should be kept as active as possible in order to maintain an effective circulation. **Wound infection** is always a potential danger, particularly in view of the proximity of the perineum. Perineal hygiene is again an important factor in the nursing management. Occasionally infection manifests itself late, e.g. after six months, and is recognised by the development of pain in the region of the artificial joint with an elevated erythrocyte sedimentation rate. If the infection does not resolve with the administration of broad spectrum antibiotics the **prostheses may have to be removed** at a revision operation and a pseud-arthrosis created.

OPEN REDUCTION AND INTERNAL FIXATION OF FRACTURES

Where a fracture is irreducible, unstable or complicated, it may require reduction by means of open operative manipulation, and fixation internally by the use of some mechanical device. In this way shortening and deformity of the limb can be avoided. Internal stabilisation of some of the fractures in multiple injuries will also allow more freedom in their general management. In other instances, internal fixation provides an alternative to plaster immobilisation with its resultant complication of stiffness of joints, and in the elderly it enables earlier mobilisation and improved general nursing care.

At operation, once the bone fragments are exposed and the bone ends freed from any intervening soft tissue, a trial reduction of the fracture is carried out to assess stability, alignment and rotation. Where possible, bone clamps are used to hold the bony fragments in the reduced position until the internal support has been fixed in place. Some examples of the types of mechanical devices used in individual fractures are illustrated on page 105.

Immobilisation. In some instances it may be considered necessary to apply the additional support of external splintage until signs of bony union are evident. A collar and cuff sling, broad arm sling or plaster splint may be used in the upper limb. In the lower limb external splintage may be provided by waterproof covered pillows, sandbags, a Thomas's splint or plaster immobilisation. A plaster bed or jacket will be necessary to give added support to the internal fixation of spinal fractures but if neurological complications are present the patient is nursed on a Stryker turning frame and the use of plaster is avoided.

Physiotherapy. Once wound healing is complete the stability at the fracture site resulting from the internal fixation allows for early and intensive re-education of the muscles and joints related to the injury. This differs from the more cautious approach to physiotherapy in the conservative management of fractures which are potentially unstable. Although internal fixation is a method of providing added stability to a reduced fracture, healing of the fracture will, nevertheless, be related to the age of the patient, the site of the injury and its complexity. The immobility of the patient, however, may be less prolonged if the fracture has been well stabilised.

Following surgery of the upper limb, once the initial tissue reaction has subsided and elevation of the limb is no longer necessary, the patient is allowed up wearing the support of a sling. In the absence of any obvious complications, e.g. pain or haematoma, he may be discharged towards the end of the first week. The patient must understand the importance of seeking medical advice should he feel any discomfort in the limb; if plaster is applied he must be instructed in the care of this limb. Regular attendance as an outpatient is necessary until union is complete.

Following operation on the lower limb mobilisation of the patient again depends on the progress of fracture healing. Partial weight-bearing may be allowed earlier in some cases particularly if internal fixation of the fracture has provided absolute stability.

The commonest example of internal fixation nursed in the orthopaedic and accident wards is that used to stabilise a fracture of the neck of femur in the elderly. As well as stabilising the fracture the operation relieves pain and allows use of the limb thus increasing the mobility of the patient. The elderly are prone to so many complications when immobilised such as pressure sores, pneumonia, deep venous thrombosis and bladder infection, that this measure is often life-saving. If such a patient is capable of sitting out of bed the operation provides the stability to allow him to do so comfortably. In other patients with a stable fracture and successful internal fixation crutches are sometimes supplied on the first post-operative day to allow **early weight-bearing. This, where practical, is an ideal method of management of the elderly patient** as the period of post-operative immobilisation is virtually eliminated.

Prognosis. This is good in uncomplicated fractures which have been treated early. Although a fracture has been internally fixed it does not follow that union will occur. Sometimes a further operation of bone grafting is necessary to establish fusion.

Complications. Infection, with the development of chronic osteomyelitis, is the main danger. This is basically why open reduction and internal fixation of fractures is not used more widely. Although in the treatment of compound fractures it is generally avoided for this reason, certain special circumstances demand its use, e.g. in complicated fractures and in certain combinations of multiple injuries. **Union may be delayed** where the blood supply to a bone is poor, e.g. in some fractures of the lower ends of ulna, tibia and humerus; indeed **non-union** may result. Bony union may also fail to occur where a fracture is comminuted and a gap exists because fragments of bone are missing.

BUNIONECTOMY

This is a simple operation done to relieve the symptoms of **hallux valgus** (a condition more common in females). The protruding part of the head of the first metatarsal (exostosis) is removed using an osteotome. Thus the contour of the medial side of the foot is restored so that normal footwear can be worn more comfortably.

Post-operative Management. Immobilisation. The foot is supported by a crêpe bandage applied from the tip of the toes to above the ankle. In order to minimise swelling the lower limb is elevated on a waterproof pillow.

Physiotherapy. Gentle foot exercises are commenced once the pain has settled. When tissue reaction has subsided the patient can sit out of bed. Between the 5–7th days she is allowed up to walk with the aid of crutches. Weight-bearing is avoided on the affected limb unless she feels the necessity to take a little weight on the heel of this foot as a means of steadying herself. The patient is often discharged at this stage. She returns at the end of a fortnight to have the stitches removed, after which she progresses from partial to full weight-bearing by about the 16th day.

Prognosis. This is good provided that the discomfort is strictly localised to the bunion. The patient's desire for the removal of the bunion must also be linked with the resolution to wear comfortable **broad-fitting shoes:** there is always a possibility that the **deformity may recur,** particularly when she persists in wearing unsuitable footwear. Unless the patient has a sedentary job she is advised that before returning to work she should continue exercises until normal function is regained in about 6–8 weeks time. During this period the temporary use of a metatarsal arch support allows some patients to walk more comfortably.

BONE GRAFTING

This is an operation used to produce union or fusion of the two fragments of bone in a fracture or osteotomy where there has been delayed or actual non-union. Although any fracture may fail to unite, the commonest sites requiring bone grafting are in the lower limb, particularly the shafts of the femur and tibia. The aim of the operation is **to place a bridge of bone between the un-united bone fragments.** This provides a scaffold on which new bone tissue is built resulting in union of the fragments.

The simplest type of bone graft is in the form of small **chips** or **slivers** of **cancellous bone.** The donor sites from which such bone is obtained are the iliac crest and upper end of the tibia. Cancellous bone chips are readily packed into bony crevices, in and around the fragments, while bone slivers are laid on the surface under the periosteum, i.e. a modified Phemister graft (*Fig. 44a*). Additional means of internal fixation such as a bone plate or Küntscher nail may be considered necessary in some cases to give extra stability.

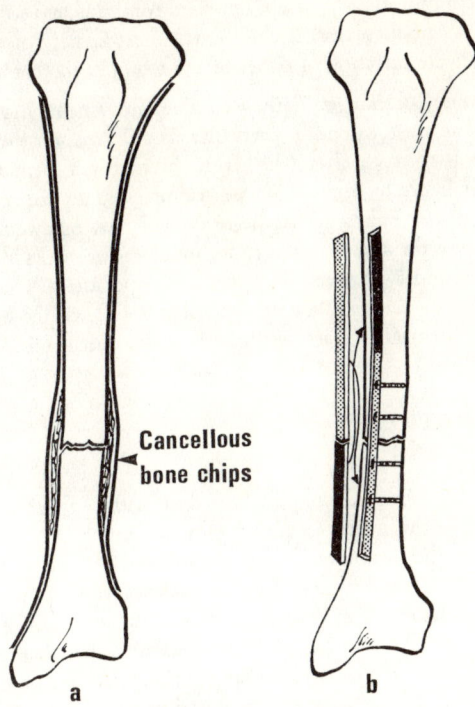

Cancellous bone chips

FIG. 44 (*a*) Phemister bone graft
(*b*) Sliding cortical bone graft

A **rectangular slab of cortical bone,** usually obtained from the tibia, may be used occasionally to strut the site which requires grafting (*Fig. 44b*). It is in the form of either an inlay or onlay graft. The graft is held firmly in position by internal screw fixation. This type of graft is strong and gives stability to the fracture. Its disadvantage is that, due to the density of cortical bone, absorption of the graft and its replacement by new bone is much slower than in the case of a cancellous graft.

Post-operative Management. Immobilisation. Once the patient has recovered from the anaesthetic he is often more comfortable if supported by pillows in the semi-recumbent position provided this is permissible; thus the tension on the iliac crest donor wound is relieved. Pain is usually more severe here than in the grafted area, particularly if the patient takes a deep breath, coughs or sneezes. It is essential that adequate analgesia is administered so that the patient can practise breathing exercises painlessly, thereby avoiding chest complications.

Physiotherapy. Maintenance physiotherapy is extremely important as these patients have often had a long period of immobilisation already and are more prone to such complications as deep venous thrombosis and stiff joints. In older patients these risks are increased. A close watch must be kept on temperature as a pyrexia may indicate infection of either of the wounds, the chest or the bladder.

Ambulation and Discharge. Early excessive movement may interfere with healing of the iliac crest wound in particular. For this reason the patient may be kept in bed for 7–10 days, after which time haematoma formation and wound infection are less likely to occur. Stitches in both wounds are removed in about 14 days and if plaster splintage has been applied it is renewed. The period of immobilisation is as for a fresh fracture, i.e. about 12–16 weeks in lower limb and spinal operations, and 8–12 weeks in upper limb operations. The patient follows the same programme of mobilisation, partial and full weight-bearing as in the management of the original fracture. Progress is dependent on X-ray and clinical assessment.

SPINAL OPERATIONS

Laminectomy

This is the surgical approach required to deal with a space-occupying lesion arising from one of the structures forming or occupying the spinal canal, e.g. an intervertebral disc, the meninges, the spinal cord or the neural arch. After incising the skin the area is exposed by reflecting the muscles from the posterior aspect of the bony ring, or laminae, and the adjacent spinous processes. The interspinous ligament connecting the laminae of two adjacent vertebrae is excised. Where necessary a small piece of each adjacent lamina is nibbled to enlarge the space, i.e. a **keyhole incision.** If wider access is required one lamina, or half of the neural arch, is removed, **hemilaminectomy. Total laminectomy,** i.e. removal of both halves, may be necessary in the exposure of larger or more obscure spinal lesions.

Post-operative management. Immobilisation. The rigid support of a plaster bed or spinal frame is unnecessary, as this operation has not interfered with the stability of the spine. The main stabilising anterior and posterior intervertebral body ligaments are not divided. The wound is covered by an occlusive dressing which remains in position until the sutures are removed in 10–14 days. Although the patient is free to adopt any position in which he feels comfortable it is important that his spine is supported. This is achieved either by placing a fracture board beneath the mattress or by nursing the patient in an orthopaedic bed in which the spring has been re-enforced. He is usually more comfortable with only one small pillow under his head.

Physiotherapy. Gentle back extension exercises are commenced on the 1st post-operative day and these are increased as pain settles.

Ambulation and Discharge. This may be early or may be withheld until later depending on the individual practice of the surgeon or the type of operation performed. In the first instance the patient is able to sit out of bed on the second post-operative day. As pain settles and posture is improved by physiotherapy he becomes gradually more active. By 10-16 days he should be able to go home. On the other hand, it may be preferred to keep the patient in bed for the first three weeks. He is then allowed up to walk wearing a lumbar support and is discharged usually within a week.

Prognosis. This depends on the type of space-occupying lesion and its amenability to surgical eradication. In a disc lesion, for example, the operation for its removal may cure completely the patient's symptoms. On the other hand the invasive nature of a malignant lesion makes it difficult to determine its margins and complete removal is often uncertain. Recurrence is therefore not unlikely.

Complications. Only when it is necessary to remove several laminae from two or more adjacent vertebrae is there any real danger of producing spinal instability, e.g. in the decompression of an enlarging tumour. Minor or major damage to a spinal nerve root or major blood vessel is a serious complication which, fortunately, rarely arises. Infection is uncommon because the muscles fill the space which might otherwise be occupied by haematoma formation.

Spinal Fusion

This may involve the local fusion of two adjacent vertebrae, or a more radical procedure in which several vertebrae are fused together. The surgical approach may be anterior, antero-lateral or posterior. In an anterior operation the adjacent vertebral bodies are fused, while in a posterior procedure the fusion is of the adjacent laminae, with or without the posterior inter-articular joints. Spinal fusion may be considered necessary where disease has significantly damaged the stability of the spine or has interfered with the function of the spinal cord and nerve roots, e.g. scoliosis, tuberculosis, disc degeneration and spondylolisthesis; trauma may also produce instability of the spine, e.g. fracture dislocation. The lumbar region is perhaps the most common site of spinal fusion.

Pre-operative Procedure. Where possible a **plaster bed** and anterior shell should be made at least three weeks prior to operation. This not only allows the plaster to dry thoroughly but also enables the patient to become accustomed to its restriction if he lies in it for increasingly long periods during the pre-operative week. During this week it is necessary to ensure that the patient is comfortable in his plaster. Any areas of local pressure should be hammered out and softened, or alternatively should be padded, whichever method gives the better result. It is also good practice prior to operation to **give the patient the experience of being turned in his plaster bed** by the method commonly used in that ward; this will give him added confidence when the procedure is carried out post-operatively.

Before operation is finally arranged this patient in particular must be free from any respiratory infection and the chest should be clear on clinical and X-ray examination. Evacuation of the bowel by an enema is an important pre-operative procedure the day before operation, as post-operative distension of the bowel by gas or faecal obstruction is a distressing complication.

Operation. The most common surgical approach used is the posterior method where the laminae and inter-articular joints are arthrodesed. The principles of surgical fusion governing other joints apply also to the spine. Once the surfaces are prepared a bone graft composed of cancellous bone chips and slivers, or a cortical bone graft, or indeed a combination of both is placed in position. In addition, internal screw fixation of the prepared inter-articular joints may be undertaken to produce stability.

Post-operative Management. Immobilisation. On completion of the operation the plaster bed must be available in theatre so that the patient is placed directly into it before being returned to the ward. Extra special post-operative observation is necessary as the patient in this plaster bed cannot be nursed in the left lateral position used commonly in the post-anaesthetic recovery period.

Physiotherapy. Breathing exercises are extremely important for a patient in this position. Obviously he will be reluctant to breathe deeply and so effective analgesia is necessary to relieve pain and allow for deep breathing exercises.

Special Points in Nursing Management. In the early stages of recovery, vomiting, if it occurs, can be a serious complication. It is useful to have a **suction machine available** should such a situation arise. **Temperature, pulse** and **blood pressure** should be recorded frequently during the first two or three days. A **record of the fluid intake and output** ensures efficient fluid balance. The more frequently a patient can be turned the less likely he is to develop complications. Ideally such a patient should be nursed on a **turning bed** (Stryker frame). Alternatively, an apparatus for turning the patient in his own bed, i.e. a turning machine, should be available. Although less convenient this latter procedure can still be accomplished by two nurses. Where such facilities are not available four or more persons are required to change the position of the patient. Consequently he is turned less regularly. In the initial post-operative period, the patient should be turned after he has been given an analgesic. Once on his front, in the prone position, the uppermost shell is removed.

As there is a tendency for the patient to perspire the **skin** should be sponged, dried thoroughly and powdered. Any areas of redness indicate **pressure** and the appropriate area in the plaster should be examined for any irregularity which must be corrected. Where dried blood has hardened on the felt lining it is removed using a sharp knife. It is important to reconstruct the contour with suitable padding, e.g. orthopaedic wool. If the cause is not obvious it is advisable to pad the area with smooth soft padding such as orthopaedic wool or felt. This will, however, require to be renewed regularly as it absorbs moisture. The wound is sealed at operation with a small occlusive dressing. If the patient complains of excessive pain, and particularly if there is a pyrexia this area is easily inspected for redness, swelling and tenderness, the signs of haematoma formation and wound infection.

Once the patient has recovered from the anaesthetic, a **feeding routine** has to be established, fluids being particularly important to promote a good urinary output. Initially the patient should be offered 3–4 fl. ozs (75–100 ml) at quarter-hourly invervals. The type of fluid given can be varied, e.g. fruit juice, milk, water, etc. As food intake is increased at regular meal times this routine can be altered accordingly. Very often a system can be evolved so that the patient can help himself. An adjustable table may be useful whereby the patient is able to obtain a drink from a feeding cup using a flexible polythene straw. Anything which gives the patient a feeling of some independence will boost his morale. The supine position is a difficult one for feeding and evacuating the bowel and bladder successfully. This can give rise to alimentary tract upsets. It should be explained to the patient that, for this reason, he will remain on a **modified diet** so that such disturbances may be avoided. The male patient can usually manage to use a urinal successfully. The plaster bed is also designed to allow for a bed-pan to be positioned satisfactorily.

Although wound healing is usually complete in about 14 days this is in no way related to the bony fusion, which may not occur for 12–16 weeks. The patient remains immobilised and therefore requires some form of **occupational therapy.** Television, radio and tape-recorder are useful means of communication with the outside world. The patient may prefer, however, to have some form of creative therapy, e.g. needlework, basketwork, painting, etc. The occupational therapist can usually find a craft suitable for such a patient confined to this position.

Other nursing procedures, e.g. **hairwashing,** are fairly easily accomplished by removing the top end from the bed, or the head support in a turning bed. The patient's head is supported by an assistant while the hair is being washed. Most patients can brush their own teeth, particularly while in the prone position. The **cutting of toenails** and the **removal of hard skin from the feet** have to be done by the nurse. Sometimes a chiropodist is available to help with the care of the feet.

Ambulation and Discharge. As signs of bony union become apparent radiologically and clinically, the patient is lifted from his plaster and nursed on a bed with fracture boards beneath the mattress. He then starts mobilising exercises. The patient continues to rest on his plaster bed as a means of support during night-time. Once muscle and joint function are satisfactory the patient progresses gradually from sitting in bed to standing out of bed. When he recovers his sense of balance he starts walking with assistance. Sometimes a plaster jacket is applied for additional support. At this stage the patient is discharged and attends as an outpatient. After a few weeks the plaster jacket is replaced by a more flexible spinal support which is later discarded.

Prognosis. When successful this operation prevents increasing deformity, e.g. in scoliosis and spondylolisthesis. In fractures and fracture dislocations it also ensures stability. Where inflammatory destruction of the vertebral bodies has occurred, e.g. in tuberculosis, spinal fusion by producing stability eliminates the chance of recurrence. This is especially so in an anterior fusion when it is possible to remove any pus, debris and sequestra prior to the arthrodesis. The main advantage to the patient is the relief of painful symptoms.

Complications. Urine retention may cause distress and may indeed require relief by catheterisation. **Abdominal distension** accompanied by vomiting is indicative of the development of paralytic ileus. The relief of **constipation** is more comfortably achieved by the use of suppositories or a small enema rather than by the frequent administration of aperients which tends to produce abdominal discomfort. **Chest complications** and **deep venous thrombosis** are always potential dangers and must be anticipated. The formation of **renal calculi** may be suggested where a patient complains of pain or a dull ache in the region of the back or pelvis but often the first indication is the presence of **haematuria. Infection,** a danger associated with any surgical procedure, is fortunately relatively uncommon. **Failure of fusion to occur** is the main complication. This necessitates a revision operation. If this is not feasible, or if after a second operation union does not occur, the patient will have to wear a spinal support permanently.

AMPUTATION

This operation means the complete removal of a limb, or part of a limb, because trauma or disease has rendered it either useless to the patient or a danger to his continued existence. The loss of a limb is a mental shock and physical handicap to a person. The **operation, post-operative management** and **rehabilitation** are carried out by a **team** consisting of surgeon, nurse, prosthetist (limb fitter), physiotherapist, occupational therapist and medical social worker. A friendly discussion with the members of this team is often reassuring and beneficial to the patient; it may help him to accept such distressing circumstances more philosophically. The object of the operation is not that he should lose his limb but that he should go home mobile and free from pain. Often it can be arranged for the patient to meet another who has been successfully rehabilitated with the aid of an artificial limb. This helps to give added confidence.

At this stage it may be opportune to give the patient some indication of **what he should expect in the post-operative period.** It is important to reassure him that he will be given pain relieving drugs so that he **should not experience pain.** He will, however, experience **the phenomenon that his limb is still there (phantom limb).** This is quite normal and may persist for weeks or even months. In an above knee amputation for example, as the limb gradually 'disappears' the knee is 'lost' first, followed by the rest of the lower limb and finally the toes. When he gets up at first he will **feel slightly 'off balance'** but this sensation also goes away gradually as he becomes more mobile.

It is worth remembering that in other conditions affecting a limb, e.g. in poliomyelitis, the patient lives in hope that the limb will recover; an amputee loses that hope; the prosthesis is his future. Therefore **he must be given encouragement** and this may be achieved by showing the patient the type of prosthesis with which he may be fitted eventually, e.g. the modular or adjustable limb, or the patellar-bearing prosthesis in the lower limb; the powered prosthesis in the upper limb.

A demonstration of how these are designed specially to provide maximum function is often helpful. A brief explanation of the **programme of retraining** and how a personal interest is taken in each individual to achieve the best results will perhaps enable the patient to adapt to the situation before it actually arises. **Morale is important** and if possible the operation is performed when the patient feels ready for it.

The **technique of operation** is aimed at fashioning a stump of the correct length and contour with good muscular control, unimpaired sensation, healthy wound healing and a non-adherent scar. Haematoma formation must be avoided. Careful aseptic technique in all subsequent dressings avoids the risk of infection.

Indications for Amputation

The main indications for amputation include peripheral vascular disease, bone neoplasm and trauma.

In **peripheral vascular disease** there are many associated problems which must be considered and carefully treated if possible before operation. Dry gangrene may exist or wet gangrene with infection; sloughing of the tissues and purulent discharge may be present. The patient may be either **diabetic** or **arteriosclerotic** and may suffer from symptoms of **mild toxaemia,** e.g. **in infected gangrene.** The **general nursing care** is therefore as important as the specific attention to the limb. Where pain is less severe and amputation less urgent it is desirable to get the **part affected** by wet gangrene **dry** and clearly defined before surgery is undertaken. This may be achieved by the use of astringent lotions and the application of an antibacterial powder. The appropriate systemic antibiotic therapy is given once the infecting organism is identified.

In **malignant bone neoplasm,** careful consideration is given to the pathology of the lesion. For example, in osteosarcoma surgery may be withheld until a course of radiotherapy has been given. Six months later, the chest is examined for signs of pulmonary metastases. In their absence amputation of the limb is carried out at the appropriate level.

In **trauma,** the injury may have produced amputation of part of a limb, e.g. amputation of a finger by some sharp instrument or machine. On the other hand the injury, although severe, may be localised interfering with the main blood supply to the rest of the limb, e.g. dislocation of the knee. In this instance it may be possible to rely on the collateral circulation to fulfil the function of the damaged artery but if this response is absent it may be necessary to reconstruct an artery using a graft. Where reparative or reconstructive surgery fails amputation will be considered necessary. If there is doubt as to the effective collateral circulation to part of a limb, e.g. through arteriosclerotic vessels or through a reconstructed artery, it is possible to ascertain a more accurate impression of the situation by means of an arteriogram.

The **level** at which amputation is performed depends on many factors which include the general condition of the patient, the degree of discomfort, the underlying disease and other complications e.g. gangrene, infection, soft tissue and arterial damage. Probably the above and below knee amputations are the most common levels nursed in orthopaedic and accident wards.

Post-operative Management. Immobilisation. A stump dressing and supporting bandage, consisting of wool and crêpe, are carefully applied in theatre. This is essential to control oedema. The stump rests directly on the bed in the extended position and in slight abduction. This position can be controlled by laying a roller towel over the stump and incorporating a sandbag on either side (*Fig. 45*). The foot of the bed is elevated. In upper limb amputations the patient is nursed flat for the first 2–3 days with the stump by his side or resting on a pillow. This avoids the dependent position and thus limits the extent of oedema.

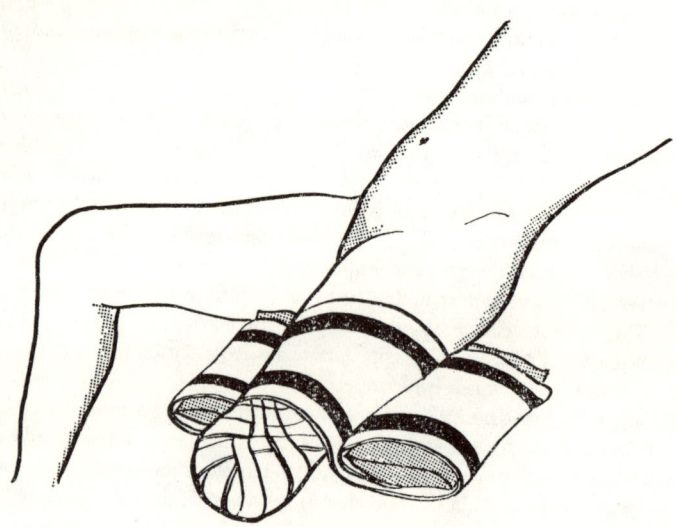

FIG. 45 Post-operative position of stump

General Points in Nursing Management. The painful limb has been removed. If the patient recovers from the anaesthetic suffering from **pain** he feels the operation has failed. Strong analgesia is recommended for at least the first 48 hours and should not be withheld. It is preferable to anticipate pain and administer the prescribed analgesic drug before the patient actually suffers the discomfort. The slight chance of addiction is less serious than the greater chance of **chronic phantom limb pain.**

Wound healing is usually complete in 14 days. Its success is dependent on the surgical technique used. The provision of adequate skin flaps, the suturing of the wound in layers without tension and with good haemostasis **preventing haematoma formation** are all important to primary wound healing. A **non-adherent dressing** is usually applied following wound closure as it is more easily removed subsequently in the ward. An **efficient drain** is particularly necessary in lower limb amputations and this drain is removed between the 2nd and 4th day. This procedure requires an absolutely sterile wound dressing technique and extreme care and gentleness in handling the stump. Although the procedure need not be painful a premedication drug may be given because the first dressing can be rather distressing for the patient. Any marked **bruising, haematoma formation** or **excessive oedema** should be noted and reported as these can predispose to tissue sloughing and infection. Any suggestion of **infection** is treated promptly by the commencement of a prolonged course of **antibiotic therapy.** The stitches may be removed over two or three consecutive days in order to make sure that wound healing is satisfactory. The first sutures are removed at about the 14th day. There should always be a **tourniquet readily available** for use in the event of a profuse haemorrhage. Unless a nurse is aware of the possibility it is not uncommon for a **pressure sore** to develop **over the skin on the heel of the unaffected foot.** This may be avoided either by elevation of this limb in a sling or by placing a thick sorbo-rubber pad behind the ankle to raise the heel from the bed.

Physiotherapy. General exercise is important. A patient helper device should be attached to the bed to enable the patient to move about. Stump exercises are started about the fourth day once wound healing is fairly well advanced. In the lower limb, abduction of the hip and extension of the knee are the important movements to be regained. Abduction and rotation of the shoulder with flexion of the elbow in upper limb amputation must be actively encouraged.

Ambulation and Discharge. Stability, balance and the mechanics of walking with an artificial limb should be taught if possible before a lower limb is amputated. The patient kneels in a prosthesis, thus simulating an amputee's gait. After the drain is removed post-operatively he is allowed up to balance and stand. Within the first week he has progressed to walking between parallel bars.

The ideal management of amputation is for the patient to recover from the anaesthetic with his amputated limb or section of limb already replaced by an artificial prosthesis. This method is not universally used because of difficulty, first in producing the artificial limb in the required time and second the problem of devising an inner socket which can be adjusted as the swelling of the stump diminishes. One method of **immediate prosthetic fitting** used is that which utilises plaster of Paris. The wound of the below-knee stump is covered with a non-adherent dressing. The stump is cushioned with fluffed lamb's wool held in position with an elasticated stump stocking which also provides a degree of tension on the stump. A plaster 'cup' is specially applied over this so that its tension is greater at the distal end and less at the proximal end of the stump. A walking pylon with removable shoe piece is incorporated in this plaster which is then allowed to set. The patient is able to stand and gradually learns to walk between parallel bars wearing this prosthesis. Full weight-bearing on the stump and prosthesis is contra-indicated. The patient, however, may find that the ability to bear weight lightly on this side gives a greater feeling of confidence and balance. The plaster cast is changed after about two weeks at which time the stump sutures are removed. Eventually it is replaced by the permanent prosthesis.

Where it is not possible to fit an immediate prosthesis the patient may be allowed home as soon as the stump has healed. He must be confident in crutch walking, as he will depend on the use of crutches for mobility until his artificial limb is fitted. Where patients, e.g. the elderly, lack confidence in the use of crutches or other walking aids they may need to spend a period of time in a convalescent unit until fitted with the artificial limb. Regular attendances at a special limb fitting centre are necessary, in order to have a good functional artificial limb fitted and to be carefully re-educated in walking with this prosthesis.

Prognosis. Although amputation seems a formidable and tragic procedure it is surprising how well patients of all ages adapt to the wearing of a prosthesis. The long term results depend on the pathological indication for amputation. A good prosthesis should not produce any discomfort, nor should skin sores or other such complications arise. The formation of a good stump is largely dependent on collaboration between the surgeon and prosthetist.

Complications. Haematoma may be seen at the first dressing of the wound either by the obvious extravasation of blood, or by the swelling of the stump and the presence of fluid on palpation. This must be evacuated, usually through the suture line, using strict aseptic precautions. If it occurs, infection of the haematoma affects the patient both generally and locally. He feels unwell, the temperature is elevated and there is throbbing pain and heat in the stump. Under premedication the infected haematoma is evacuated. Antibiotic therapy is commenced immediately. **Contractures of joints** may develop but can be avoided if adequate attention is given to the positioning of the stump (*see pp.* 202, 210). Other early complications include **haemorrhage, fat embolism** and **gas gangrene**.

Late Complications following Amputation. The following late complications may develop:

1 **Skin conditions, bursitis and cyst formation. Contact dermatitis** may occur due either to sensitivity to the materials used in finishing the socket of the prosthesis or to the antiseptics or solutions used in cleansing the skin. Recognition and avoidance of the offending substance are necessary in order to treat the condition effectively. The late development of **oedema** and **'fishmouth' ulcers** are controlled by fitting a socket which distributes and absorbs pressure as well as adequately supporting the stump, e.g. sorbo-rubber covered by plastic. **Recurrent infection** is a potential problem. There is an actual increase in the number of bacteria in the skin of the stump as compared with normal skin. Daily hygiene of the stump is therefore of great importance. Antiseptic baths are useful in preventing the development of **epidermal cysts** which result from the formation of epithelial plugs.

2 **Circulatory disturbances.** There is a potential risk of poor circulation in the stump where the amputation has been necessary to treat ischaemia or gangrene of the limb. Where the collateral vessels are also diseased, **anoxia of the tissues at the**

end of the stump may develop and **ulceration** of the stump results. **Necrosis of the skin** can occur if there is vascular insufficiency above the level of the stump.

3 **Exostoses.** Where spurs of bone form on the end of the stump fragment these may require to be removed if they are causing pressure on the inner aspect of the soft tissues.

4 **Neuromas.** These are small masses of nerve fibres which grow beyond the point of nerve division. Although not painful to touch they are often associated with pain on pressure from the artificial prosthesis. These neuromas may be excised but unfortunately they recur.

5 **Causalgia.** This is a most distressing condition in which there is severe, constant pain in the stump. It is not associated with phantom limb. The patient guards the stump carefully, resents examination of it and cannot tolerate his prosthesis. Trophic changes are seen in the skin which has a characteristic smooth glossy appearance. Treatment may be successful by **sympathetic block** but if this fails there is little hope for relief of pain. **Cordotomy** (selective division of a sensory tract in the spinal cord) may be necessary in an effort to help some patients. It must be adequate and at a sufficiently high level in order to interfere with the sensory painful stimuli before they reach the brain.

6 **Phantom Limb.** The normal phenomenon of the painless phantom limb has already been described in this chapter. Sometimes, however, the patient is afflicted by **chronic phantom limb pain.** It is another distressing complication. Often the patient feels as though the limb has not been removed. The condition can produce severe emotional stress which is also an aggravating factor in producing pain so that the patient is caught in a vicious circle. Phantom limb pain may be a result of **unsuccessful wound healing of the stump,** e.g. where there has been infection and prolonged sepsis. Involuntary twitchings or jerkings of the stump are often an additional problem. Once pain exists it is very difficult to eradicate altogether. The stump and the part of the limb proximal to it should be examined thoroughly for anything which might contribute to the pain. The patient should be assessed psychologically. Although psychotherapy may be considered beneficial **the pain nevertheless must always be regarded as real.** Local measures directed at **improving the stump or the prosthesis** may benefit some patients while others may require **cordotomy.**

22 THE POSITIONING OF PATIENTS AFTER SURGERY AND IN THE MANAGEMENT OF TRAUMA

The position in which the patient is nursed is determined by either the nature of he operation or the management of the injuries. The main considerations are:

1 Safe recovery from anaesthesia
2 Limitation of reactionary oedema resulting from trauma or operation
3 The optimum position with regard to the efficiency of plaster immobilisation or splintage
4 Avoidance of dislocation of joints
5 Prevention of joint contractures and other deformities

In general the patient in the **immediate post-operative period** is nursed in the lateral position without a head pillow until he recovers from the anaesthetic. At this stage he may feel quite comfortable due firstly to the effect of the post-operative analgesia and secondly to the fact that the reactionary oedema has not yet reached its maximum. After the patient has been washed and changed the tendency is to prop him up often using a back-rest support and three or four pillows. Although the patient's condition may seem to justify this, after more major surgery oedema and swelling may be aggravated. If, for example, a limb is encased in plaster, complications can quickly result. For this reason during the early post-operative management of such a patient it is desirable that he lies in the **recumbent position** with a firm pillow supporting the head comfortably. The initial **position of his limbs after trauma or surgery** is also important. The use of pillows placed transversely under the lower limbs should be avoided; where necessary, e.g. under a plaster, the pillow should be placed **longitudinally** under the limb in extension in such a way that pressure is avoided behind the knee and the heel is left free (*Fig. 46*).

Bedclothes should not be tucked tightly round the feet otherwise equinus deformities may be produced. Where there is any doubt, a **bed cage** should be inserted to relieve pressure on the feet. The nurse must be alert to the possibility that **flexion contractures of joints** may develop unobtrusively, particularly in the elderly and in those patients confined to bed for a long time. Treatment of established deformities presents many difficulties and for this reason they must be prevented.

Operations on the Upper Limb

Immobilisation may be by means of a complete arm plaster, a plaster shell and bandage or by a simple supporting bandage. After more minor surgery, e.g. division of the carpal ligament in carpal tunnel syndrome, the arm may be supported sufficiently on a waterproof covered pillow. Where more traumatic

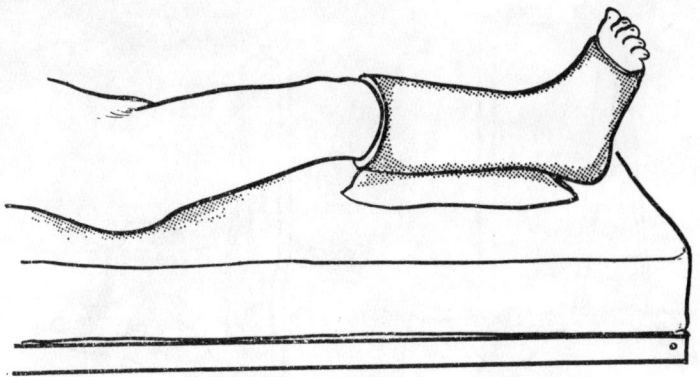

FIG. 46 Positioning of pillows under a plaster cast

operations have been undertaken, e.g. arthrodesis of the wrist, the tissue reaction anticipated is relatively more severe. It is therefore always advisable to **elevate the limb.** Where the arm is in plaster this may be achieved by means of two lengths of cotton or old bandage attached to loops incorporated in the plaster and fixed either to a stand by the bedside or to the beam of a Balkan frame (*Fig. 47a*). Where the limb is not encased in a plaster the method of elevation must include complete support of the elbow, otherwise traction on the hand and wrist occurs. The common method used is a tube gauze sling which includes the whole length of the arm and an extension with which to suspend the limb from a stand or bed frame (*Fig. 47b*). The sling must be fixed securely to the skin of the upper arm by two strips of adhesive plaster. One strip is applied anteriorly and the other posteriorly, each covering 2–3 in. (5–7.5 cm) of the sling and extending 2–3 in. (5–7.5 cm) on the skin of the upper arm. In this way the sling is not pulled off leaving the elbow unsupported. At the same time the upper limit of the sling should not cause constriction as this would interfere with circulation. The limb is suspended in a position which is comfortable for the patient, which allows free use of the fingers and which is also effective in encouraging venous circulation thus minimising swelling.

Operations on the Lower Limb

Immobilisation is by means of a partial or complete plaster cast, splintage in a Thomas's splint, or by a simple supporting bandage. Tissue reaction to injury or surgery often creates a problem in the post-traumatic or post-operative period.

This may be aggravated by the fact that patients tend to sit up in bed as soon as they feel fit, even as early as a few hours after major surgery. Venous pressure is thereby increased. There is, temporarily, some muscle inactivity in response to surgery and the venous circulation is less efficient due to loss of some degree of

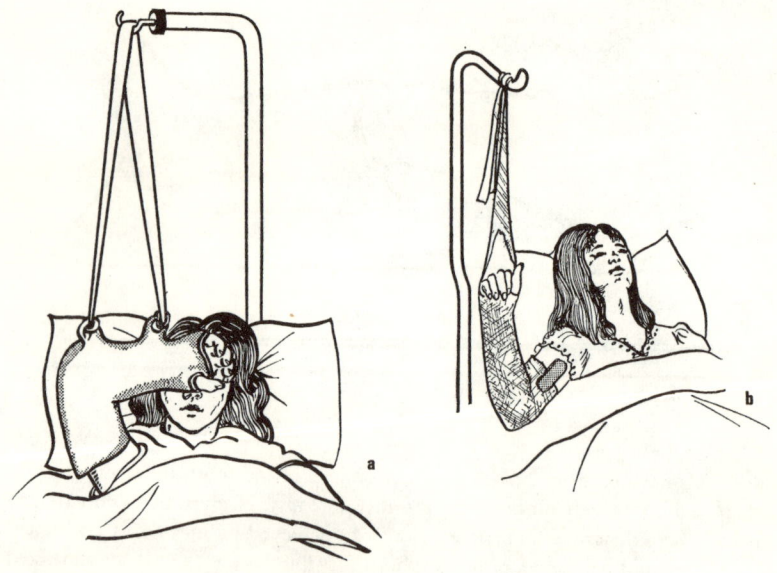

FIG. 47   Methods of elevating the upper limb
(*a*) Plaster suspension
(*b*) Tube gauze sling

muscle contraction. The tendency to develop oedema is increased and therefore it is important that the limb is elevated for the first 3–4 days after surgery. This allows for reactionary oedema to settle.

There are several methods of **elevating a lower limb in or out of plaster:**

1 A limb out of plaster may be elevated by: raising the foot of the bed; cradling the posterior aspect of the knee and ankle using sorbo-rubber supports; allowing the mattress to conform to the natural contour of the limb by placing sandbags underneath it at these levels so that the calf and heel remain free from pressure; using suspensory cords where a Thomas's splint is in position.

2 A limb in plaster may be elevated by: placing one or two waterproof covered pillows under the limb so that the heel is left free; cradling it in a suspensory sling from a Balkan frame; constructing plaster loops through which cords are passed to suspend the limb, again from a Balkan frame.

The Recumbent Position

There are obviously certain disadvantages for the patient associated with the recumbent position. **Feeding** and **toilet** are among the main difficulties. For the short time involved it is often kinder to allow the patient to sit up for food and toilet; it is important that he is helped back into the recumbent position thereafter. Where the foot of the bed is elevated some patients experience difficulty in micturition during the first 24–48 hours. The bed may be lowered for a short period until the patient voids urine satisfactorily.

Hip Spicas

Immobilisation in a single or double hip spica is practicable only where a patient can lie for a prolonged post-operative period in the supine or prone position comfortably without obvious complications. The patient is therefore usually in the younger age group and free from any disease which would contra-indicate this type of immobilisation, e.g. cardio-respiratory disease.

A hip spica is a rigid support moulded to the contour of the lower two-thirds of the patient's body. Should the patient be placed in bed on a firm mattress there would be stress on the plaster in the poorly supported areas, namely, the lumbar spine and the posterior aspect of the knee and ankle. **Waterproof covered pillows are placed under the plaster** at these levels **to give the necessary support.** On the first post-operative day the patient is turned into **the prone position** to allow the posterior aspect of the plaster to dry. In this position extra pillows are required, one under the shoulder girdle, one at the level of the iliac crests and one supporting each shin. This ensures that the chest, abdomen, knee and toes are free from pressure and that the plaster cast is relieved of stress at its weaker points.

Patients With Other Conditions Which Influence Their Position

In some instances **modifications in the position of the patient** are necessary where there is another condition present, unrelated to the orthopaedic problem, such as cardio-respiratory disease. A compromise has to be made whereby both conditions are considered and the best possible results for each obtained. This may necessitate propping up the patient. Therefore in the immediate post-operative period although an effort is made to elevate a limb as far as possible from the dependent position the comfort of the patient must be considered.

Joint Dislocations

Post-operative joint dislocation occurs most commonly in the hip joint particularly **after arthroplasty.** In an anterior or lateral surgical approach the capsular ligaments stabilising the joint are divided and the hip is dislocated by an external rotational manoeuvre in order to expose the joint surfaces to be replaced. Post-operatively, if the limb is allowed to rotate externally, redislocation of the joint may occur. After a posterior surgical approach the hip is dislocated by an internal rotational manoeuvre. Post-operatively, internal rotation of the limb predisposes to redislocation of the hip joint.

This complication may be avoided if the nurse recognises the site of the wound which indicates the rotational movement permitted. The limb is maintained either in the neutral position or in a position of rotation opposite to that likely to produce dislocation. Supporting pillows on the lateral aspect of the thigh in the first instance or between the knees in the other will provide the necessary safeguard.

Spinal Operations

In the post-operative management of spinal operations the position in which the patient is nursed will be determined by whether or not the operation produces instability of spine. In disc operations the stability of the spine may be relatively unaffected, e.g. in a keyhole approach, and the patient can rest comfortably in the lateral position until the post-operative discomfort has settled. He is then free to sit up. On the other hand, e.g. in operations of spinal fusion, the spine is temporarily unstable until union occurs. This patient is immobilised in the supine position in a plaster bed. A turning frame is used to allow his position to be changed from supine to prone alternatively.

Amputations

The patient lies supine with **fracture boards** under the mattress to give support. Joint contractures must be avoided otherwise fitting and utilisation of an artificial limb is unsatisfactory. Pillows are contra-indicated as a means of support for a lower limb stump therefore the foot of the bed is raised initially to provide the necessary elevation. If possible **the patient's position should be changed** thereafter **from supine to prone at regular intervals** throughout the post-operative period. Stiffness of the shoulder and elbow in upper limb amputation must be prevented. As soon as the tissue reaction has settled in 2–3 days, free movement of these joints is encouraged.

Multiple Injuries

Patients who have sustained serious multiple injuries, in particular those which involve injury to the chest or head, require special attention with regard to their position. It is also desirable to have some means of altering the patient's position quickly when necessary. For this reason a **special 'accident' bed** which is mechanically adjustable is useful. The ability to tilt it in any direction allows such problems as the removal of respiratory secretions, the control of bleeding and the alleviation of hypotension to be managed efficiently without further distressing the patient.

Nurses tend to be most apprehensive in the handling of the severely injured. The patient on the other hand may suffer from the complications associated with total immobility unless the nursing staff can alter his position for him. It is important that the nurse should have detailed information about the extent of the patient's injuries and the extent of movement permitted. Good liaison with the medical team caring for the patient is necessary in order that the best nursing management can be accomplished. Where it is undesirable to move the patient he should be nursed either on a **sheepskin** rug or on a special **mattress,** e.g. one which has **alternating air-filled sections** which are electrically controlled to allow for distribution of pressure, thus minimising the risk of skin sores as a result of pressure on specific areas.

23 SURGICAL AND NURSING PRINCIPLES IN THE MANAGEMENT OF WOUND HEALING

The factors which are necessary to produce successful wound healing are:

1. The general fitness of the patient
2. The technique of wound closure
3. Control of bleeding and the absence of haematoma
4. Aseptic technique in wound dressing
5. Exclusion of subsequent infection

The General Fitness of the Patient

A patient who is undergoing elective surgery has the advantage of being medically assessed with regard to his fitness for the particular operation he has consented to undergo. There may be less opportunity for the patient who has been the victim of trauma to have this detailed pre-operative investigation.

The patient is examined clinically. The blood group, cell count and haemoglobin are ascertained. Respiratory and cardiac function are examined and chest X-ray and electrocardiograph often utilised to complete this assessment. Urine analysis establishes that renal function is satisfactory and excludes the presence of abnormal constituents such as sugar and albumin.

Infection must be excluded. Sometimes this is quite obvious as in upper respiratory infection. On the other hand, only specific enquiry or examination of the patient will reveal the presence of such infection as vaginal or urethral discharge or small septic spots on the skin.

Technique of Wound Closure

The main objective in the technique of closing a wound is the exclusion of any 'dead space' where blood can accumulate. This predisposes to delayed wound healing perhaps complicated by infection. The wound is therefore closed in layers from below upwards, the cut ends of each layer of tissue being approximated accurately. The skin sutures, although tight enough to close the wound completely, should not be so tense that they cut into the skin. This results in damage to the tissue often with resultant infection.

Control of Bleeding and Haematoma

During the operative procedure the surgeon takes specific care in controlling obvious bleeding, either by ligature or diathermy of the bleeding vessels as they are incised. Where a tourniquet has been applied to control bleeding prior to operations on the limbs bleeding from small blood vessels will not be obvious. These are usually occluded naturally by the special mechanism of the body in the control of bleeding. If on completion of the operation the wound dressing and covering bandage are specially applied to exert gentle pressure, haemostasis will be increased. When a long bone is cut, e.g. in osteotomy, bleeding occurs from the medullary canal. Where such bleeding can be anticipated, or in major surgical procedures requiring a large wound, a suction drain with a closed sterile drainage system is often inserted. It is passed from within the deeper layers of the operation wound, or from any dead space which has been produced due to the nature of the surgery performed, through a separate puncture wound in the soft tissues to the exterior; the risk of introducing infection into the wound is thereby eliminated. The drain is removed within 48 hours by gentle traction. The main wound dressing is undisturbed. Elevation of a limb in the initial post-operative period also tends to minimise bleeding.

Aseptic Technique in Wound Dressing
The wound is normally left untouched until it is inspected prior to the removal of sutures. Where the patient has an unexplained pyrexia or any other relevant symptoms and signs, e.g. a rapid pulse or general malaise, it may be considered necessary to inspect the wound to exclude the presence of a haematoma or of an abscess. An absolutely sterile dressing procedure is essential. It is also important that the wound dresser, usually the nurse, is free from any infection such as a sore throat or localised infection of the fingers, hands or arms. The stage at which wound sutures are removed depends on several factors; whether the patient is a child or an adult; the site of the wound; the extent of surgery performed. Some sutures are removed as early as the third or fourth day, e.g. in facial wounds in children; others remain undisturbed for 12–14 days, e.g. in wounds in the region of the hip joint. Sometimes sutures are removed in stages. Deep tension sutures may be removed at the first stage, alternate wound sutures at a second stage and the remainder at a third stage dressing.

Exclusion of Infection
Infection may occur at one of three stages:

  1 During operation or at the time of injury
  2 In the period of post-operative hospitalisation
  3 As delayed infection, not manifest for several weeks or even months

Where an operation is prolonged or difficult the risk of infection is greater. This is because the wound is exposed for a longer period and the immediate environment, although thoroughly sterilised at the commencement of operation, is more likely to become contaminated. The patient's general resistance to infection may also be influenced by the nature or difficulty of the surgery performed. Where such a situation has arisen the patient may be given antibiotic therapy in large doses after surgery. A broad spectrum antibiotic which can attack a wide variety of organisms is normally selected. Compound wounds in accident surgery are usually treated as potentially infected and managed by early administration of antiobiotics rather than delaying until infection is obvious.

In the **post-operative period** infection may result where bleeding or haematoma has occurred and has become infected before it has been discovered. In pelvic or hip surgery there is always the danger of infection from the perineal area. The risk of wound contamination by urine or faeces can be reduced considerably if the operation wound is sealed completely by a waterproof occlusive dressing. This must be combined with thorough perineal hygiene. Cross infection from another source in the ward may still occur but is relatively less common because of the greater attention to strict asepsis and isolation or barrier nursing of patients with known infections.

The **management of an infection** at this stage is by the administration of **antibiotics** in maximum doses which are continued often for a prolonged period. The method of administration may be by intramuscular injection or in some cases, e.g. in trauma, where an intravenous infusion has been necessary, the antibiotic may be introduced intravenously. Once the patient's acute symptoms and signs have resolved he may be given his drug orally. Although 'blind' antibiotic therapy may be utilised initially it is important to **obtain a specimen of any discharge for culture** of the organism by the bacteriologist thus determining its type and sensitivity to antibiotics.

Delayed infection is more associated with trauma, although it does occur in some cases where elective surgery has been performed. Despite the immediate treatment by antibiotic therapy this type of infection may be difficult to eradicate completely. Recurrence is often a problem.

A patient reacts to unmodified pain in three possible ways. Firstly, he avoids any movement which produces pain although sometimes, reflexly, he attempts to remove a limb from the painful stimulus. Secondly, the response of the autonomic nervous system produces tachycardia, hypertension, sweating and vaso-constriction. Thirdly, there is the interpretation of pain by the higher centres and its evaluation according to the patient's past experience of this or similar pain.

Appreciation of pain is obviously subjective and what is painful to one person may be tolerable to another. There is a different threshold to a painful stimulus in different individuals and, indeed, in the one individual at different times. The patient with a high pain threshold does not feel pain readily. The individual with a low pain threshold, on the other hand, interprets probably minimal pain as intolerable. There is also a third group in which the patient feels pain but tolerates it without wishing to 'bother' anyone. Pain is, therefore, open to various interpretations and extremely difficult to measure. In the ward or recovery area it may be difficult to know if the patient is suffering pain. This is made much more difficult if he is unable to communicate, for instance, where he has multiple injuries and is on a ventilator in an intensive therapy unit. Recognition of the existence of pain is the first step in its relief.

The Attempted Assessment of Pain

Various research projects are currently being carried out in an attempt to measure pain. None of these at present is applicable clinically and so the clinician and nurse are forced to rely upon the patient's own volunteered statements where this is possible. Otherwise frequent measurements of pulse rate, blood pressure and central venous pressure are essential in order to indicate when pain is being experienced and also when the therapy is effective in its relief.

The Relief of Pain

Preliminary Preparation. A patient undergoing surgery of any kind fears two things, intolerable pain and the unknown. An important part in the preparation for surgery is an informal talk with the patient by the members of staff involved in the operation and the recovery period, i.e. the surgeon, the anaesthetist and the nurse. It is wise to give an explanation about the post-operative period, with particular mention of such things as the method of splintage and the possibility that blood transfusion, chest or bladder drainage may be required. This does not disturb the patient; conversely it makes the recovery from anaesthesia less terrifying. The patient will then realise that the presence of such rather formidable apparatus is normal.

He should realise also that he will be completely unaware of any of the operative proceedings and will not waken until these are completed. The anaesthetist will give this assurance as well as describing briefly the procedure of administering the anaesthetic. If the patient is told that he will naturally experience some discomfort post-operatively but that a drug can be given to make the pain less acute, he will tolerate it more readily when it occurs. The nurse can complete this pre-operative preparation by giving a short explanation of the post-operative management, e.g. frequent pulse, blood pressure and temperature assessments during the initial 24–48 hours, the position of the patient, the management of bladder and bowel evacuation and the type of diet to be given.

Operation. Although it is generally accepted that the more extensive the surgery or injury the more severe is the pain, relatively simple operations may be associated with a significant degree of discomfort in the post-operative period, e.g. after bunionectomy or meniscectomy. This should be carefully considered in the control of pain and sometimes it may be possible to prepare for this before the patient leaves theatre. Sometimes, for example after bunionectomy, it may be possible to introduce a local, long-acting regional block anaesthetic which will last for 4–5 hours. This provides for the complete relief of pain during the interval between the end of the anaesthetic and the stage of full recovery of consciousness. The patient does not wake up feeling discomfort but will remain free from pain for the first few hours. By this time he has more fully recovered from the effects of the anaesthetic, and other means of pain relief such as parenteral analgesia can be considered with safety. The analgesic drug can be administered before the patient actually experiences any real discomfort.

Post-operative Recovery. The crucial period is the first 48 hours when maximal pain is normally experienced. Once pain has developed it is more difficult to relieve and it will require usually a larger dosage of any drug to alleviate this discomfort than would have been required had the situation been anticipated.

Methods of Pain Relief

There are four common methods of relieving pain in the management of post-operative surgery and trauma, any one of which may be appropriate in an individual case. Occasionally a combination of these methods may be the most successful way of relieving the pain.

Parenteral Analgesics. This is the commonest method of administering a pain-relieving drug, often in the form of a narcotic, e.g. Morphine. The route chosen is of considerable importance. In a severely injured patient, for example, repeated subcutaneous or intramuscular injections are usually undesirable. Firstly, they can only add to the general discomfort of the patient and secondly, where the peripheral circulation is inadequate the rate of absorption of the drug may be unpredictable and its ultimate effect less satisfactory. In these patients the use of the intravenous route overcomes the problem of malabsorption of the drug. The peak and duration of its action with potential side-effects can be more accurately determined. The opiates are the most commonly used drugs in this situation. It is accepted practice that they should be diluted so that they can be given in small incremental doses intravenously, for instance, into an intravenous infusion which is already running. If Morphine is used as an example of such a drug given in this way it is usually diluted to the strength of 1 mg/ml and administered 1 ml at a time until relief of pain is obtained. When a patient is being mechanically ventilated, as in the case of a severe chest injury, there is no danger of the usual results of drug depression of the respiratory centre. The patient, however, may be more sensitive to the cardiovascular depressant effects of potent analgesics.

Repeated injections can lead to accumulation of the drug and may lead to over-depression of the respiratory centre and cardiovascular centres. Hepatic and renal function may be disturbed with the result that drug detoxication and elimination may be defective. There is also the risk of producing physical and psychological drug dependence, i.e. addiction through chronic exposure to narcotic analgesics, an important factor to bear in mind when such drugs are administered over a long period.

The use of this method of pain relief is most effective when the painful stimulus is anticipated and the drug is given in advance of the painful experience such as prior to physiotherapy and the changing of painful dressings or plasters.

Inhalation Analgesia. With the apparatus now available this technique of administering pain relief is relatively easy. The drugs are all volatile or gaseous agents and many of them are used in general anaesthesia in theatre. Using a fairly simple apparatus they can be administered to the patient who is breathing spontaneously, and with special vaporisers to the patient who is receiving ventilator therapy. This method is particularly useful prior to painful procedures such as rigorous physiotherapy, endotracheal aspiration of secretions and the changing of painful dressings, e.g. amputation stump dressing or plaster casts. Three main agents are used.

1 **Trichlorethylene** (Trilene) in air from a special vaporiser, either the Tecota or the Emotril, gives concentrations of 0.3 and 0.5 per cent. Although originally used specifically to relieve pain in obstetrics this agent is now widely used in general surgery. The patient breathes the vapour mixed with air for a few minutes prior to the painful procedure and intermittently during it. Pain relief is good and the method can be used repeatedly over short periods of time.

2 **Entonox** (nitrous oxide 50% premixed with 50% oxygen) has been adopted also from obstetrical practice and is widely used in post-operative pain relief and in pain therapy in the intensive therapy unit. Its continuous use over a long period of time is not without some risk of bone marrow depression.

3 Penthrane 0.5 per cent in air administered from a special vaporiser is another agent used in the relief of pain. Although this has been used extensively in obstetrical work it would appear that the method could also prove useful in the management of pain in patients in the post-operative period and in those with multiple injuries.

Regional Blockade. This is a means of producing complete analgesia in one area of the body without any danger of central depression. A local analgesic, such as Lignocaine or Prilocaine, is injected in the region of the main nerve supply to the affected part. The procedure can be repeated over a period of time, e.g. when used in intercostal or paravertebral blocks for multiple rib fractures. An alternative method is to introduce a plastic catheter into the epidural space and, by injecting the local analgesic, one can produce a regional block over a widespread area. This technique has also been used to relieve pain from abdominal wounds, thoracic wounds and rib fractures.

Sensory Blockade. This technique of pain relief is interesting. Certain drugs act not only centrally by producing sedation but also on the sensory tracts in the spinal cord so blocking painful stimuli before they reach the higher centres. These drugs produce a state resembling natural sleep. In addition to producing analgesia the drugs also abolish muscle spasm and this can be extremely useful in patients with excessive muscular tone, i.e. spasticity, and also in patients undergoing mechanical assistance to respiration.

Recognition of Other Factors Contributing to Discomfort
Where a patient becomes restless or distressed despite apparently adequate sedation after trauma or operation it should not be assumed that post-traumatic or post-operative pain is necessarily the cause. Careful examination of the patient should be carried out to exclude other causes, e.g. a full bladder, a tight bandage or plaster, pins not carefully closed or fastened through the skin. Sometimes, for example, a patient in a hip spica is cold merely because of the attempt to expose the plaster so that it may dry. So often these or other such problems can be resolved quite simply, the result being much more satisfactory than the repeated administration of analgesia.

Oral Analgesics. These have not been classified with the methods of relieving pain because during the first few days post-operatively their use is so limited. They are not sufficiently quick-acting, and in the immediate post-operative period their rate of absorption is too unpredictable. After the initial period of discomfort has passed transient, less severe pain can be effectively relieved by any one of the various preparations available.

Summary
While pain is a universal experience and there are many drugs and techniques available for its relief, the successful management of pain depends largely on the recognition of its existence. There are two extremes to be avoided: unmodified

pain in the restless patient whose condition will deteriorate unless the situation is improved; the over-enthusiastic use of particularly potent narcotic analgesics which can produce severe depression of the central nervous system and lead to grave life-threatening complications.

The series of changes involving the building up and breaking down of chemical compounds for materials and energy in the body is called **metabolism.** Tissues constantly undergo change. The process by which degenerate or worn-out tissue cells are removed is called **catabolism;** that which involves the repair or regeneration of new tissue cells is termed **anabolism.** The balance between these two processes constitutes normal metabolism. If, for example, catabolism were increased the patient would tend to lose weight; conversely, if anabolism were in excess he would gain weight. The physiology and biochemistry involved in the metabolism of the cells, tissues and organs of the body are indeed complex.

There are two ways in which injury produces a metabolic reaction in orthopaedic and accident surgery. One follows on a **planned surgical procedure,** the other results from **accidental trauma** sustained by the individual. The response of the tissues and organs varies with normal stimuli and abnormal situations. There are, however, other patterns which may be obvious in the patient recovering from trauma, disease or surgery. Some of these are quite normal while others are abnormal and may have serious consequences unless one is aware of their development and is ready to treat them promptly. This chapter is included for the nurse because there are many practical problems with which she is involved and which are directly related to the metabolic response to injury.

Tissue Metabolism

The tissues receive their required nourishment directly or indirectly from food taken in the daily diet. This includes the proteins, fats, carbohydrates, water, vitamins and minerals (largely in the form of the elements sodium, potassium, calcium, magnesium, iron and certain trace elements like copper, cobalt, zinc, manganese and iodine). The carbohydrates and fats are essentially the substances which provide heat and energy; the proteins are the body-building materials; vitamins and minerals are additional food factors necessary for the vital processes of the body to take place. These substances are processed by the various organs of the body by the chemical action of their secretions or hormones. Thus the tissues receive their individual nutrition by selecting and utilising the specific foods they require to maintain their function. This normal metabolic process requires the consumption of a large amount of oxygen taken into the lungs, absorbed into the blood stream and conveyed to the tissues where the chemical changes occur. There are as a result waste products from tissue metabolism, e.g. carbon dioxide, urea, salts, food residue and water, which are disposed of by the excretory organs, i.e. the lungs, kidneys, bowels and skin. One can understand therefore that the body fluids, the arterial and venous blood, the extra-cellular and intra-cellular fluid are full of varying quantities of these elements.

In order to maintain normal body function the amount of these substances present in the body at any one time must be carefully balanced. The balance of body biochemistry also maintains the correct alkalinity or acidity of the various fluids and secretions in the body, e.g. blood is slightly alkaline, gastric secretion is acid. Where injury or disease disrupts the normal pattern abnormal situations develop.

Normal Reaction to Injury

In the post-operative or post-traumatic period there are certain changes which occur and these are considered normal in this particular phase. For example the nurse will be familiar with such findings as a moderate elevation of temperature, a raised pulse rate, a low intake of fluid and food and a diminished urinary output. There are other less obvious changes, e.g. the oxidising of fat, a transient loss of body weight, a temporary imbalance in electrolytes due to certain losses from the body, hyperglycaemia and glycosuria. These changes are influenced to some extent by the short period of starvation following injury, by some readjustment of pituitary and adrenal function in response to injury and by the period of immobilisation of the patient. This period of normal metabolic response to injury should only last 5–7 days during which time return to normal should be evident. The patient's temperature and pulse settle, the caloric intake in the diet is increased and urinary excretion returns to normal.

In the management of this initial period it is important that this natural response is not upset. The tendency to treat an early fever with immediate antibiotic therapy must therefore be avoided. Any attempt to compensate a diminished urinary output with copious fluids orally or intravenously should be delayed at this stage. Electrolyte balance is not usually assessed meantime but if it is, the temporary imbalance must be regarded as physiological during this period. Caloric intake is relatively unimportant during the first three days following operation or trauma.

These facts may suggest that the clinical observations made during the early treatment of injury or operation should be ignored. On the contrary they are extremely important as they first of all indicate that this natural response has occurred and secondly that a pattern of normal convalescence is taking place.

Abnormalities of Response

These may be related to:

1 The type of injury
2 The degree of fitness of the patient and his nutritive state
3 Adrenal insufficiency
4 Other uncontrolled extra-renal fluid losses

The Type of Injury. There is usually an excessive response to excessive trauma or major surgery or indeed sometimes after more moderate trauma. Where surgery is planned it is important that a careful technique is used to minimise trauma. If necessary, it may be possible to programme the operation into stages so that the patient can recover fully from one stage before further surgery is undertaken. At operation, provision for the complete replacement of blood loss must be made to avoid oligaemic shock. Similarly the management of severe trauma must be considered so that treatment does not temporarily increase the catabolic reaction, e.g. by an operation which could probably be delayed until the patient's body has had time to correct some of the deficiencies which have occurred in response to the injury. Where there has been excessive injury, the post-operative or post-traumatic course must be watched carefully. All fluid loss must be measured and correlated with intake. If there is any deficit, particularly after the sixth day, early replacement is essential. The patient's biochemistry otherwise becomes grossly unbalanced and this can produce adrenal depression, severe hypotension and collapse of the patient.

The Degree of Fitness of the Patient. Where a patient has had a poor caloric intake, e.g. an elderly person living alone, someone with an existing disease which upsets the normal function of the affected system such as diabetes, or an individual having had previous trauma or operation, he is generally depleted in some of the essential elements of body function. These patients are much more liable to electrolytic imbalance, phlebothrombosis and wound infection. Where possible, such as prior to elective surgery, it is of the utmost importance to correct any deficiency in order to avoid a complicated convalescence. This is done by the administration of intravascular blood, plasma or electrolytic fluid substitute. Where this has not been possible, e.g. in a malnourished elderly patient admitted with a fracture of the neck of femur, it is vital that recognition of the depletion response is made early and corrected before irreversible damage occurs. The nurse must record all intake and output accurately and note any signs of imbalance, e.g. dehydration or oedema, a smell of acetone from the breath, etc. Blood pressure, pulse and temperature readings four-hourly are essential in this general assessment.

Adrenal Insufficiency. Sometimes the adrenal glands fail to respond to a decrease in the level of circulating pituitary hormone (A.C.T.H.). This may be functional, e.g. due to underlying disease, or anatomical, e.g. after adrenalectomy. In such a situation the blood pressure remains subnormal and this hypotension leads to an oliguria. There is a marked loss of salt from the body. These patients cannot therefore tolerate trauma or infection. The diminution in the normal catabolic response to injury can be alleviated by adrenal hormone therapy. Blood and urine analyses determine the amount of cortisone given. A.C.T.H. is substituted when the initial reaction is under control and this is gradually reduced in dosage until it is eventually discontinued during the convalescent period.

Extra-Renal Fluid Loss. This involves the loss of fluid from the body other than by way of the renal tract. The loss may be brought about by a deficient intake, e.g. post-operative starvation, or by actual fluid loss as in vomiting and diarrhoea or by bleeding in major surgery or multiple injuries. As well as the loss of water there is a depletion of the essential elements in solution in the fluid, such as potassium and sodium in gastric or intestinal loss and of plasma proteins in bleeding. If during the period of normal response to surgery or trauma, i.e. during the first week, the patient develops a complication such as paralytic ileus, e.g. in fractures of the pelvis, this immediately converts the normal pattern to an abnormal one. Early recognition of such a complication (at the stage of its development) is an important step in its effective management. The exact nature and amount of fluid lost must be known so that the immediate replacement of the depleted substances can be made in a form in which they can readily be utilised, namely by intra-vascular administration. The patient again becomes more susceptible to the complications of convalescence, and clinical observations with if necessary repeated biochemical analyses will be important until complete recovery is achieved.

Factors which Influence the Normal Response to Injury

1 Immobilisation
2 Diet
3 Environmental temperature

Immobilisation. Although immobilisation is usually a relatively minor factor in the metabolic response to injury in orthopaedic and accident surgery in particular it may often be prolonged and radical allowing the patient very little freedom of movement. There is some interference in calcium and phosphorus metabolism. This may be reflected in the fact that patients on prolonged complete immobilisation tend to develop renal calculi. Biochemical analyses at intervals during this period may be an important means of recognising the development of such complications.

Diet. In the management of patients in the post-operative or post-traumatic period the advancement to a well-balanced diet is usually achieved by the end of the first week. Where, however, this period has been complicated by a condition such as paralytic ileus, or if the patient is unconscious due to a head injury, attention to the composition of diet, its caloric content and the method of feeding the patient is extremely important. The patient otherwise becomes rapidly depleted and biochemically unbalanced. The surgeon, dietician and ward sister may require to discuss the problem together so that an accurate diet can be given for the individual patient.

The route of administration, where oral diet cannot be given, is usually by a nasogastric tube. The diet must be nutritious but at the same time it must be easily digestible and palatable otherwise the patient's system may not tolerate it. Feeding by this method is usually better divided into smaller feeds given 3-hourly during normal waking hours. Clinical assessment of the patient will indicate whether the diet needs to be adjusted, i.e. either increased or decreased. Supplementary vitamins and iron are usually necessary because the foods given in fluid form tend to be deficient in these elements.

Sometimes it is necessary to replenish a patient by prolonged intravenous feeding. This is only employed where for some reason the patient fails to tolerate gastric feeding. Such a diet may consist of: fat emulsion which yields the most energy; amino-acids in solution to compensate for excess protein metabolism; electrolytic substances in solution to correct any mineral deficiency.

Environmental Temperature. This appears to have some influence on the metabolic response to injury. By increasing the temperature of the area in which the injured patient is nursed, there is a likelihood of reducing the hypermetabolic response associated with trauma. The breakdown and liberation of protein from skeletal muscle giving rise to an excess urinary excretion of nitrogen and a rise in heat production are the main factors in the response to injury. The reason for the response may be that reduction in the demand on the patient's own tissues is needed at a time when he is unable to feed and drink adequately himself. The reaction may be modified where the environmental temperature is raised and a diet with normal protein content is tolerated.

How Metabolic Response to Injury Involves the Nurse

As science advances it is not sufficient for the nurse to be aware only of the well-known problems in relation to pain, position of the patient and wound healing. She must understand the patient who does not progress normally. Investigations with regard to the assessment of the metabolic state of balance involve the nurse in the careful measurement and recording of fluid balance, urine collections, special diets, endocrine function tests and sometimes the nursing of patients in a controlled environmental temperature.

NURSING OF CHILDREN

The children's orthopaedic ward is generally the noisiest ward in the hospital but it is also the happiest. This happy atmosphere is most important as the treatment of many orthopaedic conditions requires either a lengthy period of hospitalisation or numerous short stay visits.

Although perhaps immobilised in various forms of splintage as part of their treatment for either a congenital abnormality or following an accident, most of the children are otherwise healthy and naturally noisy. They need to be **kept occupied** throughout their stay in the ward and this demands a great deal of ingenuity and participation from the nursing staff. The period during which they are confined to bed is undoubtedly the most trying time and unless they are **stimulated into using up their excess energy** in some way they will very soon become frustrated and difficult to handle. The nurse should ensure at all times that a small child is not left sitting in his cot without toys or without someone to play with him. If the child's condition requires long periods lying in the prone position it is preferable to have the head of the cot facing the centre of the ward where he can see other children and watch the nursing staff moving around. If he is immobilised in the recumbent position his toys may be strung across the cot or tied to the cot sides within his reach.

It is much more practical for children who are not acutely ill to be dressed in day clothes rather than pyjamas and most hospitals now provide clothes for this purpose.

Education

Most children now receive a certain amount of education while in hospital. This is most important for those who are physically handicapped as they may have to depend on a sedentary job to earn their living. The children are usually taught in the ward during normal school hours and although it may make the management of nursing duties more difficult, the teachers are understanding and can plan a successful programme with the co-operation of the nursing staff.

Visiting

Open visiting in many children's hospitals enables parents to spend longer periods with their child and where possible they should be encouraged to take an active part in nursing the child.

The mother may wish to arrange her visits to coincide with mealtimes or 'tucking-down time', and when leaving she should tell the child she is going home. It is inadvisable and unkind to tell the child she is just going out for a few minutes and will be back shortly. If the child is old enough to understand the mother may tell him when she will return, e.g. after dinner or tea-time. The mother should be asked to bring to hospital any **special toy or piece of blanket** of which the child is especially fond and to leave it with him as this may provide a source of comfort and a link with home.

A note should be made of any child who does not have regular visitors or correspondence from home and in these cases the nurse should ask the social worker to make enquiries regarding the home circumstances. This information may help in deciding when to dismiss the child.

While parents are in the ward visiting, the nurse in charge should be available to answer any questions. Although the opportunity should be given to parents to see the doctor it is the nurse's responsibility to keep them informed of the child's day to day progress. Having this constant contact with the parents the nurse may find she is able to reassure and advise them on the problems of handling the child when he is ultimately discharged. As the doctor is usually unable to communicate directly with the patient because of the age of the child the parents often depend on the nurse as the 'communication link' between them and the medical staff. For this reason the nurse should be well informed of the child's condition and progress.

If the parents are interviewed by the doctor it is advisable that the nurse in charge is present. Parents are often over-anxious when being interviewed and may be unable to comprehend, or may indeed misconstrue what is said to them. This practice leaves the parents free to ask the nurse for explanation of any point they may not have appreciated fully because of their natural anxiety.

Feeding
Many of the children may be lying in the recumbent or semi-recumbent position and may encounter difficulty in feeding themselves. Plates with a raised outer rim are available and with this simple feeding aid most children manage very well. Cups with spouts or lips are also useful and are readily available in unbreakable plastic. Care must be taken that hot plates are not placed on paralysed limbs as sensation may be totally absent and a severe burn may result.

Care of Children in Traction
The particular care of a patient in traction as described in Chapter 19 is important. It should be remembered, however, that often a child is either too young to communicate or too frightened or bewildered to give a reason for his discomfort. In the management of fractures of the femur immobilised in traction a child's crying may not be due entirely to pain related to the injury but rather to discomfort associated with pressure from the apparatus used in the immobilisation. In these circumstances the nurse should examine carefully all the possible areas of pressure, i.e. the ring of the splint in the groin and the slings or pads particularly beneath the knee or ankle.

Care of Children with Paralysis and Sensory Loss of Lower Limbs

In Plaster. On return to the ward a careful note should be made of the **position of the child's toes and foot in the plaster.** This position should then be checked frequently to ensure that the toes do not withdraw upwards inside the plaster. In children with sensory loss extra special care should be taken to prevent **plaster sores** developing as the child will not make any complaint. Care should therefore be taken in the initial handling of the cast to ensure that indentations do not occur which may cause pressure. **Rough edges should be trimmed or protected by adhesive tape.** The child must also be prevented from inserting foreign bodies, e.g. coins or beads, down inside the plaster as these can easily cause sores if undetected. **Where one limb only is enclosed in plaster care should be taken that it does not rest on top of the unprotected one.** If the child is capable of **crawling around the toes must be protected** as they may be scraped and the skin removed without his being aware of it. **Special care must be exercised when removing plasters from children.** A child is always apprehensive, especially at the sight of a plaster saw or shears. A pleasant conversation with the child will often allay his fears and gain his co-operation. Removal must be carried out in complete confidence by one experienced in the art.

In Calipers. All calipers must be inspected daily for signs of **wear and tear** and to ensure that they **continue to fit properly.** Any necessary repairs are carried out promptly. The wearing of ill-fitting calipers gives rise to sores. If the ring is too tight a sore may develop due to pressure; if too large, sores due to friction may occur. Careless handling of the calipers must be avoided. **They should not be left on top of radiators as this may warp the metal, or in the bathroom where they may become wet.** If the aim in fitting the caliper is to allow the child to bear weight nothing is gained by applying the caliper and then seating the child in a wheelchair all day. He should be given the opportunity to **stand at a specially adapted standing table or, if capable, allowed up to walk with a suitable walking aid.**

Advice on Discharge

The mother should be familiar with the fitting and removal of the calipers. She must realise the reason why the child wears them, what the surgeon hopes to achieve by this treatment, and if possible, for what period they will remain necessary. She must be aware that it is her responsibility to inform the hospital if the calipers are damaged in any way or if the child outgrows them. **To avoid tripping accidents** all rugs should be removed from the floor thus enabling the child to move around safely. When attending orthopaedic clinics or physiotherapy departments these children require to have transport provided and this is usually arranged through the Women's Voluntary Service before the child leaves hospital.

NURSING OF THE ELDERLY

Orthopaedic problems are not peculiar to any one age group but those most commonly seen in the elderly patient are fracture of the neck of the femur, osteoarthritis and rheumatoid arthritis. Special mention should be made of the treatment of fractured neck of femur in the elderly person. It is a common injury, often the outcome of a comparatively simple fall. In the majority of patients there is underlying osteoporosis. The shock of the accident may cause mental confusion and incontinence may be a problem. The patient avoids movement because of pain and unless preventative measures are taken pressure sores can develop rapidly. Whenever possible, operative treatment is carried out thus avoiding prolonged nursing in bed.

When treating the elderly patient it must be kept in mind that the **aim of all treatment is the eventual rehabilitation of the patient,** i.e. the process whereby he is restored to a state of optimum efficiency and given an opportunity to regain his place in the community. The achievement of this aim requires a team effort on the part of the medical and nursing staff, physiotherapists, occupational therapists and medical social workers.

Nursing the elderly requires **patience**—patience to take time to understand the individual's needs, to humour the slightly disorientated, to listen, to watch and encourage the patient while he laboriously carries out some task which the nurse could do much more quickly. Old people can be temperamental and difficult but once they become acclimatised to the hospital environment they respond to a regular routine carried out by staff they have come to know.

Whenever possible **patients should be out of bed** for at least part of the day. They should be **dressed in their own clothes** and women patients should be encouraged to take an interest in their appearance. When patients start to bear weight they should wear firm walking shoes. Where, however, a patient cannot make use of the advantages of being allowed to sit in a chair, it is preferable to continue bed nursing with regular changing of position and intensive physiotherapy so that early walking can be attained. Otherwise the patient who is unfit to sit in a chair adopts a slumped position with such complications as deformity and pressure sores. These are as detrimental to recovery as the other complications one is trying to avoid.

Bladder and bowel problems often accompany illness in the elderly. Urinary incontinence may be controlled by regular emptying of the bladder. Only very rarely is catheterisation indicated. Regular bowel habits should be developed. Faecal incontinence may be due to inadequate emptying of a loaded bowel. A well-balanced diet is essential but maintenance of an adequate fluid balance is even more important.

Pressure sores develop easily in an elderly bed-bound patient, particularly if he is confused, incontinent and taking little nourishment. A patient in this category is termed **'at risk'** and should be nursed on some type of air mattress to help prevent the breakdown of the pressure areas. Despite the use of a mechanical aid, regular turning and changing by the nursing staff is still necessary.

The discomfort experienced by a patient, e.g. with rheumatoid arthritis, when several nurses attempt to move him during the process of nursing care can be minimised by the **use of a patient-lifting device,** e.g. the Ambulift. Once nurse and patient become familiar with its use many procedures can be carried out easily even where the patient is heavy or crippled, e.g. immersion bathing, transferring from bed to chair or chair to commode.

The patient's progress, although controlled by the doctor and physiotherapist, is also dependent on the observations and advice of the nursing staff. Together they decide at which stage he is able to sit in a chair, to bear weight using a walking aid and eventually to walk unaided. They are also concerned with his progress in normal daily living activities, i.e. feeding, dressing and toilet.

The elderly patient confined to hospital for a long period becomes dull and apathetic if his mental and spiritual needs are not considered. The **occupational therapist** fills a vital rôle here by organising group activities, e.g. singing and action groups and discussions often aided by voluntary workers. Every member of the staff can help, if only by exchanging a few words with some lonely person. The regular visits of the hospital chaplain give opportunities to discuss spiritual matters and short religious services provide comfort and reassurance. The occasional film show or entertainment by a local group brings the outside world into the hospital, as do the visitors. It may even be possible to arrange an outing, either with the patient's own visitors or with a group from the hospital.

The decision to dismiss the patient is made only after careful consideration of his ability to carry out the normal activities of daily living and the **medical social worker's report** on his home circumstances and relatives available to give support.

If the services of a home help are required or if the provision of the Women's Voluntary Service 'Meals on Wheels' is necessary, such arrangements should be made before the patient leaves the hospital. In order to assess his ability to live alone it may be necessary for him to be taken on a 'home visit' by the medical social worker.

After dismissal, follow-up visits by a district nurse, who maintains contact with the hospital and who knows the patient's past history, provide a useful link between hospital and home. If there is a Day Hospital in the area the patient may attend once or twice a week, thus maintaining the progress made in hospital, making regular social contacts and relieving relatives at home for a regular period each week.

PHYSIOTHERAPY AND OCCUPATIONAL THERAPY

PHYSIOTHERAPY

The physiotherapist is an important member of the Orthopaedic and Accident team. On her careful instruction and supervision depends the patient's rapid return to normal function. This is achieved by her regular ward visits throughout the day when the patient is either given individual tuition or participates in class therapy, and by her continued interest and encouragement when he attends as an outpatient, perhaps for several weeks or even for months after his discharge.

In the management of the patient following surgery or trauma the physiotherapist provides a planned programme of exercises designed to prevent complications, to maintain function and to re-educate parts in which function has been impaired.

Prevention of Complications

Chest complications, circulatory sluggishness or failure, and deformities are among the problems which may occur in patients following trauma or surgery. **Breathing exercises,** during which the lungs are fully expanded and cleared of any accumulated secretions by coughing, are extremely important in the prevention of collapse of the lung and hypostatic pneumonia, particularly in the ill or the elderly. **Active exercises** or **passive movement of limbs** may help alleviate the tendency to the development of deep venous thrombosis. Deformity should be avoided if all **joints are put through their normal range of movement** either actively, if the patient can co-operate, or passively where the patient is incapable of exercising the parts.

Maintenance of Function

Where a part of the body has been injured by trauma or if an operation has been performed its function is temporarily impaired. The patient may be confined to bed or his activity restricted by various types of immobilisation. Therefore, as well as planning specific active or passive exercises for the individual patient the physiotherapist has to organise a programme of **maintenance exercises;** the patient usually takes part in group therapy whereby all muscles and joints uninvolved in his particular type of immobilisation are kept functional. Active exercises can be practised by the patient himself at regular intervals throughout the day and for specified periods. The nurse can co-operate in this respect by turning back the bedclothes and giving the patient encouragement with these exercises between the regular visits of the physiotherapist. It is also desirable that springs and sandbags should be left within easy access of the patient. If muscle strength is to be improved these must be used not only at specific exercise sessions but at intervals throughout the day.

Re-education of Parts with Impaired Function. Where for example a limb has been immobilised, perhaps in extension, for a prolonged spell, e.g. fracture of the lower end of femur, the muscles allowing flexion movement of the knee are inactive and the knee joint becomes stiff. The process of re-education requires encouragement from the physiotherapist and enthusiasm and effort on the part of the patient; the patient, assisted by the physiotherapist, needs to spend a considerable time exercising at regular intervals throughout the day in order to restore normal muscle tone and knee flexion. If the patient is finding difficulty in initiating contraction of his muscles, electrical stimulation may be necessary to do this. Once some muscle activity has been achieved he must continue to use these muscles to improve tone until the process of re-education is well advanced. When this stage has been reached the patient will be allowed out of bed. He then has to be re-taught the process of walking, first using crutches and later unaided.

Crutches

Patients who require crutches must be able to use them safely and competently before returning home. A few short periods of instruction are sufficient for the majority to attain this but for others, including the elderly, infirm and nervous, more practice is necessary. In these cases, when the physiotherapist is not available, the nursing staff can help shorten a patient's stay in hospital by supervising his walking with the aid of crutches. The patient must always wear sensible low-heeled footwear to ensure stability while walking.

Measuring for, and Care of, Crutches. Although the easiest way to measure a patient for crutches is to deduct sixteen inches from his height it is inadvisable to accept this vague estimate. Alternatively, a measurement is made from the axillary fold to the external malleolus on the side of the weight-bearing limb. It is important to check that all the nuts on the crutches are tight and that the rubber ferrules are not worn out.

Crutch Walking

Standing Up. A most important part of the patient's treatment is to ensure that he can rise confidently from a chair and return to it safely. The nurse should place herself in front and to the side of the affected limb. Her feet should be apart to give her a comfortable and stable position. The patient holds a crutch vertically in either hand by the handpiece. He places the two crutches approximately shoulder distance apart in front of his chair. Next he is encouraged to slide his weight to the front half of his chair and to bend the knee of the weight-bearing leg so that the foot may be placed in a position where it is flat on the floor and the toe is in line with the crutches. The patient now leans forwards to bring his shoulders into line with the crutches from which position he stands by extending this knee and hip. The crutches are now slipped into position with the padded tops in the patient's axillae and gripped firmly between the arms and the ribs. The hand grips should be at such a level as to allow the patient to have a few degrees of flexion at his elbows but no weight should be carried on the crutch tops in the axillae.

Walking. The first move is to lift both crutches clear of the floor and place them approximately a foot ahead of their previous position. The patient now swings his trunk forwards and is able to straighten his elbows and bear his weight on the crutch grip. Simultaneously he steps with his unaffected foot to its new position in front of the crutches and so completes a step. If the patient is unable to attain the position beyond the crutches it is acceptable for him to ground his foot in line with them.

Turning. When turning right, the patient should lift his right crutch backwards and the left forwards alternately. Six inches is an adequate distance for the crutches to move at a time and both should not be clear of the floor together. When turning left the reverse movements are performed.

Sitting Down. It is stressed that the patient should advance to his chair and only turn when he has sufficient space, so obviating awkward steps backwards. When he has turned with his back to his chair he steps backwards until his leg is in contact with the front of the seat. The crutch tops are now slipped forwards from under the axillae and he lowers himself by flexing the weight-bearing knee and both elbows until seated.

Stairs. The patient progresses to stair climbing when he has mastered the activities already described. On ascending a flight of steps the crutches and the weight-bearing foot all start in a straight line a few inches from the bottom step. The patient then swings his body so that his weight is transferred to the crutches thus allowing his foot to be lifted on to the first step. The crutches can now be brought on a level with the foot before the operation is repeated. Descending a flight of steps is performed in the reverse manner with the weight-bearing points a few inches from the edge of the top step where the crutches can be lifted and placed on to the next. The weight is again taken up by the crutches to allow the foot to step down to their level. The cycle can now be repeated. If a bannister is available it can substitute for a crutch thus making the negotiating of stairs easier for the patient.

The nurse should always be behind the patient on ascending stairs and in front of him on descending so being in a position to help should he slip. If the end of a crutch is placed on a small object such as a rug or a blanket it will slip when the weight of the patient is carried on it. It is also worth mentioning that crutches are in the category of equipment which should be within reach of a patient who is incompetent to walk unaided.

Passive Movements

The physiotherapist uses passive movements where the patient is unable to perform his normal joint range of movement actively. If passive movements are not carried out regularly, soft tissues shorten and contractures are allowed to form which are not easily corrected. It is also possible to perform passive movements beyond their limit so damaging joints or producing fractures of porotic bones especially in the elderly; great care is therefore necessary.

To Perform Passive Movements. The operator should stand with her feet apart so that she is in a stable and comfortable position throughout the range of movement. The palmar aspects of her hands should be moulded accurately to the surface of the limb and pressure over bony prominences avoided. The joint should be taken through its range slowly and smoothly.

Common Sites at which Deformities Develop and their Correction. When the patient is unable to maintain the leg in the normal position at the hip, the leg usually rolls into external rotation. This fault should be corrected by rotating the leg into the mid-position with one hand on the thigh proximal to the patella and the other controlling the leg and foot. The position of the leg can then be retained by sandbags or pillows.

Tightening of the structures behind the knee causes it to become flexed and this must be prevented by full extension of the joint. This is performed with one hand placed in front of the thigh proximal to the patella and the other firmly holding the ankle with the forearm lying along the sole of the foot. The forearm maintains the foot fully dorsi-flexed and so ensures that the gastrocnemius muscle is stretched.

When correcting a dropped foot deformity the hands are in the same position as described in the previous movement. The knee is kept in full extension and the ankle and foot are carried from the plantar flexed position into full dorsiflexion. It is important to take the ankle and foot together so that individual joints of the foot are not strained. The nurse should note that this is only a general outline and in each individual patient modifications are necessary.

Hydrotherapy

Hydrotherapy, or the use of water in the treatment of patients, has a history reaching far back to the days of the Roman Empire. In Britain it reached its climax with the development of Spas in the 18th and 19th century where the water was taken for its supposed curative properties and a variety of either hot or cold jets, sprays or douches was applied to the patient. Investigation has shown that much of the benefit derived from 'taking the waters' was due more to the regular regime imposed on the patient rather than to any curative properties possessed by the water.

Modern hydrotherapy treatments are primarily concerned with the use of the deep pool. In such a pool the patient may be totally immersed in warm water so relieving pain and muscle spasm; he becomes almost weightless due to the buoyancy of the water. As a result a severely handicapped patient achieves a freedom of movement quite impossible on land.

Patients who obtain benefit from pool treatment fall into two main groups:
(i) those severely handicapped by such conditions as paraplegia, anterior poliomyelitis and rheumatoid arthritis;

(ii) others in the early stages of treatment where pain and muscle severely restrict free movement. For example: following a period of immobilisation in plaster; after joint surgery to enhance the results, as in hand and hip arthroplasty, osteotomy or synovectomy; where there has been recent injury to muscles, tendons or peripheral nerves.

As the patient progresses and improvement occurs it is usually more satisfactory to transfer to 'dry' treatment and reserve the use of the pool for recreational purposes.

The trained nurse does not play an active part in the actual hydrotherapy treatment and the unskilled task of preparing the patient for immersion is adequately performed by orderlies. However, in many instances the patient is returned direct to the ward from the pool. The nurse should appreciate that these patients have been immersed in water above body temperature and are therefore hot; they have undertaken unaccustomed exercise and are tired. Patients must be made to rest, wrapped in blankets, for half an hour to allow slow cooling of their bodies thus avoiding the dangers of chill and fatigue.

The nurse may never be asked to treat a patient in the hydrotherapy pool but some knowledge of this type of treatment enables her to make a greater contribution to the total care of the patient.

OCCUPATIONAL THERAPY

Occupational therapy is **treatment by physical or mental activities,** prescribed by a doctor and supervised by a qualified occupational therapist, for the purpose of hastening recovery from disease or injury. It is primarily a psychological treatment because its treatment value depends on the patient's interest being diverted from preoccupation with his disability to some useful activity and achievement. The occupational therapist is therefore an important member of the team involved in the total care of the patient. Like the medical social worker and the physiotherapist, her interest in the patient begins while he is in the ward and continues for many weeks or months after his discharge. In this way she enables him to recover the manual skills and the mental concentration necessary to return to a normal way of life. The type of occupational therapy prescribed may be classified under four headings.

1 **General Therapy.** This is usually prescribed for long term patients, during the period before active exercises can be commenced. The purpose of such treatment is to maintain morale, to stimulate respiratory and circulatory function and to provide for maximum physical activity within the limits of the patient's condition; thus invalidism is avoided. The patient can be given some form of occupation which can be done in bed within the limits of his restriction by whatever form of immobilisation is used. Patients who are disinterested in craft work may enjoy studying subjects of further education, e.g. languages, art, etc. which can also be done while in bed. Group activities such as play reading, games and singing are most beneficial.

2 Specific Therapy. This is probably the most important form of occupational therapy. The aim in treatment of all patients is that ultimately they can return to work as soon as possible. Early restoration of function in the part or parts affected is therefore essential. If possible an occupation is selected which is in some way related to the patient's normal job. It must be interesting so as to provide an incentive for the patient, i.e. he will wish to achieve certain results in the work prescribed. The exercises involved in the specified work are then carried out voluntarily. These are suitably selected to develop the tone and power of muscle, the range of joint movement, the neuro-muscular control and work tolerance, for example:

(a) **Mobilising an upper limb.** Work such as weaving or basketry is suitable in this instance. It is placed so that the patient requires to elevate his limb, to reach out for wool or cane and to use fine movements of the fingers in the process of weaving. Flexion and extension of the elbow, pronation and supination of the hand, and abduction, adduction and circumduction of the shoulder are the important movements to be regained.

(b) **Mobilising a lower limb.** Quadriceps function, knee flexion and mobility of the hip are the important features in restoration of function in the lower limb. Non-weight-bearing exercises on a foot-operated loom or printing machine help to develop quadriceps muscle tone. Other machinery using a bicycle motion in its operation is necessary for hip and knee flexion exercise, e.g. the 'rehabilitation bicycle'.

In both the upper and lower limb the occupations selected provide graduated resistance which is important in improving muscle tone and joint function. This is achieved by the aid of adapted tools and by the attachment of springs, slings or weights to the equipment used in order to graduate the amount of effort needed.

3 Assessment. When a patient starts therapy the work will only occupy 1–2 hours per day. Gradually he progresses to longer hours and perhaps more strenuous work as this can be tolerated, i.e. work tolerance. In order to provide information for the doctor or resettlement officer, with regard to the patient's fitness to attempt a full working day or his need for retraining, it may be necessary to assess his capabilities beforehand. Bench, machine, industrial, catering and domestic work are examples of some of the activities which can be assessed and graded in the occupational therapy department.

4 Personal Activities in Daily Living. These include feeding, toilet, washing, dressing and the freedom of mobility necessary to perform these tasks. Many occupational therapy units have apartments which contain a bedroom, kitchen, bathroom and lounge where patients with mobility problems can be retrained before going home. These are basically 'self-care' units where the staff can assess the patient's fitness to live independently. They can detect the need for aids for the disabled which the patient can often obtain before going home. Assistance, e.g. 'home help', 'meals on wheels', etc., may be considered necessary. Advice can also be given with regard to adjustments to clothing, e.g. zips instead of buttons. The occupational therapist can also discuss the layout of the patient's home, what his normal day involves and can offer suggestions by which the daily routine is more easily accomplished.

Physiotherapy and Occupational Therapy

These two departments work closely together and are often in the same area of the hospital. The patient oftens attends physiotherapy for heat and exercise and thereafter goes to his occupational therapy class. As the physiotherapist helps to improve movement in stiff joints and to strengthen weak muscles, the occupational therapist's work is complementary by providing work which will use the function of these muscles and joints.

The co-operation of all members of the team consisting of surgeon, ward sister, physiotherapist, occupational therapist and medical social worker is essential if the patient's treatment is to be ultimately successful. Before being discharged from hospital the patient should be placed in the care of an outside authority so that a personal interest in his progress can be maintained and follow-up therapy continued. Such services are provided by the Local Health Authorities.

The work of the radiographer is skilled and technical. Close co-operation among the medical, X-ray and nursing personnel is essential, particularly in the accident wards and operating theatre where portable X-rays are required frequently. **There are certain hazards associated with repeated exposure to radiation.** These include destruction of blood cells, bone marrow depression, and sterility by depression of the function of the ovaries or testes. Radiation is measured in units called 'rads' and the dosage of each exposure is carefully calculated so that the patient receives the minimum. Although the radiographer is subjected to repeated amounts of radiation, the accumulated dose is still within the limits of safety. The radiography staff, however, are required to wear special protective lead aprons and badges which register the amount of radiation accumulated from repeated exposures. For these reasons it is obviously important for the nurse to have some knowledge of this speciality.

Radiographs in the Ward
Where a patient is unfit to be moved, either because he is ill or because he is immobilised by complicated apparatus, it will be necessary for portable radiographs to be done in the ward. The nursing staff are often involved in assisting the radiographer with the positioning of the patient and the film cassettes. A nurse may indeed be asked to hold a cassette in position while a film is being taken. This is generally avoided where at all possible, nevertheless in certain circumstances she may be the only person available. She is then exposed to direct radiation and must protect herself by wearing a lead apron. It is important for everyone uninvolved in the radiographic procedure to leave the area or at least stand five feet clear of the path of radiation.

Radiographs in Theatre
The operating theatre is a sterile area and so the radiographic technique used in theatre has to conform to the highest possible standard of sterility. The radiographer, like other members of theatre staff, dresses in special theatre clothing. The X-ray machine is positioned so that it is clear of the sterile area and at least four feet distant from any anaesthetic equipment. This excludes the danger of ignition of gases from a stray spark which, although highly unlikely, cannot be ignored completely. Many operating tables incorporate a special tunnel into which the X-ray cassette can be placed to obtain an antero-posterior view. The operation site is left undisturbed. The radiographer is careful to touch only the under

surfaces of sterile drapes during this procedure to avoid contamination. She will require the co-operation of the surgeon and his assistants in the positioning of the patient, tube and cassette for the required X-ray views. Where a lateral X-ray view is necessary the X-ray is held in a special film holder during the exposure. The theatre nurse or assistant covers the part of the patient to be X-rayed with an additional sterile drape for this procedure. Sometimes it is impossible to get the correct view by placing the X-ray in a film holder. It is then necessary to improvise and support the cassette against the patient, for example by using sterile rolled up towels. The cassette is first of all dropped into a sterile cover held by one of the operation team and is then, according to the instruction given by the radiographer, positioned against the part to be X-rayed. The members of the operating team retreat from the area during the exposure of the film. If the anaesthetist requires to control the patient's breathing during the procedure he must be provided with a protective lead apron.

The patient can suffer burns of the skin unless special care is taken in the positioning of the X-ray machine. If it happens to contact the patient's bare skin in the region of a diathermy pad which has become dry, leaving it unearthed, an electrical burn may result. Another danger arises when the light beam diaphragm attached to the tube head has been left on. Considerable heat can be generated in the diaphragm casing, and the skin on which it is focused can indeed be burned.

Radiographic Equipment. The X-ray machine, the tube head, supporting arm and cones are wiped using a cloth wrung out in an antiseptic solution. Moisture must not, however, be allowed to penetrate to the inner parts of the machine. Lead aprons, film holders and cassette tunnels are also treated with the antiseptic solution. This duty is normally the responsibility of the radiography staff.

Preparation of Patients for X-ray

Unless any special X-ray examination of the patient is requested there is generally little preparation required prior to the procedure. It is advisable for the patient to empty his bladder before going to the X-ray department. The part being examined should be free from radio-opaque articles, e.g. buttons, zips, rings, etc. The patient should be clad in a warm dressing gown with, if necessary, an extra blanket round his shoulders as he may have to wait until the film is developed and found to be satisfactory.

Special X-ray investigation such as a **myelogram** is sometimes necessary. The patient is usually given an aperient two nights prior to the procedure and light meals for the preceding 24 hours. After the procedure the patient rests in the recumbent position for two or three hours to allow the spinal fluid to settle after the introduction of the contrast medium (Myodil). Otherwise, if the patient sits up suddenly, he may feel quite dizzy and suffer from headache.

When an appointment for X-ray is arranged it is important to give clear written details of the patient's name, his hospital number, the region to be included on the X-ray and, if possible, the specific views required. The reference to right or left limbs must be stated definitely. This not only avoids confusion in the X-ray department but also, in the event of surgery, is an important factor in the prevention of an operation being carried out on the wrong limb.

Care of X-ray Films. A patient's X-ray films are part of his case record and must therefore be preserved and filed in sequence. They are usually contained in a special film cover bearing a label with the patient's name and hospital number; the dates and region of X-ray are listed in sequence. In the assessment of the patient's progress, reference to such X-rays may be made over subsequent months or even years.

There are certain **social problems** which are more common among patients attending or admitted to the Orthopaedic and Accident Unit. This is perhaps because of the particular nature of the patient's condition. The problems include those concerning **readjustment, mobility, work** and **finance.**

PATIENTS IN THE ACCIDENT WARDS

These patients are emergency admissions. This creates immediate psychological as well as practical difficulties. The patient has not had any time to make arrangements for children to be looked after, debts to be paid or employers to be notified. All these patients are suffering from some degree of shock and for many it may be their first experience of hospital. Their injuries usually necessitate their being confined to bed for some time. As they lie thinking about their problems daily, these although perhaps basically trivial become magnified out of proportion. It is very often the nurse who first realises that a problem exists but she does not necessarily understand the significance of a patient's anxious look, his withdrawn manner or his odd behaviour. The following paragraphs should help her to understand some of the social problems with which her patients may be extremely concerned.

Injuries Resulting in Disfigurement

In a young patient in particular a disfiguring injury can cause deep psychological anxiety. Amputation of a limb for example is not only a most shattering experience to a patient but also a source of concern as to how his family and friends will react when he goes home. His second concern is usually his job, which may involve climbing or heavy labouring. What kind of work will he now be able to do; what about his hobbies, e.g. football, hill-walking and dancing? Added to all this is the general discomfort following amputation. It is therefore not surprising that such a patient can become considerably depressed. The medical staff can try to reassure the patient that he will be able to lead a fairly normal life with the use of an artificial limb. It may take some time, however, before the prosthesis can actually be worn. By this time the patient may have been discharged. In the meantime he may become acutely embarrassed by his disability particularly once he leaves hospital and he feels he is a source of curiosity to those around him. It is often helpful for the medical social worker to see the immediate relatives in order to discuss their reaction to the disability. The support of his family may be all that is necessary to give him confidence. Once he gets his artificial limb and realises how mobile he is then, his disability no longer seems to be a serious problem.

Paraplegia
The adult paraplegic has similar problems of adjustment. He is, however, usually transferred early to a paraplegic unit for specialised care. In this situation the patient does not often fully understand the permanence of his paralysis although it has been explained to him. He feels that in being transferred to a special unit there is still hope. It is often the relatives who benefit more from a talk with the medical social worker. She can discuss the practical problems concerning the care of the patient in the future, e.g. rehousing to ground floor accommodation.

Shorter Term Problems
These are often of a more practical nature. For example, a patient in hospital with a fractured femur has to accept that he is incapacitated for several months. His main concern may be how his wife will cope on a considerably reduced income. The medical social worker can discuss the financial position with both him and his wife. She can give advice on budgeting, approach hire purchase firms to reduce payments and arrange for rent to be paid weekly. Financial assistance is only given in cases of extreme hardship but relatives may be given help with fares to and from the hospital.

Another immediate problem is whether or not a patient is going to lose his job. The medical social worker can approach his employers and, although it is clear that the patient will not be fit for his original job, provision can very often be made for a lighter one.

Elderly Patients
There is always a large proportion of elderly people in the accident unit. Their injuries are usually the result of a road accident or of one sustained in the home. Their problems while in hospital tend to be concerned with their pensions or the paying of their rent and these are easily resolved. The difficulty arises when these people are ready for discharge. They are quite often unable to continue living alone and the medical social worker can sometimes help them to accept the idea of spending the rest of their lives with relatives or in an old folks' home. Occasionally the relatives are aggressive and find it difficult to accept that the patient cannot be completely cured. This may be an expression of their own guilt; they may feel they could perhaps have been more helpful. Where a patient is able to return to his own home it is important that adequate help and supervision are arranged for him. Community resources provide such services as 'home help', 'meals on wheels' and the 'health visitor'; these can be arranged by the medical social worker to help the patient on his discharge.

The Severely Handicapped Patient
Where patients are so severely handicapped that they are unable to be looked after

at home, e.g. the confused or incontinent, they are transferred either to a young chronic sick unit or to a geriatric ward. The relatives, especially of a younger patient, are often extremely shocked and worried about his future. The medical social worker provides them with the vital link with the hospital so helping to share in their problems.

Suicide and Assault

Occasionally patients who have attempted suicide are admitted. The events leading to the incident can be discussed in confidence with the medical social worker. She then aims at supporting the patient throughout his period of hospitalisation and at helping him to develop the more enjoyable aspects of life. Loneliness, predisposing to depression, is often a contributory factor so that the patient must be guided into helping himself develop positive interests in order to occupy his time.

In the case of wife assault the patient requires much support and understanding to overcome the shock of what has happened. Although the situation has perhaps happened before, she often returns to her home after she is discharged from hospital. A patient may, however, wish to start a completely new life. She can be assisted in making plans for her future while still in hospital and can continue her contact with the medical social worker after her discharge.

Aggressive Behaviour

Accident patients may be very aggressive and difficult in the wards, often an expression of guilt and worry—guilt that the accident may have been caused by their own carelessness and worry about their home, family and job. It is most important that these patients are given a chance to analyse the reasons for their aggressive behaviour in order to help them to adjust to hospitalisation. Often the first few days are the most anxious for the patient during which time he generally appreciates the extent of his injuries, the length of time he will be in hospital and the treatment involved. It may involve lying on his back for several weeks, unable to move. He has difficulty in getting to know the other patients and his mind therefore dwells on his various problems. The medical social worker aims at helping him to become adjusted to his enforced stay in hospital by discussing such anxieties with him.

Children

Children who are involved in accidents also require assistance. Many of the parents feel guilty about the accident which they believe might not have happened had they been watching the child more carefully. Mothers in particular find relief in talking to the medical social worker. In many cases the accident can reveal various family stresses: there may be a large family; difficulty in making ends meet; a husband who does not give a great deal of support to his home and family. The medical social worker can help by: **giving support; helping to plan a better family budget; putting the parents in touch with more appropriate social work agencies** such as Family Welfare Units which can give closer supervision.

If a child's injuries are permanent, e.g. if he is paraplegic as the result of an accident, the problems to be faced by the parents are very much greater. During the time the child is in hospital the mother, especially, requires a lot of preparation to face the problems likely to arise when the child goes home. Once again the practical problem of housing must be discussed in order that suitable ground floor accommodation is obtained before the patient is discharged. The financial situation of the family is also investigated as the worry and upset in normal equilibrium due to the accident often results in arrears of rent and other regular payments. Help with fares is given to enable the parents to visit as often as possible.

Many are the psychological problems of such a case. The parents feel very sorry for their child; they shower him with gifts so spoiling him thoroughly and when he goes home he expects the same attention. If a child is in hospital for any length of time it is inevitable that he will become fond of its artificial atmosphere and the parents must be prepared to cope with difficult behaviour when he is discharged. The child may have difficulty in adjusting to being one of the family again especially if he has been in an adult ward. Although unable to express his feelings in words he may envy other children who are able to move about freely while he is confined to a wheelchair. The child's mother must be helped to face these problems and may require continued contact with the medical social worker over a long period.

PATIENTS IN THE ORTHOPAEDIC UNIT

Adjusting to Disability

One of the main problems in an orthopaedic unit is helping a patient to adjust to and accept a disabling condition so that he can lead as normal a life as possible. The period of adjustment may take a long time. The patient is first visited by the medical social worker while in the ward and he continues to receive guidance and assistance during and perhaps after the 'follow-up' period as an outpatient. A patient suffering from a condition such as arthritis may have attended the Ortho-paedic clinic on several occasions before being admitted for operative treatment. His condition may have deteriorated quickly over a period of months impairing his mobility and causing him considerable pain. Although after operative treat-ment he will require to spend some time in hospital it is hoped that as a result he will become more mobile.

Loneliness is a problem particularly connected with immobility and also with the adjustment to a disabling condition. It is very easy to lose touch with friends and relatives if one is confined to the house. When a patient who feels lonely at home is in hospital for any length of time he often dreads leaving behind the companionship of everyone in the ward. If the medical social worker sees the patient before he goes home she can help him to look on the brighter aspects of life, to adjust to his disability and to accept help from community resources. If he is unable to get out, he can be put in touch with centres for the disabled or with 'visiting' organisations both of which are usually run by local authorities and voluntary bodies. Where the patient is younger it may be possible for him to get an invalid car. This allows opportunities for employment. In many other respects an invalid car permits a disabled person to lead a more normal life. He is free to visit friends, to go to the cinema and to attend church organisations. When a patient suffers from a mobility problem it is important that he lives in suitable housing. If he lives in an upstairs flat and has difficulty in negotiating stairs it is better for him to be moved to ground floor accommodation, or to live in a flat serviced by a lift so that he can get out from time to time. In most cases this can be arranged on medical grounds through the local authority if the patient is agreeable.

Problems of Compensation and Retraining
Some patients who have sustained an injury for which they have received initial hospital treatment may require further surgery to relieve symptoms. This may not be undertaken for several months. Future employment is essentially their main concern and although this can be discussed the patient cannot be offered a job until he is pronounced fit for work. Some are reluctant to express their feelings and often one finds it is due to the fact that they have a compensation claim against their firm if the accident happened at work. Others, however, cannot face the reality of having to change their type of job. Here the medical social worker can have a talk with the patient, outlining the facilities available and how rehabilitation and retraining can be arranged. The patient is often comforted by the knowledge that such help is obtainable.

Psychological Causes of Pain
On occasions a patient is admitted to the ward suffering from pain, e.g. backache. Investigations are carried out but no organic cause is found for his symptoms. It may therefore be thought that he has some deeper psychological worries which are being expressed in back pain. The medical social worker is often asked to investigate his case before the clinician refers him for a psychiatric opinion. By talking to the patient she tries to build up a good relationship with him and so gain his confidence. Often many stresses in home life are revealed and the medical social worker can help the patient in resolving such problems.

Aids for Disabled Patients
Patients who have a permanent disability have difficulty in being completely independent at home. There are many devices available to help such people who for example are unable to pick something off the floor, have difficulty in putting on shoes and stockings and in tying shoelaces. These people can be put in touch with the Red Cross or the local authority occupational therapists who supply such devices. Sometimes alterations have to be made to a patient's home, e.g. a rail to enable the patient to manage a few steps, a ramp where there is a wheelchair and handles fixed to the bath to allow the patient to get out of it more easily. These

are problems which come to light in the ward when patients are talking amongst themselves or with the nursing staff.

A medical social worker in a general hospital is often asked to arrange convalescence for patients. This type of request is very common in the orthopaedic wards as many of the patients are so disabled that it is not easy for them to arrange for a holiday. Their disability may mean they are unable to manage stairs and there are some convalescent homes designed to cope with this problem. Those who have an operation on the leg or the hip must learn to walk again after a period of immobilisation. Often they lack confidence and a short holiday before going home makes the break from hospital less upsetting.

SUMMARY

It is interesting to note that there is a difference in the adjustment processes of the accident and orthopaedic patients. Those who have been involved in an accident are forced to adjust to a situation which has already happened, e.g. a patient admitted unconscious from a road accident who has to have a limb amputated. When he becomes aware of what has happened he needs help and understanding to face the reality of the situation. It may be easier however for him to adjust to the disability simply because it has already happened. The orthopaedic patient who is suffering from a deteriorating condition affecting his mobility has a more difficult problem. Perhaps he realises that the pain in his legs is getting worse and that he is not able to walk as far as he did before. He may feel that some day he will require a wheelchair although he cannot openly express these fears. Understanding and support over a period will help him to talk about his anxieties and gradually he may be able to face the future rather than turn his back on it pretending that his condition will not deteriorate.

The rôle of the medical social worker in hospital is to act as the link between patients in hospital and their homes. She tries to help them adjust to a long spell in hospital and, in many cases, to a disabling condition and a new way of life. Her contribution to the total well-being of the patient is extremely important. After the medical and nursing management is complete it is her objective to befit these patients for reintegration into society and to restore their confidence in a brighter future than perhaps they had ever anticipated.

APPENDIX: COMMON ORTHOPAEDIC APPLIANCES

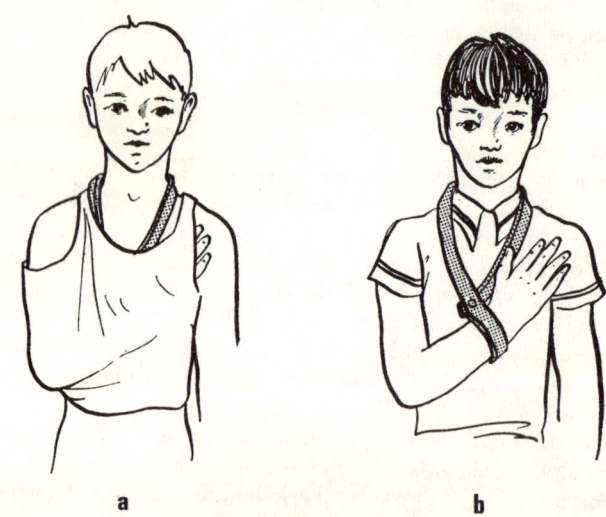

FIG. 48   (a) Inside collar and cuff sling
(b) Outside collar and cuff sling

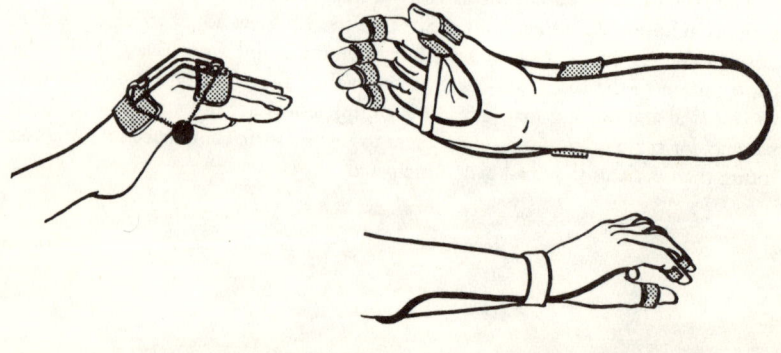

a

b

FIG. 49   (a) 'Knuckle-duster' splint. Used in ulnar nerve palsy to correct clawing of the fingers
(b) Radial nerve splint. Used in radial nerve palsy to correct drop wrist deformity

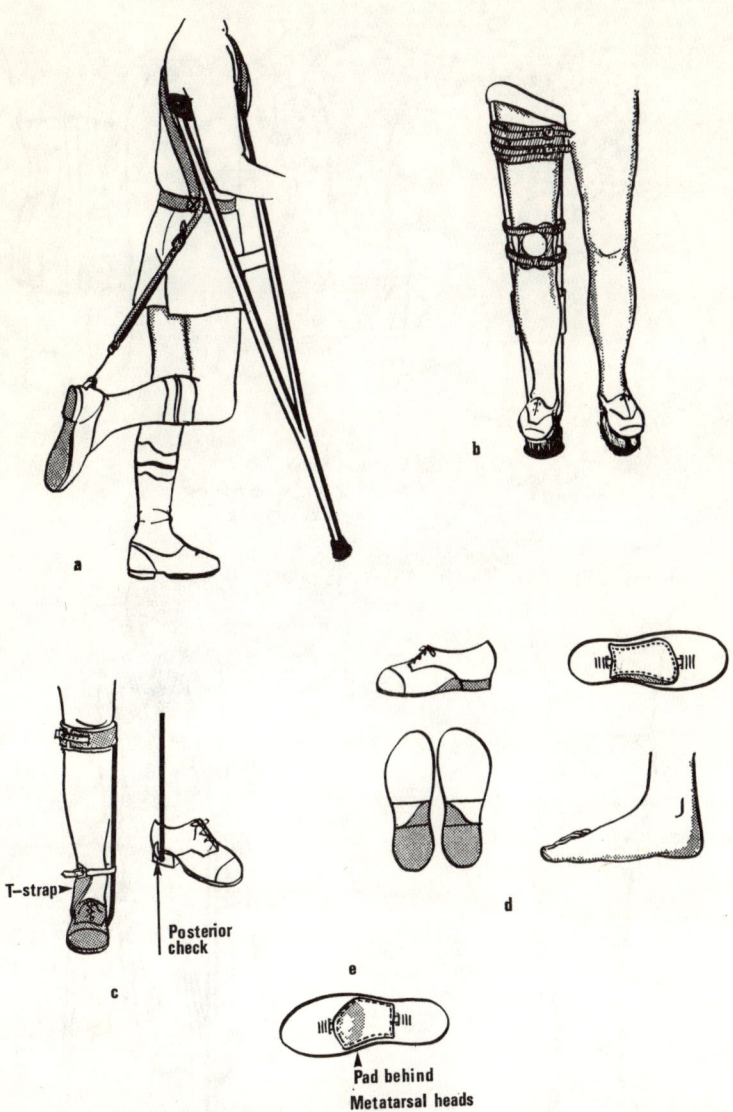

FIG. 50   (a) Pelvic sling
(b) Weight-relieving caliper and patten
(c) Below-knee caliper (inside iron and outside T-strap). Posterior
check device used in the correction of drop-foot deformity
(d) Crooked and elongated heel; longitudinal arch support (used in
the correction of flat foot deformity)
(e) Metatarsal arch support (used in the treatment of metatarsalgia)

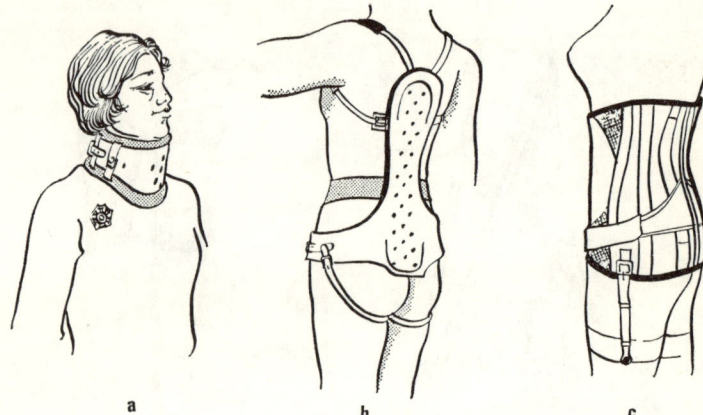

FIG. 51 (*a*) Cervical collar
(*b*) Spinal brace (Robert Jones)
(*c*) Lumbo-sacral support

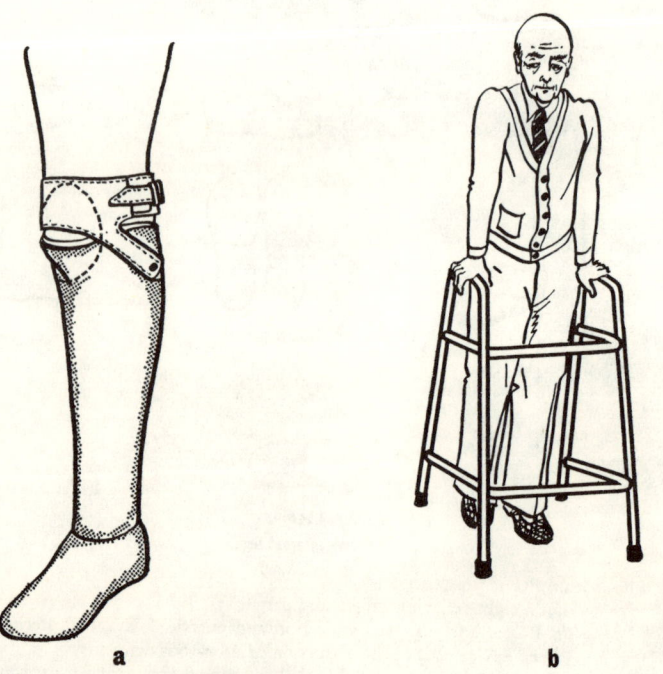

FIG. 52 (*a*) Patellar tendon bearing prosthesis
(*b*) A walking aid

INDEX